A History of Population Health

Clio Medica

STUDIES IN THE HISTORY OF MEDICINE AND HEALTH

VOLUME 101

The titles published in this series are listed at *brill.com/clio*

A History of Population Health

Rise and Fall of Disease in Europe

By

Johan P. Mackenbach

BRILL
RODOPI

LEIDEN | BOSTON

Cover image: A mother appeals to a tuberculosis nurse to save her baby son ("save him for me") from tuberculosis. Poster made for the Italian National Fascist Federation for the Fight against Tuberculosis (1932). Colour lithograph by N. Rettroni (?). Wellcome Collection (CC BY 4.0).

The Library of Congress Cataloging-in-Publication Data is available online at http://catalog.loc.gov
LC record available at http://lccn.loc.gov/2020003235

Typeface for the Latin, Greek, and Cyrillic scripts: "Brill". See and download: brill.com/brill-typeface.

ISSN 0045-7183
ISBN 978-90-04-42582-8 (hardback)
ISBN 978-90-04-42913-0 (e-book)

This book is printed on acid-free paper and produced in a sustainable manner.

Contents

PART 3
Synthesis and Outlook

Preface

This is a book about long-term trends in the health of Europeans, and about how and why diseases have come and gone. It is about the role of politics and biology, and about everything in-between, from religion to medical care and from tobacco control to the Industrial Revolution. Starting in the early 18th century and ending in the 2010s, it puts the spectacular changes in life expectancy and morbidity patterns into perspective, and tries to identify the deeper causes of the dramatic variations between European countries. Its main conclusion is that most diseases are man-made, that 'human agency' accounts for both the rise and fall of disease, and that between-country differences in political, sociocultural and economic conditions have profoundly influenced population health.

The idea for a book like this arose long ago, in 1984, when I read Fernand Braudel's *La Méditerranée* – an integrated history of the whole Mediterranean area during the reign of Philip II of Spain (1527–1598) – while I was sitting under a cypress tree in the South of France. Full of admiration I thought by myself: how wonderful would it be to paint such a broad canvas on the history of health? It took more than three decades before I felt capable of giving it a try, and even now it is easy to see the enormous gulf between Braudel's depth and breadth and my more modest achievement. Nevertheless, I hope readers with a similar interest in 'big picture' histories will be interested in the result.

While working on this book, I received generous support from many colleagues. After stepping down as head of the Department of Public Health of Erasmus MC in Rotterdam, I was allowed to spend the years remaining until my retirement on writing a book (I actually wrote two ... the other one appeared in 2019 under the title *Health inequalities: persistence and change in European welfare states*). The *Stichting Maatschappelijke Gezondheidszorg* financially supported the production of this second and more ambitious book.

A special word of thanks goes to Marina Karanikolos (London) who helped me with collecting and analysing the mortality data. David Leon (London), Mart van Lieburg (Rotterdam), France Meslé (Paris) and Frans van Poppel (The Hague) read the manuscript and provided me with lots of detailed and useful comments. In various stages of writing, I also received useful suggestions from (in alphabetical order) Evgeny Andreev (Moscow), Virginia Berridge (London), Timo Bolt (Rotterdam), Francisco Bolumar (Madrid), Jan Willem Coebergh (Oegstgeest), Martin Gorsky (London), Martin McKee (London), Wilma Nusselder (Rotterdam), Şevket Pamuk (Istanbul), Diego Ramiro (Madrid), Enrique Regidor (Madrid), Paula Santana (Coimbra), Sergey Shishkin (Moscow),

Sergey Timonin (Moscow), Jacques Vallin (Paris), Anatoly Vishnevsky (Moscow), and Vasiliy Vlassov (Moscow). I am also grateful to three anonymous reviewers for their comments.

Of course, all the remaining errors – and there are likely to be some, in view of the vast terrain I had to cover – are entirely mine.

Rotterdam, December 2019
Johan Mackenbach

Illustrations

Plates

Figures

Supplementary Figures

Tables

Supplementary Tables

CHAPTER 1

Introduction

Utopia Come True?

Are we living in Utopia? This may seem a strange question – our television news with its footage of disaster does not immediately suggest we do – but today's world is much more similar to our ancestors' utopian dreams than most people realize. 'Utopia' – a newly invented word meaning 'nowhere' – was the title of a book by Thomas More (1478–1535), published in 1516. It describes an imaginary and perfectly organized kingdom, located just off the coast of America. A few decades before, the 'New World' had been discovered, and this had sparked the idea that an ideal society did not have to await the hereafter, but could be created here and now.

The perfect organisation of Utopia guarantees its citizens complete happiness. Private property and the privileges of the nobility have been abolished, everybody works only 6 hours a day, and the head of state is chosen in free, representative elections. In More's Utopia, people live in spacious and ventilated houses, and the government inspects their food and supplies them with clean drinking water. A system of social security prevents those who fall ill from becoming poor, and those who are poor from falling ill – and people who despite all countermeasures still fall ill, have the right to be treated in excellent public hospitals. No wonder that, as More notes, "[not] anywhere are there healthier men and freer from diseases."[1]

Although the term 'utopia' has become synonymous for unattainable ideals of perfect societies, it is remarkable how much of More's utopian health vision has been realized in the 20th century, and mostly without the draconic reorganization of society that More thought necessary. Through the centuries, utopian visions have served as a source of inspiration for those who believed that a better world could be created, in which nobody would suffer from avoidable or remediable ill-health. This is even more clear in the case of a number of 19th

1 Thomas More, *De Optimo Rei Publicae Statu Deque Nova Insula Utopia* [*On the Best State of a Republic and on the New Island Utopia*] (Leuven, 1516). The sentence in the text was cited from the Open|Utopia edition, edited by Stephen Duncombe, p. 135 (www.theopenutopia.org, accessed 25/08/2019). For commentaries on the health aspects of More's Utopia, see Phil Withington, "Utopia, Health, and Happiness," *Lancet* 387, no. 10033 (2016): 2084–085; Johan P. Mackenbach, "Thomas More, Etienne Cabet and the Paradoxes of Utopian Thinking," *European Journal of Public Health* 14, no. 2 (2004): 113.

century Utopias. The novel *Voyage et Aventures de Lord William Carisdall en Icarie* by Étienne Cabet (1788–1856) is a good example. This book, published in 1840, describes a communist utopia in which prevention of illness had a high priority (Plate 1).

The following quote gives an idea of Cabet's utopian dream:

> Within the city there are no cemeteries, no noxious products manufactured, no hospitals: all these establishments are on the outskirts, in open places, near swift-flowing streams or in the country. [...] You would see here neither cabarets, nor roadhouses, nor cafés, nor smoking joints, nor the stock-exchange [...] just as there are no prostitutes or pickpockets, no drunkards or mendicants; but instead you would find everywhere PRIVIES, as elegant as they are clean and convenient, some for women, others for men [...].[2]

Cabet's work attracted considerable support, and in 1848 a group of 1500 followers set off from France to America to establish a colony on the model of *Icarie*. However, practice proved to be more difficult than theory: the group split, and Cabet himself died in St. Louis shortly thereafter. Nevertheless, many 19th century readers must have felt attracted by the prospect of living in a cleaner, safer, more equitable, and healthier city. And it only required social justice and good government![3]

Rising Life Expectancy

Over the past three centuries, health of Europeans has improved enormously. This can most clearly be seen in the spectacular increase in the length of life (Figure 1). Around the middle of the 19th century, life expectancy at birth fluctuated around an average of less than 40 years, but in the last decades of that century life expectancy began to rise rapidly, to reach the current values of between 65 and 80 years among men, and between 75 and 85 years

2 The original publication is Étienne Cabet, *Voyage et Aventures de Lord William Carisdall en Icarie* (Paris: H. Souverain, 1840). The quote is cited from an extract at http://urbanplanning.library.cornell.edu/DOCS/cabet.htm (accessed 20/08/19).

3 Some philosophers have argued that striving for utopia inevitably leads to totalitarianism, because the realization of utopian societies is incompatible with human freedom (e.g., Melvin J. Lasky, *Utopia and Revolution* (Chicago: University of Chicago Press, 1976)). More's Utopia is indeed far from a liberal society, and even needs slavery for its functioning. Also, seriously ill, but incurable patients are persuaded to commit suicide or have themselves euthanized. See Chapter 7 for the Soviet Union as a 'realized utopia', and Chapter 8 for the need to 're-think Utopia'.

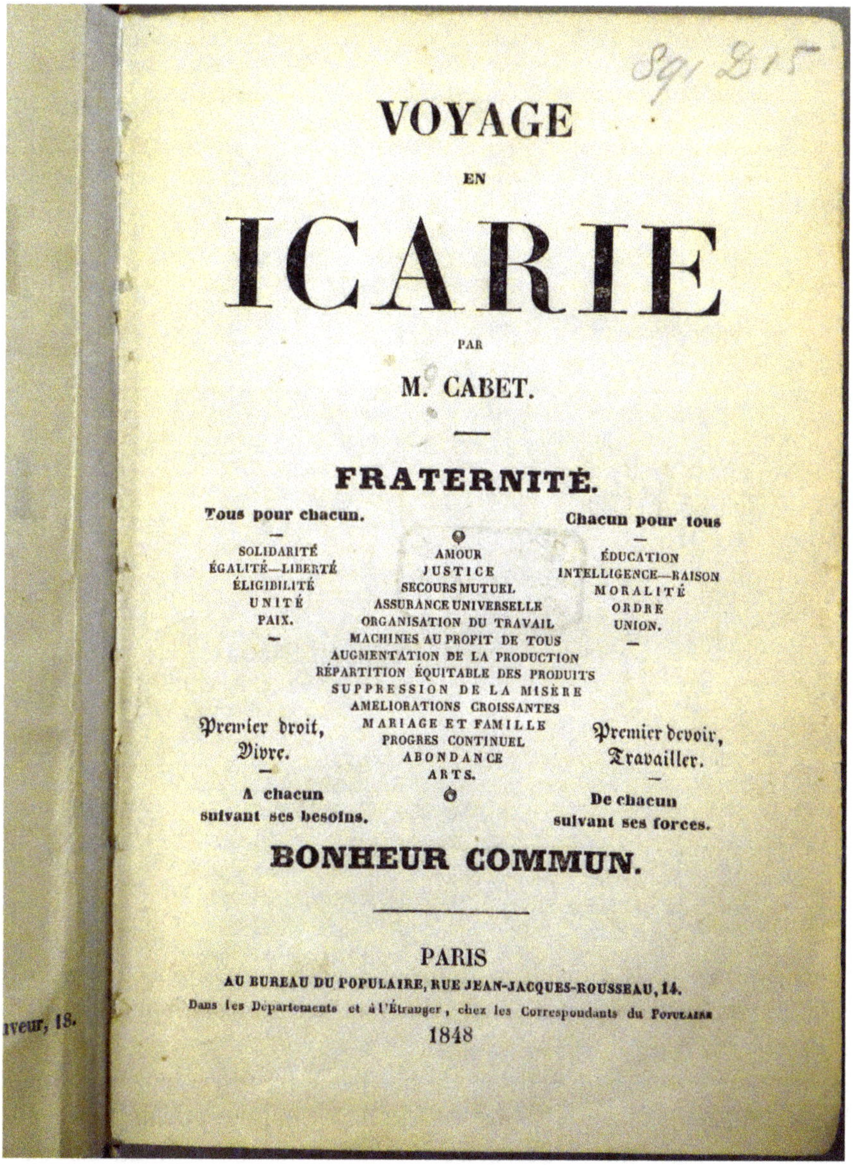

VOYAGE

EN

ICARIE

PAR

M. CABET.

FRATERNITÉ.

Tous pour chacun. — Chacun pour tous

SOLIDARITÉ
ÉGALITÉ—LIBERTÉ
ÉLIGIBILITÉ
UNITÉ
PAIX.

AMOUR
JUSTICE
SECOURS MUTUEL
ASSURANCE UNIVERSELLE
ORGANISATION DU TRAVAIL
MACHINES AU PROFIT DE TOUS
AUGMENTATION DE LA PRODUCTION
RÉPARTITION ÉQUITABLE DES PRODUITS
SUPPRESSION DE LA MISÈRE
AMÉLIORATIONS CROISSANTES
MARIAGE ET FAMILLE
PROGRÈS CONTINUEL
ABONDANCE
ARTS.

ÉDUCATION
INTELLIGENCE—RAISON
MORALITÉ
ORDRE
UNION.

Premier droit, Vivre. — Premier devoir, Travailler.

A chacun suivant ses besoins. — De chacun suivant ses forces.

BONHEUR COMMUN.

PARIS
AU BUREAU DU POPULAIRE, RUE JEAN-JACQUES-ROUSSEAU, 14.
Dans les Départements et à l'Étranger, chez les Correspondants du POPULAIRE
1848

PLATE 1 Cabet's utopian principles. Title page of *Voyage en Icarie*, 1848

Title page of the 5th edition of Cabet's Voyage en Icarie, published in 1848. It lists a number of principles summing up Cabet's philosophy, such as Fraternité [Brotherhood], Tous pour chacun – Chacun pour tous [All for everyone – everyone for all], Premier droit, Vivre – Premier devoir, Travailler" [First right, to Live – First duty, to Work], and Bonheur commun [Common happiness]. After settling his utopian community in Nauvoo (Illinois), Cabet announced that the common dining room would be decorated with wall inscriptions listing the principles of the community. These ranged from the abolition of private property to the duty to work, and from the duty of mutual assistance to the prohibition of tobacco.

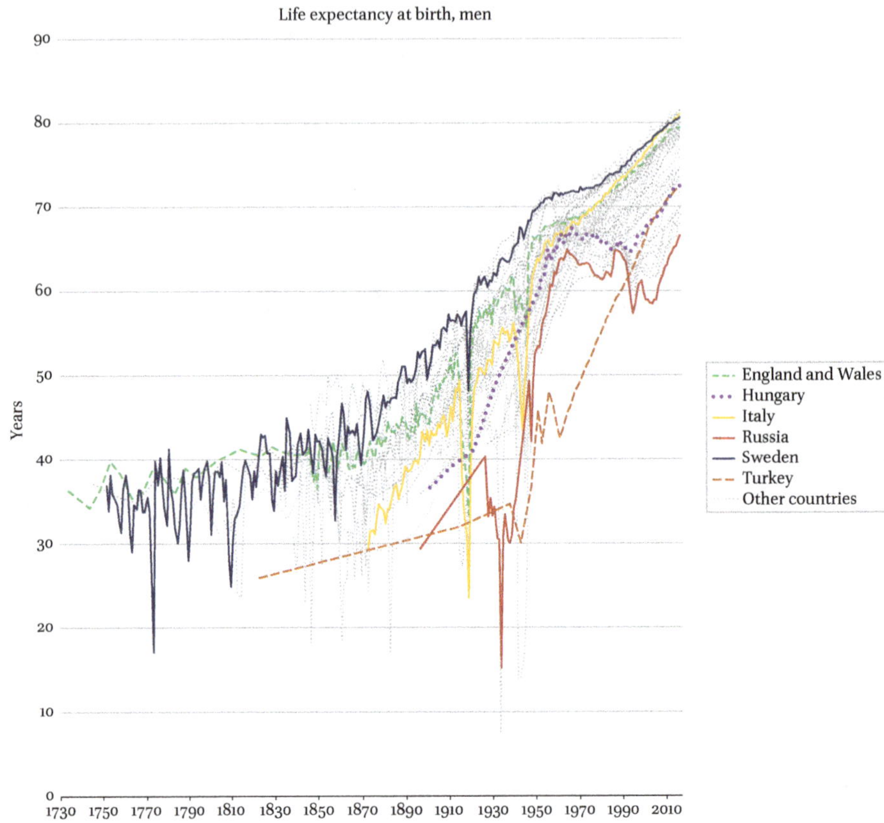

FIGURE 1 Trends in life expectancy in Europe, 1730–2015
Notes: For women, see Suppl. Figure 1
SOURCE OF DATA: SEE SUPPL. TABLE 1

among women. It is difficult to think of a more important change in the whole of human history – unimaginable even for the most utopian among our predecessors.

This increase in the length of life has been accompanied by enormous changes in people's health. Many diseases have disappeared, and while other diseases have taken their place, these occur at higher ages than the diseases of the past, so that most health problems now occur among older people. And because the greatest advances have been made by preventing diseases from occurring, not only has the total number of life-years increased, but so has the number of years that Europeans can expect to live in good health.

It is only more recently that the number of years that we can expect to live in *ill*-health has also increased. Since the middle of the 20th century, medical treatment of chronic conditions has made an increasing contribution to improvements in life expectancy. As a result of increased survival of patients with chronic diseases, total life expectancy has increased faster than 'healthy life expectancy', and years of life spent with disease have increased rather strongly.

Although the improvements in population health have been spectacular everywhere, European countries have followed very different trajectories. Health improvements have occurred at different times and with different speeds, resulting in the very broad band of upward moving life expectancies that can be seen in Figure 1. The width of this band has been indicated by the highlighted curve for Sweden, which for a long time had the highest life expectancy, and the curve for Turkey, which until recently was the country with the lowest life expectancy.

The gap in life expectancy between Sweden and Turkey increased from around 10 years in the beginning of the 19th century to around 25 years in the 1930s, and then narrowed again to around 8 years in the beginning of the 21st century. More generally, for most of the time Northern and Western Europe have taken the lead, later joined by Southern Europe, and with most parts of South-eastern and Eastern Europe consistently staying behind.[4]

Using a unique collection of historical data and recent research findings, this book shows that these trends and variations did not arise spontaneously, but were mostly man-made. This does not only apply to health improvements – which often resulted from increases in the human capacity to address the causes or consequences of disease – but also to temporary setbacks. Throughout European history, health and longevity were therefore closely related to economic, political and sociocultural conditions.

The Rise and Fall of Disease

Talking about setbacks: the rise of life expectancy has not been a smooth process, as can be clearly seen in Figure 1. Some of the dips in the life expectancy curves were very deep indeed – the deepest dip occurred during the 1933 famine in Ukraine when average life expectancy at birth briefly declined to below 10 years. Below the surface of rising life expectancy and declining total mortality the trends are even more irregular. Specific causes of death have risen and

4 For more detailed studies of convergence and divergence of life expectancy between European countries, see Johan P. Mackenbach, "Convergence and Divergence of Life Expectancy in Europe: A Centennial View," *European Journal of Epidemiology* 28, no. 3 (2013): 229–40; David A. Leon, "Trends in European Life Expectancy: A Salutary View," *International Journal of Epidemiology* 40, no. 2 (2011): 271–77.

fallen over time, and it is only because 'falls' ultimately had the upper hand that life expectancy could rise.

This is one of the main findings of this book, which reviews the history of around 40 health conditions. These range from famine and plague to motor vehicle injuries and suicide, and from maternal mortality and cholera to diabetes and cerebrovascular disease. Seen in a long-term perspective the trends for these health conditions often follow a striking pattern of 'rise-and-fall'. Most diseases which were common at their peak, were uncommon centuries or decades before, and their rise was usually followed by an equally impressive decline.

Although each disease has its own specific causes, we will see that the general explanation for rises of disease is that human efforts to improve their living conditions often required or allowed them to undertake new activities, which later turned out to be health-damaging. Just like long-distance trade brought the plague from Central Asia into Europe, so did education and reading increase the risk of myopia, and just like urban living increased the likelihood of tuberculosis infection, so did an affluent diet increase the risk of ischaemic heart disease.

Similarly, declines of disease had many specific explanations, but when one takes a bird's eye view it becomes crystal-clear that it is highly unlikely that most declines occurred spontaneously. The general explanation is that the drive for better living conditions not only brought new health risks, but also created the necessary conditions for reducing these risks. For example, prosperity brought better nutrition and better housing, and economic growth made it possible for countries to invest in science and technology, safe drinking water, vaccinations, cholesterol-lowering drugs, and road traffic safety measures.

Nevertheless, it would be too simple to see economic development as the only, or even the main, driver of changes in population health. The history of Europe is full of examples where economic development and population health did not move in parallel. This shows that economic growth was usually not a sufficient condition for health improvement. For example, at various points in time Sweden, the Netherlands and Albania were over-performers in health as compared to their level of economic development, whereas Portugal and Russia were under-performers.

Closer inspection of these and other examples reveals that acceptance of measures to reduce health risks also often required sociocultural change, and that effective implementation required institutions able to deliver them on a large scale, such as an effective public health sector and an accessible health care system. Throughout European history, creating these conditions was a profoundly political enterprise. This is illustrated by the fact that national boundaries and political events, such as revolutions and dissolutions of empire, often coincided with sharp break-lines in population health.

These are the issues that this book is about. Using a wide range of quantitative data, from life expectancy to infectious disease notification rates, and from lung cancer mortality to average heights of recruits, we will look through the 'telescope of history' to discern some of the deeper causes of the rise of life expectancy since the 18th century. The results will be used to reflect on contemporary theories of determinants of population health, and the first of these is the theory of the 'epidemiologic transition'. Because this has proven such a powerful organizing concept we briefly introduce this theory up-front in this introductory chapter.

The Epidemiologic Transition Theory

The 'epidemiologic transition theory' was originally proposed in a paper by Egyptian-American epidemiologist Abdel Omran (1925–1999). This paper, published in 1971, has since become a 'citation classic', with more than 4000 citations in later scientific publications. The epidemiologic transition describes the mortality component of the 'demographic transition': the long-term decline of (first) mortality and (then) fertility that accompanied socioeconomic modernization around the world.[5]

Omran characterized the epidemiologic transition as a "long-term shift [...] in mortality and disease patterns whereby pandemics of infection are gradually displaced by degenerative and man-made diseases as the chief form of morbidity and primary cause of death." This shift occurs in three stages: the "age of pestilence and famine" in which life expectancy "vacillat[es] between 20 and 40 years" and "mortality [is] high and fluctuating"; the "age of receding

5 The 'demographic transition' theory was introduced around the middle of the 20th century. Its intellectual history has been traced in Dudley Kirk, "Demographic Transition Theory," *Population Studies* 50, no. 3 (1996): 361–87; Jean-Claude Chesnais, *La Transition Démographique* (Paris: Presses Universitaires de France, 1986). More critical assessments can be found in Dennis Hodgson, "Demography as Social Science and Policy Science," *Population and Development Review* 9, no. 1 (1983): 1–34; Simon Szreter, "The Idea of Demographic Transition and the Study of Fertility Change," *Population and Development Review* 19, no. 4 (1993): 659–701. Like Omran and others, and despite its ambiguity, we will sometimes use the term 'modernization' in this book, usually accompanied by the adjective 'socioeconomic'. For an interesting commentary on this somewhat dubious term, see AHR Roundtable, "Historians and the Question of 'Modernity'," *American Historical Review* 116, no. 3 (2011): 631–751.

pandemics" in which life expectancy "increases steadily from about 30 to about 50 years" and "epidemic peaks become less frequent or disappear"; and the "age of degenerative and man-made diseases" in which life expectancy "rises gradually until it exceeds 50 years" and mortality "eventually approaches stability at a relatively low level."[6]

In his 1971 paper Omran did not define 'degenerative and man-made diseases', but in a later update he mentioned cardiovascular disease, cancer, stroke, diabetes, and metabolic disorders as examples of 'degenerative diseases'. "Radiation injury, accidents, occupational hazards, carcinogens in the environment and in industry, and food additives" are examples of "diseases introduced by man."

Omran recognized that in Western Europe and North America the shift started early and took approximately 100 years. This is the 'western' or 'classical' model of the epidemiologic transition. In a number of other countries, notably Eastern Europe and Japan, the transition started later but proceeded much more quickly (the 'accelerated' model). He considered rising living standards to be an important driver of population health change in the western model, and public health and medical technologies to be relatively more important in the accelerated model.[7]

Although the notion of an 'epidemiologic transition' has stuck in the demographic and epidemiologic literatures, it has since become clear that Omran's picture of these long-term changes in population health is less than accurate, both conceptually and factually. The characterization of the shift as one from 'pandemics' of infectious diseases to 'degenerative and man-made diseases' is imprecise, as is the distinction between the three 'stages'. Furthermore, just when Omran published his theory a renewed decline of mortality contradicted his idea that the transition had ended in new stability.

These and other problems have shown that Omran's theory is in need of repair, but a satisfactory replacement has not yet been agreed on. Can the

6 Abdel R. Omran, "The Epidemiologic Transition: A Theory of the Epidemiology of Population Change," *Milbank Memorial Fund Quarterly* 49 (1971): 509–38; the citations are from pages 518–20. The original paper was republished twice: in 2001 in the *Bulletin of the World Health Organization*, and in 2005 in the *Milbank Quarterly*. For the history of this 'citation classic', see George Weisz and Jesse Olszynko-Gryn, "The Theory of Epidemiologic Transition: The Origins of a Citation Classic," *Journal of the History of Medicine and Allied Sciences* 65, no. 3 (2009): 287–326.

7 Omran revisited his original ideas several times, without making substantial changes. See Abdel R. Omran, "The Epidemiologic Transition Theory. A Preliminary Update," *Journal of Tropical Pediatrics* 29 (1983): 305–16; Abdel R. Omran, "The Epidemiologic Transition Theory Revisited Thirty Years Later," *World Health Statistics Quarterly* 51, no. 2–4 (1998): 99–119.

stages simply be relabelled or is a more fundamental revision in order? Can more recent changes simply be accommodated by adding a fourth stage, as some authors have proposed, or should these be seen as the start of an entirely new transition?

The McKeown Debate and the Preston-Curve

There can be little doubt that the modern rise of life expectancy is related to improved living standards. It cannot be a coincidence that both life expectancy and national income showed steep rises over the 19th and 20th centuries – but how exactly are the two related? Two scientific studies, both published in the 1970s, still form the anchor-points of present-day discussions of this question.

The first is a series of publications by British professor of social medicine Thomas McKeown (1912–1988). McKeown made a detailed analysis of the history of cause-specific mortality in England and Wales since the 1840s, and summarized his conclusions in *The Role of Medicine – Dream, Mirage or Nemesis* (1976). His analyses showed that the decline in mortality was the result mainly of a decline of infectious diseases, and that infectious disease mortality decline for the most part antedated the introduction of specific medical interventions, such as vaccinations and antibiotics. In other words: the role of medicine can only have been marginal.

McKeown also showed that most of the decline of mortality from infectious diseases in England and Wales was due to a decline of air-borne diseases, particularly respiratory tuberculosis, and not to the water-borne diseases to which most public health interventions were targeted. He therefore concluded that neither medical care nor public health interventions could account for the decline in mortality. This must therefore have had another explanation – which he thought was improved nutrition, due to improvements in agricultural productivity and food transportation.[8]

8 McKeown published his findings first in a series of papers: Thomas McKeown and Robert G. Brown, "Medical Evidence Related to English Population Changes in the Eighteenth Century," *Population Studies* 9, no. 2 (1955): 119–41; Thomas McKeown and Robert G. Record, "Reasons for the Decline of Mortality in England and Wales During the Nineteenth Century," *Population Studies* 16, no. 2 (1962): 94–122; Thomas McKeown, Robert G. Record, and R.D. Turner, "An Interpretation of the Decline of Mortality in England and Wales During the Twentieth Century," *Population Studies* 29, no. 3 (1975): 391–422. These were followed by two books, both published in 1976: Thomas McKeown, *The Role of Medicine: Dream, Mirage, or Nemesis?* (London: Nuffield Provincial Hopsitals Trust, 1976); Thomas McKeown, *The Modern Rise of Population* (London: Edward Arnold, 1976). The title of the first book reminds us of Ivan Illich (1926–2002), who argued that iatrogenic side-effects posed "limits to medicine" (Ivan Illich, *Medical Nemesis: The Expropriation of Health* (London: Calder & Boyars, 1975)).

Although his viewpoint that the rise of life expectancy is just a by-product of socioeconomic progress, and not of human intervention, is still commonly held, McKeown's conclusions must be considered at least partly obsolete in the light of more recent findings. We will have a look at the results of more recent studies in various chapters of this book, and argue that public health and medical care have had a more important role than McKeown thought.[9]

Another influential paper, published in 1975 by American demographer Samuel Preston, also dealt with the explanation of the rise of life expectancy, but came to rather different conclusions on the role of rising living standards. This paper is mainly famous for the introduction of the so-called 'Preston-curve', which relates national income to average life expectancy at birth. It shows that people living in richer countries on average live longer than people in poorer countries, and that although the relation is steeper at lower levels of income, it holds at higher levels as well.[10]

However, an equally important finding in this paper was that when Preston compared these curves for different points in time (i.e. the 1900s, 1930s and 1960s), he found that the curve had shifted upwards from the 1900s to the 1930s, and again from the 1930s to the 1960s. At any given level of national income (adjusted for inflation), life expectancy was higher in the 1930s than in the 1900s, and in the 1960s than in the 1930s. Furthermore, the upward shift in the curve explained more of the global rise in life expectancy between these points in time than rising national incomes.[11]

Preston interpreted this as indicating that other factors than income growth, such as public health programs, maternal and child health services, and

9 The literature about the 'McKeown thesis' is massive. One of the most influential critiques of McKeown's dismissal of public health was written by British historian Simon Szreter; see Simon Szreter, "The Importance of Social Intervention in Britains Mortality Decline c. 1850–1914," *Social History of Medicine* 1, no. 1 (1988): 1–37. For a critique on McKeown's dismissal of medical care, see Johan P. Mackenbach, "The Contribution of Medical Care to Mortality Decline: Mckeown Revisited," *Journal of Clinical Epidemiology* 49, no. 11 (1996): 1207–213. In 2005, the International Journal of Epidemiology published a series of commentaries on the 'McKeown debate', one of which concluded that it was "time for burial": Emily Grundy, "Commentary: The Mckeown Debate: Time for Burial," *International Journal of Epidemiology* 34, no. 3 (2004): 529–33.

10 An example of a 'Preston-curve' will be presented in Chapter 3 (Figure 6).

11 Samuel H. Preston, "The Changing Relation between Mortality and Level of Economic Development," *Population Studies* 29, no. 2 (1975): 231–48. The importance of Preston's paper is illustrated by the fact that, like Omran's 1971 paper, it has twice been reprinted as a 'classic': first in the *Bulletin of the World Health Organization* (2003) and then in the *International Journal of Epidemiology* (2007).

antibiotics probably accounted for a sizable part of the rise in life expectancy between the 1930s and 1960s. Although these interventions were mostly developed in richer countries, health breakthroughs spread rapidly to poorer countries. This allowed them to reach high levels of life expectancy at lower levels of income than the richer countries before them.

It is important to note that Preston's conclusion is, like McKeown's, by exclusion. Rising income can explain only a small part of the rise in life expectancy, so there must be something else, i.e. public health and medical care. Direct evidence for the impact of public health and medical care is not given. Nevertheless, Preston's findings warn against simple economic determinism. This will also be the conclusion of a review of more recent studies in Chapter 3 of this book.

The Role of Human Agency

The big question underlying this 'battle of ideas' is: what has been the role of 'human agency' in achieving long-term improvements in population health? Have these improvements been a by-product of other developments which happened spontaneously? Or have population health improvements been the result of actions explicitly intended to improve health outcomes?[12]

As this book will demonstrate, most long-term health improvements did not arise spontaneously, but were in one way or another man-made. This is already strongly suggested by the 'rise-and-fall' pattern that can be seen for so many diseases. It is highly unlikely that all the declines of disease that have occurred over the past three centuries happened spontaneously. Nevertheless, in order to demonstrate a role of 'human agency' it will be necessary to look at the evidence in a lot more detail: disease-by-disease, and factor-by-factor.

It will also be important to clarify what we actually mean by 'spontaneous', which is a deceptively simple term. Classifying the developments that underlie long-term improvements in population health into 'spontaneous' and 'intentional' is not trivial. What some further reflection reveals is that this distinction is not black-and-white. There is black, then there are various shades of grey, and then there is pure white. Here is a possible classification:

1) Changes in human health as a result of changes in living conditions which happen without any human involvement. Examples include

12 The term 'human agency' – a term that has very specific meanings in, e.g., philosophy and sociology – will be used throughout this book to loosely refer to 'humans acting intentionally'. We will not assume that these acts always arise out of free will, or are always based on consciously made decisions. 'Human agency' occurs at many levels, from single individuals to international organizations.

changes in climate as occurred at the end of the 'Little Ice Age', or changes in the virulence of micro-organisms.

2) Changes in human health as a result of changes in human behaviour or of man-made changes in living conditions, which are actively pursued but for reasons completely unrelated to health. Examples would be changes in behaviour pursued for 'social distinction', or shifts from an industrial to a service economy which coincidentally reduced exposure to hazardous working conditions.
3) Changes in human health as a result of changes in human behaviour or of man-made changes in living conditions, which are pursued for reasons indirectly related to health. Examples would include changes in behaviour pursued for reasons of cleanliness, or changes in agricultural methods aimed at increasing harvest yields. Both cleanliness and large harvest yields are important in themselves, but also have indirect health benefits.
4) Changes in human health as a result of public health interventions. These are changes in human behaviour or living conditions, which are pursued for reasons directly related to health, but involve actions outside medical care. Examples are changes in smoking in response to health education campaigns, or changes in injury risk as a result of road traffic safety measures.
5) Changes in human health as a result of medical care. These are, like the previous category, by definition pursued for reasons directly related to health, but involve actions in an individual contact between a health care professional and a patient seeking care. Examples are changes in pneumonia mortality as a result of the introduction of antibiotics, and changes in survival rates from cancer due to improvements in cancer treatment.

Of these, only the changes under (1) are completely 'spontaneous', and only those under (4) and (5) are definitely 'intentional', but (2) and (3) are somewhere in-between. Nevertheless, even the population health improvements resulting from (2) and (3) should be considered 'man-made'. The multifaceted nature of all these 'man-made' changes also explains why population health is so closely related to economic, political and sociocultural conditions: these conditions do not only determine (4) and (5), but also (2) and (3).[13]

13 The scale of 'intentionality' is, of course, more continuous than these five 'positions' suggest. For example, changes in human health as a result of changes in individual behaviour, if informed by knowledge of the health effects of this behaviour, lie somewhere

How to Read This Book

This book consists of three main parts: a general overview of long-term trends in population health; a second part zooming into the detailed history of around 40 specific health conditions; and a final part in which the disease-specific story-lines are woven together again to reach some general conclusions.

In the first part we take the increase in life expectancy as our starting-point. We follow its trail back by looking at the underlying shifts in disease patterns, to discover a fascinating sequence of 'rises-and-falls' of almost all health conditions whose long-term course we can follow through time. After an attempt to revise Omran's epidemiologic transition theory, we then consider possible explanations of these changes. Starting from an understanding of disease as mostly originating from the interaction between human organisms and their environment, we review the evidence on what actually caused long-term changes in population health. These mostly did not occur spontaneously, but were driven by various forms of 'human agency'. This is reflected in strong parallels between population health change and changes in economic, political and sociocultural conditions, and in identifiable impacts of public health and medical care.

In the second part we zoom in to look at the history of a wide range of diseases and other health problems. Although it is impossible to cover everything, the many health conditions covered in Part 2 ensure that we get a good overview of the diversity of factors that have played a role in the 'rise-and-fall' of disease. This book brings together a collection of data which sometimes go back as far as the early 18th century, and often reach into the second decade of the 21st century. These are presented in a series of graphs that – even for those familiar with the history of medicine and public health – hold many surprises. These data are combined with a review of what we know about the explanation of these long-term trends, to explore in detail what their immediate and ultimate causes were.

In the third part we return to the broader perspective of the first part, and synthesize our findings into a few general conclusions on the role of 'human agency' in long-term improvements in population health. We review the historical experience of a few carefully selected countries from around Europe, in an attempt to create a coherent story of how economic, political and sociocultural change and the rise of public health and medical care shaped these countries' health trajectories. These lessons from the past are then finally used to

---

in-between (3) and (4), and advocacy for sanitation and other public health measures by 19th century medical doctors lies somewhere in-between (4) and (5).

reflect upon the challenges of the future, and to discuss the sustainability of current levels of population health.

All in all, this will be a story of tremendous progress. Who can deny the value of a longer life, and the benefits of living many more years in good health? Yet, this story also has darker sides to which we cannot close our eyes. One 'inconvenient truth' is that some of the fastest advances occurred under conditions of political oppression, suggesting that the politics underpinning population health improvement are not always innocent. The same applies to the economic underpinnings: economic growth was partly dependent on the exploitation of Europe's colonies in other parts of the world, and on the massive burning of fossil fuels which is now changing the world's climate. Furthermore, human population numbers have soared and as a result other living species have suffered. These darker sides will have to be acknowledged, if only because some of them are linked to the challenges of the future.

This book is different from many others. Let me briefly mention a few other books of medical history, to clarify what this book is and what it is not. First of all, this is not a history of 'public health', but of 'people's health'. George Rosen's *A History of Public Health* (1958) is the most widely known history of the field of 'public health'. This is still a good general introduction to the development of the knowledge base, institutions and professions in this field. More recent is Dorothy Porter's *The history of Public Health and the Modern State* (1994). This is one of the very few books explicitly focusing on the development of public health in different European countries, but like Rosen's book has very little on the actual development of the object of public health: population health.[14]

Important, but more encyclopaedic than story-telling, is the *Cambridge World History of Human Disease* (1993), which has histories of no less than 158 specific health conditions. Examples of more compact histories of disease, which are now outdated but can still be informative as a general introduction, are Erwin Ackerknecht's *History and Geography of the Most Important Diseases* (1965) and Folke Henschen's *The History of Diseases* (1966). Closer to this book comes Mark Harrison's *Disease and the Modern World – 1500 to the Present Day*

14 Rosen's *A History of Public Health* was originally published in 1958 (George Rosen, *A History of Public Health* (Baltimore: Johns Hopkins University Press, 1958 [expanded edition 1993])). In addition to the book mentioned in the text (Dorothy Porter, *The History of Public Health and the Modern State* (Amsterdam: Editions Rodopi, 1994)), Dorothy Porter has published several other important books on the history of public health: Dorothy Porter, *Health Citizenship* (Berkeley etc.: University Of California Medical Humanities Press, 2011); Dorothy Porter, *Health, Civilization and the State* (London and New York: Routledge, 2005). A compact and recent history of public health is Virginia Berridge, *Public Health: A Very Short Introduction* (Oxford etc.: Oxford University Press, 2016).

(2004). This is a synthetic history of diseases, chronologically presented, and placed in their socioeconomic and political context, but with a strong emphasis on communicable diseases and no quantitative data.[15]

The quantitative character of this book is more closely matched by a number of histories of demography, although the latter usually focus on the rise of life expectancy without paying much attention to the decline of specific diseases. Accessible to a wide readership is James Riley's *Rising Life Expectancy: a Global History* (2001). This provides a short introduction to the rise of life expectancy since the 1700s, with extensive quantitative illustrations, including a comparison between countries and a synthesis of what we know about its explanation. Similar in scope, but limited to Europe, is Massimo Livi Bacci's *The Population of Europe: a History* (1999). Another source of inspiration for this book was Jean-Claude Chesnais's *The Demographic Transition* (1992), which has an in-depth analysis of differences between European countries in mortality decline. Needless to say, in view of the publication dates of these books they do not cover the most recent, and sometimes quite dramatic, trends in population health in Europe.[16]

Concepts, Sources, Data and Methods

This book is an attempt to describe and understand the 'big picture' of population health change, pulling together insights from many disciplines. As will be clear from the (rather long) list of references at the end, it relies on the work of many specialists. Historical demographers have laid the basis for the study of long-term trends in life expectancy. Economic historians have provided many new insights into the determinants of modern economic growth and its impact on human welfare, including population health. Medical historians have told the often detailed histories of medical discovery and medical invention that laid the basis for many improvements in population health. Finally, epidemiologists have often given us a better understanding of the determinants of

15 Kenneth F. Kiple, ed., *Cambridge World History of Human Disease* (Cambridge etc.: Cambridge University Press, 1993); Erwin H. Ackerknecht, *History and Geography of the Most Important Diseases* (New York & London: Hafner, 1965); Folke Henschen, *The History and Geography of Diseases*, trans. Joan Tate (London: Longmans, Green & Co., 1966); Mark Harrison, *Disease and the Modern World* (Cambridge: Polity, 2004). For a recently published history of 10 epidemic diseases and their impact on Western societies, see Frank M. Snowden, *Epidemics and Society: From the Black Death to the Present* (New Haven: Yale University Press, 2019).

16 James C. Riley, *Rising Life Expectancy: A Global History* (Cambridge etc.: Cambridge University Press, 2001); Massimo Livi Bacci, *The Population of Europe: A History* (Oxford: Blackwell, 1999); Chesnais, *Transition Démographique*.

the rise and fall of specific diseases. All this needed to be blended together in a single story-line, which implies that I often had to prioritize consistency over originality. To the extent that there is originality in this book, it is in the synthesis of these massive amounts of information, and in the comparisons across time and space that this allows.

This book is unashamedly 'Eurocentric'. Although there is a legitimate tendency in many historic sub-disciplines to replace a focus on European history with a more global perspective, the challenge of writing a global history of population health simply seemed too overwhelming. Even for Europe – where countries like Sweden and Britain were the first to start collecting statistical data on population health – it is often impossible to construct reasonably complete time-series covering the whole trajectory of health improvement since its very beginnings. On the other hand, there are great benefits in focussing on Europe: this allows us to exploit its fascinating variations in economic, political and sociocultural conditions over the past three centuries, and to discover how these have influenced population health.[17]

Whenever convenient, European countries will be grouped into a number of geographically contiguous and historically related regions. 'Northern Europe' will refer to Finland, Sweden, Norway, Denmark, and Iceland. 'Western Europe' includes England & Wales, Scotland, Northern Ireland, Ireland, the Netherlands, Belgium, Luxembourg, Germany, Austria, and Switzerland. 'Southern Europe' is France, Spain, Portugal, Italy, Malta, Greece, and Cyprus. 'Central-eastern Europe' is Czech Republic, Slovakia, Hungary, and Poland. 'South-eastern Europe' is Albania, Slovenia, Croatia, Bosnia & Herzegovina, Serbia, Montenegro, North Macedonia, Romania, and Bulgaria, and sometimes also includes Turkey. 'Eastern Europe' is Estonia, Latvia, Lithuania, Belarus, Ukraine, Moldova, and Russia. When the term 'North-western Europe' is used, it refers to Northern and Western Europe taken together.

It is important to be aware from the outset, however, that over the period covered by this book the political map of Europe has changed repeatedly (Plate 2). Many of these currently existing countries have only recently emerged as independent states. Many came into existence after the collapse of the Soviet Union and Yugoslavia in the 1990s, or after the dissolution of the Habsburg and Ottoman Empires immediately after World War I. Others emerged in the 19th century, after the coagulation of many smaller units into the unified German

17 In this book, Europe is the European subcontinent as usually understood. It (of course) includes Russia, but not the former Soviet republics of the Caucasus and Central Asia. Because South-eastern Europe has long been part of the Ottoman empire, the experience of Turkey will sometimes also be included in the analysis.

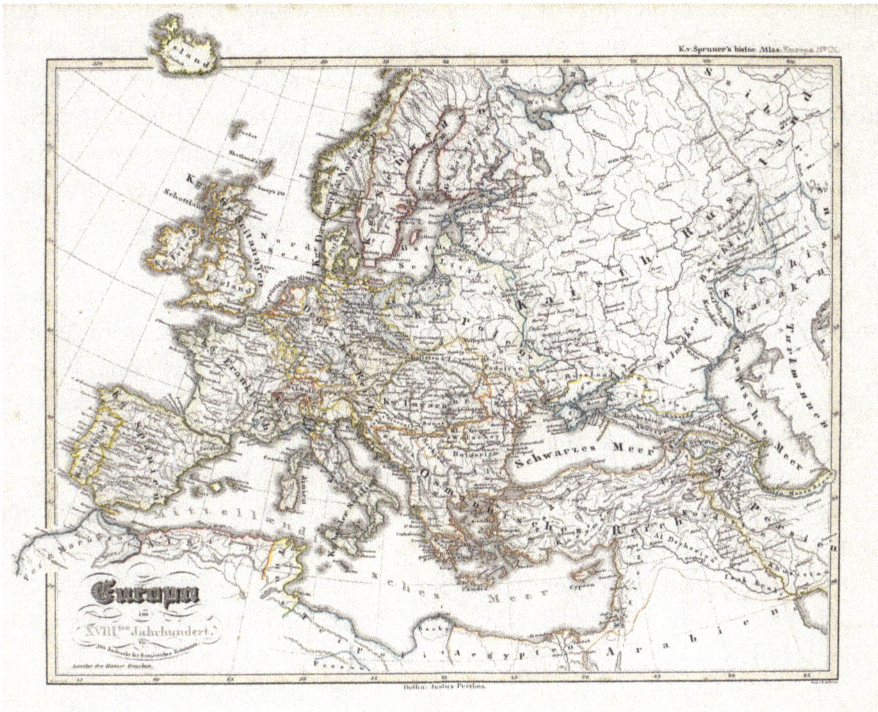

PLATE 2 Europe in the 18th century

This map shows Europe's political divisions at the start of the period covered by this book. Ireland was still part of the United Kingdom, and Finland of the Kingdom of Sweden; France was considerably smaller than it is now, after its expansion in the 18th and 19th centuries; Germany and Italy were still a patchwork of smaller political entities; Poland and Lithuania still clung together in a Commonwealth; and South-eastern Europe was still part of the Ottoman Empire. Collection Koninklijke Bibliotheek, The Hague. Reproduced with permission

KARL VON SPRUNER, *HISTORISCH-GEOGRAPHISCHER HAND-ATLAS ZUR GESCHICHTE DER STAATEN EUROPAS VOM ANFANG DES MITTELALTERS BIS AUF DIE NEUESTE ZEIT* (*ZWEITE AUFLAGE*). GOTHA: JUSTUS PERTHES, 1854.

and Italian states. This implies that it is often difficult to trace the historical development of a current population's health, but these changes also have advantages for the study of population health. Shared destinies have emerged over time, whereas others have dissolved, with sometimes profound consequences for population health.

Finding a good starting-point for this book has not been straightforward. After considering several possibilities, I settled for the early 18th century. This allows us to cover the entire trajectory of improving population health in Europe (although some improvements may already have occurred previously), and to use complete time-series of statistical data (although exceptionally some data go back even further). Several important time-series start somewhere in the first half of the 18th century, and although they cover a limited number of countries they are often very illuminating, and help us to interpret the trends seen in the increasingly complete time-series starting in the 19th and 20th centuries.

As mentioned above, the term 'population health' is to be understood as – literally – 'the people's health', and needs to be distinguished from 'public health', which has been defined as 'the art and science of preventing disease, prolonging life and promoting health through the organized efforts of society'. Public health includes activities such as food inspection, vaccination programs, tobacco control policies, and road traffic safety measures, to mention just a few. Public health is one of the two main things societies do to protect and enhance 'the people's health', the other one being the delivery of medical care. The term 'population health' thus refers to the actual state of health of the people, which is determined by public health and medical care – and by many other factors.

Population health will be measured by a range of indicators, including measures of life expectancy at birth and years lived in good health, and measures of the frequency with which specific diseases occur and give rise to morbidity and mortality. Unfortunately, historical coverage of dimensions of population health is more complete for mortality than for aspects of health among those who are alive. In some European countries, routinely collected data on mortality go back as far as the 18th century, in many others to the 19th century. Relatively abundant data are available for long-term trends in life expectancy, crude mortality rates, infant mortality rates, and (largely limited to the 20th century) causes of death.

The sources of data on population health are listed in Suppl. Table 1. Particularly useful compilations that have been used in many illustrations are the Human Mortality Database, the Human Lifetable Database, Mitchell's International Historical Statistics 1750–2010 (Volume 3: Europe, published 2013), Alderson's International Mortality Statistics (published 1981), the WHO International Mortality Database, and the WHO Health for All Databases. Alderson's mortality data were used for cause-specific mortality trends up to 1960, and WHO data for cause-specific mortality trends from 1960 and onwards. Please note that Alderson presented his data by five-year period, which smooths out annual fluctuations. Also very useful were the data compiled for the OECD 'How was life' project (e.g., on long-term trends in height and literacy). In principle, trends will be shown on a gender-specific basis. This often implies choosing between men and women, but where trends differed this will be mentioned explicitly.

All these data have limitations in terms of comparability between countries and over time, despite the fact that variations and changes in registration have often been repaired in the international compilations just mentioned. Changes in understanding and classification of disease – not to mention the possibility of real changes in the manifestation of disease – represented an obvious issue to be addressed. Wherever disease-specific data from the 18th or 19th century have been used, such as in the few pre-20th century series of mortality by cause of death, I therefore had to follow the (published) insights of specialists in the field who have assessed the comparability of modern disease concepts with older diagnostic terms.[18]

It is only with the advent of the International Classification of Diseases (ICD) in the early 20th century that a basis was laid for better comparability of disease-specific mortality data, both across countries and over time. Among other things, the ICD provided a standard form for certifying the cause of death, and a set of harmonized rules for selecting and coding the 'underlying cause of death' from the conditions mentioned on this death certificate. While this system has dramatically improved the usefulness of cause-of-death statistics, it comes at the price of ignoring co-morbidity. If two or more diseases are involved in causing the death of a person, selecting one 'underlying cause' is often somewhat arbitrary. This was already problematic in the past, when people weakened by one infectious disease would more easily succumb to the following one, and has to be kept in mind even more today, when many elderly people die from the combined effect of several diseases.

For the analyses in this book, time-trends have been reconstructed by carefully selecting the code numbers from each edition of this classification, which changed approximately every 10 years to reflect new insights in nosology (see

18 A theoretical discussion of what 'disease' is, is beyond the scope of this book, but for an introduction see Chapter 3, and for a historical overview, see, e.g., Karl E. Rothschuh, "Der Krankheitsbegriff (Was Ist Krankheit) ," in *Was Ist Krankheit?*, ed. Karl E. Rothschuh (Darmstadt: Wisenschaftliche Buchgesellschaft, 1975). It is likely that, over the three centuries covered by this book, many diseases have changed their manifestation, either spontaneously or under the influence of treatment; see Kurt Kohn, Hans H. Jansen, and Karl Freudenberg, *Gestaltwandel Klassischer Krankheitsbilder*, ed. Wilhelm Doerr (Berlin etc.: Springer-Verlag, 1957). Recent advances in 'palaeomicrobiology' may help to better interpret historical evidence: DNA testing of human remains buried during epidemics has sometimes confirmed the presence of the putative micro-organisms; see, e.g., Michel Drancourt, "Finally, Plague Is Plague," *Clinical Microbiology and Infection* 18, no. 2 (2012): 105–06.

Suppl. Table 2). In a few cases, it has been necessary to adjust cause-specific mortality trends for changes in coding, by using differences in adjacent or overlapping years to bring the rates in previous periods up or down to the level in the more recent period. Despite these careful reconstructions, there is no guarantee that the changes over time and the differences between countries that we see in the data are all real. In addition to changes in understanding and classification of disease, we must also reckon with the greater likelihood of detection of disease in modern times.

As a result of people's more frequent contacts with the health care system, and of diagnostic methods' greater accuracy, less disease goes undetected now than in the past. This should warn us against taking the 20th century rise of diseases like ischaemic heart disease and cancer at face value. In such cases, it will be important to check for supporting evidence, for example an increase in people's exposure to established risk factors of the disease in question. More generally, an important remedy against all these uncertainties is to focus on 'the big picture'; many of the trends and patterns that we see in the following chapters are simply too big and too consistent to be due to artefacts in data collection.[19]

Which diseases to include was another important choice to be made. It was clear from the outset, that this book could cover only a small fraction of the total number of diseases that affected Europeans over these three centuries. Leaving out rare diseases, that number must be at least several hundred. As one of the purposes was to compare long-term trends between countries, which can only be done with mortality data, many of the diseases selected for review have been, or still are, important causes of death. To these have been added a few less fatal diseases, for which some quantitative data are available in the literature, such as pellagra and rickets. Together, the 40-or-so diseases covered provide a broad picture of the factors driving the development of population health in Europe.[20]

---

19 Efforts to systematically 'repair' periodical changes in cause-of-death classifications are progressing slowly (e.g., France Meslé and Jacques Vallin, "Reconstructing Long-Term Series of Causes of Death: The Case of France," *Historical Methods* 29, no. 2 (1996): 72–87). The Human Cause-of-Death Database currently contains harmonized data from around 15 European countries, mostly from Central & Eastern and Eastern Europe (www.causesofdeath.org). Because these data cannot be compared with unadjusted data from routine data sources, and often cover only a limited period of time, they could not be used for this book. However, wherever relevant, results have been checked against trends as seen in the Human Cause-of-Death Database.

20 The *International Classification of Diseases* (10th revision, Clinical Modification) includes around 69,000 codes for diagnostic entities. The Global Burden of Disease study distinguishes 354 different diseases (GBD 2017 Collaborators, "Global, Regional, and National

Nevertheless, a few limitations need to be mentioned. First, the over-representation of potentially fatal diseases should be kept in mind when interpreting this book's main findings. For example, improvements in medical treatment reducing the case fatality of diseases have become more salient than would otherwise have been the case. Second, some determinants of population health cannot satisfactorily be captured when using a disease-specific lens. Diarrheal diseases give us a view of the history of unsanitary living conditions, and lung cancer and diabetes inform us about secular trends in smoking and obesity. But the health effects of environmental pollution, which are spread out over a wide range of diseases which also have many other determinants, risk to remain in the background when specific diseases are the main entry-point to the history of population health. I have partly remedied this by highlighting the health effects of air pollution in a section devoted to the lung diseases caused by occupational and environmental exposures.

I have tried to represent the European experience by including all available data in each graph, but with most countries represented by small-dotted lines in light grey. Visually, this produces a narrower or broader band showing developments in Europe as a whole. Within this band, some countries have been highlighted to illustrate the main patterns of variation. Usually Sweden (or one of the other Northern European countries) has been highlighted as a benchmark for best performance, and one country from each of the other larger regions has been marked as well, using the same colour in all graphs to ease recognition. Northern European countries are in dark blue, Western European in light green, Southern European countries in yellow, Central-eastern European countries in purple, South-eastern European countries in brown, Eastern European countries in red.

Wherever possible, mortality and morbidity rates have been age-standardized to take away the effect of variations in age-distribution between countries or over time. In order to facilitate comparisons between different graphs, most mortality rates have been expressed as deaths per 100,000 person-years, even if this is unusual (as in the case of the crude mortality rate, which is usually expressed as deaths per 1000). In the graphs, I have tried to avoid the use of logarithmic vertical axes, so that absolute magnitudes of change and variation can be compared more easily between diseases, countries and time-periods.

Incidence, Prevalence, and Years Lived with Disability for 354 Diseases and Injuries," *Lancet* 392, no. 10159 (2018): 1789–858). The *Cambridge World History of Human Disease* reviews 158 diseases, with a bias towards infectious diseases, and without entries for many other important health conditions (Kiple, *World History*).

The long-term trends shown in these graphs, which form the core of this book, will be combined with a digest of the – as mentioned above: massive – literature to understand how and why population health in Europe has changed as it has. I will present (almost) no statistical analyses of my own, in which putative determinants are related to health outcomes, but I will instead rely on what others have found. In contrast to the data presented in this book, which are almost exclusively national in character, some of the more recent studies of the determinants of mortality decline have used micro- instead of macro-level data, which is very useful because micro-level data are more suitable for addressing causal questions.[21]

As a complement to the graphs with secular changes in population health I have added a small number of illustrative pictures – historical maps, paintings, photographs, pages from influential books, etc. These are intended to remind the reader of the reality underlying the quantitative data, and somewhat abstract analyses, that form the core of this book. Finally, I hope that the very long reference list does not only serve its purpose of documenting the scientific basis for the statements made, but will also give readers who want to know more a good entry-point to the literature.

Readers who would like to have a closer look at the quantitative data used in the trend graphs, e.g. in order to check out the experience of non-highlighted countries, can find these online.[22]

---

21 On the relative merits of macro- and micro-level analyses, see, e.g., S. Ryan Johansson, "Macro and Micro Perspectives on Mortality History," *Historical Methods* 33, no. 2 (2000): 59–72. In the last two decades, micro-level analyses have become more prominent in historical demography, particularly for studying the determinants of secular changes in infant mortality; for a digest, see Lucia Pozzi and Diego Ramiro Fariñas, "Infant and Child Mortality in the Past," *Annales de Démographie Historique*, no. 1 (2015): 55–75. See also Chapter 5.

22 An excel file with the data underlying the graphs can be found at dx.doi.org/10.6084/m9.figshare.11774652.

PART 1

Long-term Trends: a Bird's Eye View

CHAPTER 2

Long-term Trends in Population Health

That the people's health has improved importantly over the 300 years since the early 18th century is well-known, but how has the pace of improvement varied over time, across health conditions and between European countries? In this chapter we will give a broad-brush picture of these changes and variations, in order to have firm ground under our feet when we review the more detailed disease-specific trends.

Changes in Over-all Population Health

The best way to start our analysis is by looking at trends in mortality. This may sound illogical: how can counting the dead inform us about the health of the living? However, the reason is simple: death usually follows disease or another health condition, and mortality rates therefore often tell us something about the frequency of disease. Furthermore, mortality data are the only health data going back to the 18th century, and are also available for a far larger number of countries than morbidity data.

Declining Mortality

The increase in life expectancy that we saw in Figure 1 is, of course, due to a decline in the mortality rate. When life expectancy at birth was below 40 years, as it was in the 18th century, the annual death rate was around 30 per 1000. This is equal to saying that each year 3 out of every 100 European citizens died. Now that life expectancy has nearly doubled, the annual death rate is around 10 per 1000. (Because of population aging, the real decline in the risk of death has actually been much greater than the two-thirds suggested by this simple comparison of crude mortality rates.) Figure 2 shows that this decline of the death rate has actually been very bumpy.

Over the three centuries for which data are available, the European experience is punctuated by enormous spikes of mortality, which have only recently diminished in amplitude. Previous studies have suggested that the amplitude of these spikes gradually diminished during the 18th and 19th centuries, but this is not immediately obvious from our data which cover an unusually large number of countries. Previous studies focused on the trend of mortality in

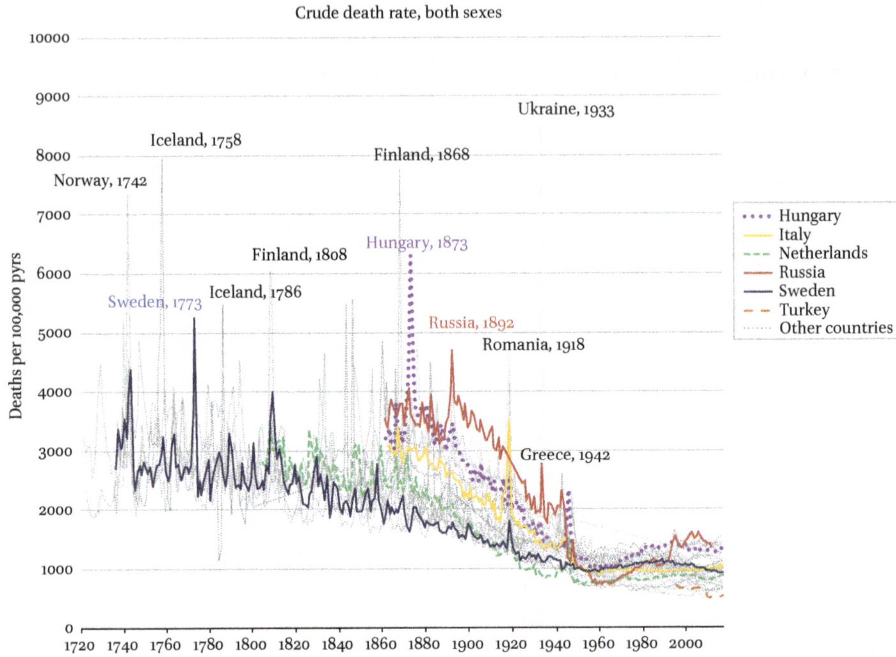

FIGURE 2 Trends in over-all mortality in Europe, 1720–2015
Notes: Norway 1742: famine. Iceland 1758: unknown epidemic. Sweden 1773: famine. Iceland 1786: smallpox. Finland 1808: war, typhus, dysentery. Finland 1868: famine. Hungary 1873: cholera. Russia 1892: famine. Romania 1918: war, influenza. Ukraine 1933: famine. Russia 1933: famine. Greece 1942: war, famine
SOURCE OF DATA: SEE SUPPL. TABLE 1

countries like Sweden, France and England, and in these countries the swings in mortality did indeed diminish in an early stage, as can be seen for Sweden which has been highlighted in Figure 2.[1]

Yet, for other countries mortality fluctuations during the 19th century are not necessarily less than during the 18th century, and some dramatic upswings of mortality even occurred in the first half of the 20th century. When all countries are taken together there was a gradual decline of the average amplitude of mortality fluctuations, but this decline reversed in the first half of the 20th

1 Alfred Perrenoud, "The Attenuation of Mortality Crises and the Decline of Mortality," in *The Decline of Mortality in Europe*, ed. Roger S. Schofield, David Reger, and Alain Bideau (Oxford: Clarendon Press, 1991).

century, and it was only in the second half of the 20th century that the trends really calmed down.[2]

What were the causes of these mortality spikes? The highest peak in Figure 2 is for Ukraine in 1933, when more than 8% of the population died in a famine. Many other spikes were also caused by large famines, such as the 1758 peak in Iceland, the 1773 peak in Sweden, the 1868 peak in Finland, the 1933 peak in Russia, and the 1942 peak in Greece. The more widely known famine of the 1840s (due to the 'Potato Blight', see Chapter 4) is invisible. This is partly because it is hidden below other, more dramatic mortality elevations, partly because there are no national mortality data from the 19th century for Ireland, where this famine caused a very strong increase in mortality rates.[3]

Large-scale epidemics are another important cause of mortality spikes. Smallpox epidemics caused cycles of mortality fluctuations on a time-scale of 5 – 15 years in many European countries. The 1918/19 influenza pandemic can also clearly be seen in Figure 2. Of all the epidemics in the 19th century, cholera is by far the most publicized, but the excess mortality involved is generally less than that of other mortality 'crises'. The main exception is the 1873 cholera epidemic in Hungary which caused a huge mortality peak.[4]

The spikes caused by famines and epidemics are more prominently visible in Figure 2 than spikes in mortality caused by wars, but this is partly due to interruption of data collection in war-time. Nevertheless, the Franco-Prussian War (1870–71) coincided with a visible spike in France's mortality trend, and so did World War I (1914–1918) and World War II (1939–1945) in the mortality trends of the countries involved that kept their vital registration systems running.

As can be seen in Figure 2, not only have mortality spikes gradually diminished in amplitude, but 'normal' levels of mortality have declined as well. Around 1870, European countries' annual death rate in 'normal' years still ranged between 20 and 35 per 1000. This rapidly declined to between 10 and 20

2 The average coefficient of variation (i.e., the average of all available countries' standard deviation of their yearly mortality rates, as a fraction of their average mortality rate over the same period) was 22% in 1720–1749, 15% in 1750–1799, 12% in 1800–1849, 11% in 1850–1899, 15% in 1900–1949, and 7% in 1950–1999.

3 Cormac Ó Gráda, "Ireland," in *Famine in European History*, ed. Guido Alfani and Cormac Ó Gráda (Cambridge etc.: Cambridge University Press, 2017).

4 Some of the highest spikes occurred in Iceland: a country with less than 100,000 inhabitants in which infection with diseases like small-pox and measles could not sustain, so that epidemics imported from abroad would subside, sometimes for decades, and then flare up again when the virus returned to infect a largely non-immunized population.

in 1930, and even further to between 7 and 13 in 1960. Many countries in Northern and Western Europe passed below the 15 per 1000 level in the 1900s or 1910s, whereas most countries in Southern, Central-eastern, South-eastern and Eastern Europe reached this low level only in the 1930s or 1940s.[5]

Because, during the 'demographic transition', mortality decline preceded fertility decline, European population numbers increased enormously. In the beginning of the 19th century, Europe had around 200 million inhabitants, and this number almost tripled to around 550 million in 1950, despite massive emigration and a series of bloody wars.

Young and Old, Men and Women

Mortality has declined at all ages, indicating that health improvements have occurred throughout the lifespan. The largest percentage declines in mortality occurred among infants and children, but even among the elderly reductions in mortality have been substantial. When we take all European countries together, and calculate average percentage declines of mortality between 1870 and 2010, we find the following astonishing figures.

Among men, mortality declined by 98% among infants, by 99% among children (ages 1 to 15 years), by 88% among young people (ages 15 to 45 years), by 67% among middle-aged people (ages 45 to 65 years), and by 55% among elderly people (ages 65 to 85 years). These declines are almost incredible, particularly in the youngest age-groups. Among women, the corresponding figures are 98%, 99%, 94%, 81%, and 71%, indicating that with the exception of infants and children the mortality declines among women have been even greater than among men.[6]

As always, these over-all averages hide important variations (see Suppl. Figure 2). Among infants and children, mortality decline first accelerated, to reach its maximum speed in the period 1930–1960, and then slowed down again. This is probably because after 1960 mortality had reached such low levels, that it became increasingly difficult to lower it further. Among the elderly, however, mortality decline accelerated over time, and reached its maximum speed in the last period (1990–2010), suggesting that the end of mortality decline is not yet in sight.

5 After the early 1960s, population ageing caused the crude mortality rate to stabilize, and to even increase somewhat. Turkey's mortality rates in this period, which stand out as very low in Figure 2, are explained by its very young population.

6 These percentage declines are based on data in the Human Mortality Database and the Human Lifetable Database, and were calculated from simple arithmetic averages of the age-adjusted mortality rates (in each of the age-groups mentioned) for 13 countries in 1870, and 25 countries in 2010.

For young and middle-aged women, the time-pattern of mortality decline is like that seen for infants and children: acceleration followed by deceleration. For young and middle-aged men the time-pattern is different, with a clear dip in the speed of mortality decline between 1960 and 1990. This caused a temporary interruption of the secular increase of male life expectancy at birth, which we already saw in Figure 1. It was due to a rise of ischaemic heart disease and other 'diseases of affluence' that we will discuss in more detail below.

Generally speaking, these time-patterns can be observed in all European countries, but the dips in the speed of mortality decline among young and middle-aged men in the 1960–1990 period have been much more prominent in some countries than in others. In Northern, Western, and Southern European countries this was just a deceleration of mortality decline, whereas in Central-eastern, South-eastern and Eastern Europe mortality among adult men actually increased between 1960 and 1990.

A striking acceleration of mortality decline in recent decades can also be seen among the oldest-old, i.e., those above 85 years of age. As a result of declining mortality remaining life expectancy at the age of 85 has recently increased rapidly. Until the early 1950s, remaining life expectancy from the age of 85 hovered between 3 and 4 years among men and between 3.5 and 4.5 years among women, but then it started to increase, gaining speed along the way (see Suppl. Figure 3).

In 2016, the highest average life expectancy from age 85 among women in Europe, 7.7 years, was found in France. France is also the country with the oldest living European (Plate 3), and the country where Jeanne Calment (1875–1997) lived. She holds the world record with a documented age-at-death of 122 years and 165 days.[7]

These trends in mortality at advanced ages are followed closely, not only by demographers but also by gerontologists, economists and many others. It was once thought that average life expectancy would not increase beyond age 85, and that age 85 even represented something like the average maximum lifespan of the human species. If this were true – so the reasoning went – not only

7 On Jeanne Calment, see Jean-Marie Robine and Michel Allard, "The Oldest Human," *Science* 279, no. 5358 (1998): 1831–831. Recently raised doubts on the true age of Jeanne Calment have been refuted in Jean-Marie Robine et al., "The Real Facts Supporting Jeanne Calment as the Oldest Ever Human," *Journals of Gerontology: Series A* 74, no. S1 (2019): S13–S20. In Europe, several small areas with an unusual concentration of centenarians have been found (e.g., on Sardinia). These are usually isolated communities that have retained a traditional life style, but that also benefit from modern hygiene, health care and living standards; see Michel Poulain, Anne Herm, and Gianni Pes, "Blue Zones: Areas of Exceptional Longevity around the World," *Vienna Yearbook of Population Research* 11 (2013): 87–108.

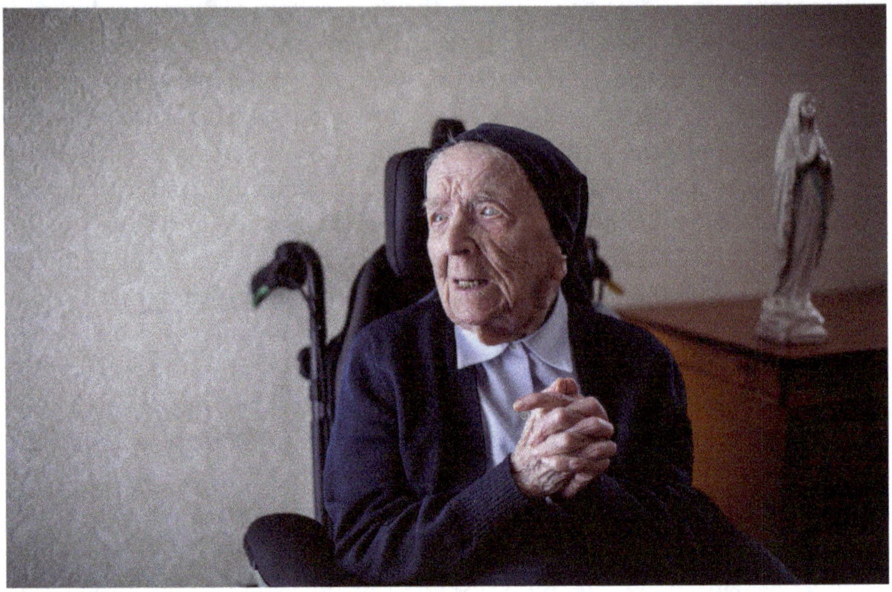

PLATE 3 Lucille Randon, a.k.a. Soeur André. The oldest person in Europe, 2019
At the moment of writing this book (October 2019), Lucille Randon was the oldest person is Europe, and the second oldest person in the world as verified by the Gerontology Research Group. She was born in 1904 in Alès, in the South of France, and entered a religious order in 1944. Since 1979, she has lived in a nursing home. At her 115th birthday, her mind was still clear, but she spent her time in a wheel-chair and had lost most of her eye-sight.
PHOTOGRAPH BY FRANCK BESSIÈRE. REPRODUCED WITH PERMISSION

would a 'compression of mortality' around this age of 85 occur, but a 'compression of morbidity' in a few years before death would also be inevitable.[8]

However, this is not what happened. The almost-doubling of remaining life expectancy from age 85, and more generally the rapid declines of mortality among the oldest-old, have belied the idea that human life expectancy is approaching a maximum. And even if there would be such a maximum, it is unlikely to be near: average life expectancy at birth among women in France, Spain, Italy, and Switzerland already exceeds 85 years. There is very little tendency for a 'compression of mortality' in a narrow age-range around the

8 This was famously argued in 1980 in James F. Fries, "Aging, Natural Death, and the Compression of Morbidity," *New England Journal of Medicine* 303 (1980): 130–35.

average age-at-death. Whether or not a 'compression of morbidity' has occurred will be discussed below.[9]

Regional and Social Inequalities

Below the surface of national levels and trends in mortality, there have always been substantial regional and social variations within countries, to the extent that some observers have claimed that for the history of mortality one cannot rely on the "misleading mean." While that may be an exaggeration, it is certainly true that studies of subnational variations are important for our understanding of the causes of mortality decline.

In the long run, all geographical areas and all social groups within European countries have benefitted from health improvements, but timing and speed usually differed between areas and groups. This has not only created opportunities for identifying determinants of population health change, but has also often led to widening health gaps. French demographers Jacques Vallin and France Meslé have even suggested to use a divergence of health indicators between regions and social groups as an indicator of new epidemiologic transitions.[10]

One of the most illuminating examples of these within-country differences are the disparities in health and health improvement between socioeconomic groups, as defined by level of education, occupational class, or income. The massive literature on this topic, which has grown explosively since these 'health inequalities' were 're-discovered' in the early 1980s, indeed shows that

9 Some studies have found evidence for compression of mortality (e.g., John R. Wilmoth and Shiro Horiuchi, "Rectangularization Revisited: Variability of Age at Death within Human Populations," *Demography* 36, no. 4 (1999): 475–95; Wilma J. Nusselder and Johan P. Mackenbach, "Rectangularization of the Survival Curve in the Netherlands, 1950–1992," *Gerontologist* 36, no. 6 (1996): 773–82), but this has not been the general tendency in high-income countries since 1980 (Colin D. Mathers et al., "Causes of International Increases in Older Age Life Expectancy," *Lancet* 385, no. 9967 (2015): 540–48). On "broken limits to life expectancy," see Jim Oeppen and James W. Vaupel, "Broken Limits to Life Expectancy," *Science* 296 (2002): 1029–031.

10 The expression "misleading mean" is from a paper by S. Ryan Johansson and Alice B. Kasakoff, "Mortality History and the Misleading Mean," *Historical Methods* 33, no. 2 (2000): 56–8. Using divergence as a signal of new transitions was proposed in Jacques Vallin and France Meslé, "Convergences and Divergences in Mortality: A New Approach of Health Transition," *Demographic Research* 2 (2004): 11–44. Regional variations in trends in mortality or other health indicators within European countries cannot be summarized in terms of one or a few generalized tendencies; see, e.g., Sebastian Klüsener et al., "Spatial Inequalities in Infant Survival at an Early Stage of the Longevity Revolution," *Demographic Research* 30 (2014): 1849–864.

inequalities in mortality and other health indicators by socioeconomic position tend to widen during over-all health improvement.[11]

Historical evidence suggests that socioeconomic inequalities in health are not a recent phenomenon. Inequalities in mortality between persons with higher and lower social positions were probably already present in the 17th and 18th centuries, at least in European urban areas. Yet, recent studies found that inequalities in infant mortality only emerged, when health started to improve at the end of the 19th century. This indicates that a higher socioeconomic position (i.e., more money or knowledge) only started to make a difference after the causes of high mortality had been discovered, and after effective interventions had been developed.[12]

During the first half of the 20th century, only few countries kept registers of socioeconomic inequalities in mortality. In England and Wales, inequalities in infant mortality declined substantially between the 1920s and 1970s, suggesting that, after a temporary widening at the end of the 19th century, inequalities in infant mortality narrowed again. However, over the same period inequalities in adult mortality remained largely stable in absolute terms, and even increased in relative terms.[13]

We are much better informed about trends in health inequalities over the last half-century. In most European countries, mortality has steadily declined among both lower and higher socioeconomic groups. Nevertheless, because

11 It was for some time believed that health inequalities had disappeared after World War II, due to higher living standards, social security and universal access to health care. In the early 1980s, the Black report in Britain (Douglas Black et al., *Inequalities in Health (the Black Report)* (London Department of Health and Social Services, 1980; repr., Penguin Books, 1982)) and similar reports in other European countries shattered this illusion. For an analysis of socioeconomic inequalities in health in Europe, see Johan P. Mackenbach, *Health Inequalities: Persistence and Change in European Welfare States* (Oxford etc.: Oxford University Press, 2019).

12 The empirical evidence on health inequalities before the 1970s is very fragmented; see Tommy Bengtsson and Frans van Poppel, “Socioeconomic Inequalities in Death from Past to Present: An Introduction,” *Explorations in Economic History* 48, no. 3 (2011): 343–56. For studies finding emergence (or widening) of inequalities in mortality at the end of the 19th century in Sweden and England, see Tommy Bengtsson and Martin Dribe, “The Late Emergence of Socioeconomic Mortality Differentials,” *Explorations in Economic History* 48, no. 3 (2011): 389–400; Robert Woods, *The Demography of Victorian England and Wales* (Cambridge etc.: Cambridge University Press, 2000).

13 For analyses of long-term trends of inequalities in mortality in England and Wales, see Elsie R. Pamuk, “Social Class Inequality in Mortality from 1921 to 1972 in England and Wales,” *Population Studies (Cambridge)* 39, no. 1 (1985): 17–31; Elsie R. Pamuk, “Social-Class Inequality in Infant Mortality in England and Wales from 1921 to 1980,” *European Journal of Population/Revue Européenne de Démographie* 4, no. 1 (1988): 1–21.

percentage declines were usually faster among the higher educated and the higher occupational classes, relative inequalities have generally increased considerably, even in the most advanced welfare states. Inequalities in life expectancy between people with primary and tertiary education now amount to between 5 and 10 years in North-western and Southern Europe, and more than 10 years in Central-eastern and Eastern Europe.[14]

A widening of relative inequalities in mortality is generally seen whenever mortality declines, regardless of country or cause of death. The same applies to several other health indicators, such as the incidence of cancer or injury. This results from the fact that higher socioeconomic groups have less difficulty following health advice (e.g., stop smoking), more often participate in prevention programs (e.g., cancer screening), and have better treatment outcomes (e.g., higher survival after myocardial infarction). Apparently, a higher socioeconomic position provides the individual with 'flexible resources', such as knowledge, money, power and social connections, which can be used to avoid disease or to minimize the consequences of disease.[15]

While the trend description above applies to North-western and Southern Europe, the story is rather different for Central-Eastern and Eastern Europe. Even under communism there were socioeconomic inequalities in health, but after the fall of the Berlin Wall these health inequalities exploded. Whereas higher socioeconomic groups soon took advantage of liberalized economic conditions and new access to medical technologies from the West, with declining mortality as a result, mortality among the less well-off rose. This dramatic widening of the gap in mortality was only reversed when, in the early 2000s, mortality in lower socioeconomic groups finally started to decline.[16]

14 For an overview, see Johan P. Mackenbach et al., "Socioeconomic Inequalities in Health in 22 European Countries," *New England Journal of Medicine* 358, no. 23 (2008): 2468–481. For the distinction between relative and absolute inequalities, see Johan P. Mackenbach et al., "Changes in Mortality Inequalities over Two Decades," *British Medical Journal* 353 (2016): i1732.

15 This paragraph is based on the 'fundamental causes' theory of health inequalities; see Bruce G. Link and Jo Phelan, "Social Conditions as Fundamental Causes of Disease," *Journal of Health and Social Behavior* Spec No (1995): 80–94. This theory finds considerable support in the European experience; see Johan P. Mackenbach et al., "Fundamental Causes of Inequalities in Mortality," *Sociology of Health and Illness* 39, no. 7 (2017): 1117–133.

16 On recent trends in mortality inequalities in Europe, see Johan P. Mackenbach et al., "Recent Trends in Health Inequalities in 27 European Countries," *Proceedings of the National Academy of Sciences* 115, no. 25 (2018): 6440–445.

Rising Height

Partly inspired by controversies about the role of living standards in the rise of life expectancy, many studies have been made of trends in body height – Europeans have grown considerably taller since the 19th century. American economist and Nobel laureate Robert Fogel (1926–2013) has used the positive correlation between people's adult height and their risk of mortality to argue that improvements in nutrition (as reflected in increasing body height) made an important contribution to increases in life expectancy.[17]

However, things are less simple than that. Height reflects growth, and growth reflects nutrition, but growth also reflects health during the first two decades of life, and is negatively affected by the extra nutritional demands during episodes of infectious diseases. Trends and variations in height thus capture the effect on growth of *both* nutrition *and* disease. This is reflected in the ambiguous term 'biological standard of living', which is commonly used in the economic-historical literature to denote what height actually measures.[18]

For many European countries, data on average height of military recruits are available since the 19th century or even earlier (see Suppl. Figure 4). (In the case of compulsory medical service, these recruits will be men of ca. 20 years old.) During the 19th century height of military recruits fluctuated in a pattern suggesting that the early phase of industrialization was sometimes associated with a temporary decline in the 'biological standard of living'. For example, in England there was a decline in height from the 1820s to the 1840s, in which the average recruit lost a few centimetres.[19]

---

17 Robert W. Fogel, *The Escape from Hunger and Premature Death, 1700–2100* (Cambridge etc.: Cambridge University Press, 2004).

18 For an analysis along these lines, see Roderick Floud et al., *The Changing Body* (Cambridge etc.: Cambridge University Press, 2011). Fogel has also argued that better health contributed to accelerated economic growth; see Robert W. Fogel et al., "Secular Changes in American and British Stature and Nutrition," *Journal of Interdisciplinary History* 14, no. 2 (1983): 445–81.

19 Time-series data on height show that, at least in England, the early phases of industrialization had negative effects, partly through the side-effects of rapid urbanization; see Roderick Floud and Bernard Harris, "Health, Height and Welfare: Britain 1700–1980," in *Health and Welfare During Industrialization*, ed. R.H. Steckel and R. Floud (Chicago & London: Chicago University Press, 1997); John Komlos, "The Secular Trend in the Biological Standard of Living in the United Kingdom, 1730-1860," *Economic History Review* 46, no. 1 (1993): 115–44. This was, however, not observed in some other European countries, such as Sweden and the Netherlands; see Lars G. Sandberg and Richard H. Steckel, "Was Industrialization Hazardous to Your Health? Not in Sweden!" in *Health and Welfare During Industrialization*, ed. Richard H. Steckel and R. Floud (Chicago & London: University of Chicago Press, 1997); J.W. Drukker and Vincent Tassenaar, "Paradoxes of Modernization and Material Well-Being in the Netherlands During the Nineteenth Century," in *Health and Welfare*

Starting in the late 19th century, height of recruits gradually increased by a staggering 10 – 15 centimetres, from around 165 cm to between 175 and 180 cm in most countries. Detailed analyses have shown that declines in infant and childhood mortality are generally followed by increases in height in the same birth cohorts. This suggests that increases in height were indeed not only due to improved nutrition, but also to reduced exposure to infection.[20]

As in the case of the increase in life expectancy, European countries also differed in the timing of the increase in height, roughly following the pattern in which their national incomes started to grow. Height of recruits in the Nordic countries was already relatively high in the 19th century, perhaps because of proximity to protein in the form of cattle and milk. They also passed the 170 cm level relatively early: this already happened in recruits born around the turn of the 20th century. The same early rise is seen in recruits from, among others, Great Britain, the Netherlands and Switzerland. Southern, Central-eastern, South-eastern and Eastern European countries generally passed this 170 cm threshold much later: here, this happened in recruits born in the 1930s, 1940s or 1950s. Portugal was the last (together with Turkey) to pass the 170 cm level, by recruits born in the 1970s.[21]

Many European countries abolished compulsory military service in the 1990s, after the collapse of the Soviet Union and the end of the Cold War, so that time-series data of recruit heights stopped abruptly. By then, most countries had passed the 175 cm level. In a few (Sweden, Denmark, the Netherlands, Germany), the average recruit was even taller than 180 cm. Fortunately, studies of growth of children have continued, showing that the secular trend towards

---

During Industrialization, ed. R.H. Steckel and R. Floud (Chicago & London: Chicago University Press, 1997). In later phases the effects of industrialization on living standards and health became largely positive; see Joerg Baten and Matthias Blum, "Growing Tall but Unequal," *Economic History of Developing Regions* 27, no. Suppl. 1 (2012): S66–S85.

20 See, e.g., Timothy J. Hatton, "How Have Europeans Grown So Tall? ," *Oxford Economic Papers* 66, no. 2 (2014): 349–72; Ida M. Schmidt, M.H. Jørgensen, and Kim Fleischer Michaelsen, "Height of Conscripts in Europe: Is Postneonatal Mortality a Predictor? ," *Annals of Human Biology* 22, no. 1 (1995): 57–67.

21 For the association between growth in national income and rise in height, see, e.g., Timothy J. Hatton and Bernice E. Bray, "Long Run Trends in the Heights of European Men, 19th–20th Centuries," *Economics & Human Biology* 8, no. 3 (2010): 405–13; Baten and Blum, "Growing Tall but Unequal." For the relationship between height and access to protein, in the form of cattle, meat and milk, see Joerg Baten and Matthias Blum, "Why Are You Tall While Others Are Short? ," *European Review of Economic History* 18, no. 2 (2014): 144–65. Proximity to protein may also partly explain the extraordinary heights of Dutch recruits (Suppl. Figure 4). For height trends in Portugal, see Yvonne Stolz, Joerg Baten, and Jaime Reis, "Portuguese Living Standards, 1720–1980, in European Comparison," *Economic History Review* 66, no. 2 (2013): 545–78. For height trends in Russia, see Chapter 7, note 60.

greater height is still on-going – but not in the world's tallest nation, the Netherlands, where the trend seems to have stopped in the early 2000s.[22]

More Years in Good Health, More Years in Bad Health?

Data on long-term trends in morbidity, instead of mortality, are scarce before the 1970s. It is only around that time that several European countries started to conduct nation-wide surveys of (self-reported) chronic disease, disability and general health status. The most important earlier source of information is sickness insurance claims of workers in Britain during the 19th century. This is, admittedly, a narrow basis for making claims about long-term trends in morbidity, but for lack of something better we will briefly summarize the findings of these studies.

The source of information for these studies are the records kept by British 'Friendly Societies'. Before the modern welfare state developed, these mutual societies provided income replacement and medical attendance during sickness to their members, who were mostly men in manual occupations. Some studies have found a rise of sickness insurance claims coinciding with the decline of mortality in the last decades of the 19th century. This has been attributed to the fact that "[i]f more people survive, then individuals who would have died live longer, although their health remains poor." Yet, the findings of these studies are far from consistent, so it is difficult to reach firm conclusions.[23]

Were declines in mortality accompanied by a rise in morbidity or not? It is easy to imagine that they were, if mortality declines were mostly based on

---

22 Yvonne Schönbeck et al., "The World's Tallest Nation Has Stopped Growing Taller," *Pediatric Research* 73, no. 3 (2013): 371–77. In the Nordic countries, the secular trend is still continuing; see Anton Holmgren et al., "Nordic Populations Are Still Getting Taller–Secular Changes in Height from the 20th to 21st Century," *Acta Paediatrica* 108 (2019): 1311–320.

23 The quote is from George Alter and James C. Riley, "Frailty, Sickness, and Death: Models of Morbidity and Mortality in Historical Populations," *Population Studies* 43, no. 1 (1989): 25–45, p. 43. Some of the main studies have been done by American historian James Riley; see James C. Riley, *Sickness, Recovery, and Death* (London: MacMillan Press, 1989). The purported rise of morbidity seen in these studies has been criticized for the sensitivity of morbidity rates to 'cultural inflation', due to rising health expectations and institutional pressures (S. Ryan Johansson, "The Health Transition: The Cultural Inflation of Morbidity During the Decline of Mortality," *Health Transition Review* 1, no. 1 (1991): 39–68). However, an empirical study of changing 'thresholds' for declaring oneself unable to work did not find much evidence for this (Martin Gorsky et al., "The 'Cultural Inflation of Morbidity' During the English Mortality Decline," *Social Science & Medicine* 73, no. 12 (2011): 1775–783). Other studies than Riley's have not found much change in age-specific incidence or duration of sickness episodes between the 1870s and 1940s (Bernard Harris et al., "Long-Term Changes in Sickness and Health," *Economic History Review* 65, no. 2 (2012): 719–45).

increased survival for sick individuals, as suggested in the quote in the previous paragraph. But it is equally easy to imagine that they were not, if mortality declines were mostly based on declines in the incidence of disease, or if increased survival of sick individuals was due to factors that also increased their recovery rates. In all likelihood, all these mechanisms played a role, but in unknown quantities.[24]

This lack of precise insight in trends in morbidity even applies to more recent time-periods. Despite the increased availability of survey data, and despite attempts at harmonization of survey questions across European countries, the picture that arises from studies of trends in morbidity is far from consistent. A recent comparative study found a decline in severe disability among elderly people in four European countries (Denmark, Finland, Italy, the Netherlands) and an increase in two (Belgium and Sweden) over the last two decades of the 20th century. Why some countries should have experienced a decline and others an increase is a complete mystery.[25]

Combining survey data with data on life expectancy, it has become possible to calculate measures of 'healthy life expectancy', or 'disease-free life expectancy', or 'disability-free life expectancy'. Time-trends can only be calculated over the period for which survey data are available, and for an illustration of what this looks like we have prepared Figure 3. This shows trends in the Netherlands, one of the few European countries with survey data reaching back to the early 1980s (and life expectancy data reaching back to the 1850s).

Life expectancy without moderate or severe disability has increased in parallel with total life expectancy, implying that years lived with disability have remained more or less constant during the last three decades. Apparently, the effect of increased survival of people with diseases causing disability has been offset by a decreased risk of these people becoming moderately or severely disabled. Both are probably the result of more effective medical care.

---

24 The prevalence of different levels of disability represents an equilibrium between 'inflow' (incidence) and 'outflow' (death or recovery). Improvements in medical care reduce the risk of death among disabled individuals, and at the same time shift severely disabled persons to lower levels of disability, so that declines in mortality may go together with declining levels of severe disability and increasing levels of mild disability (Kenneth G. Manton, "Changing Concepts of Morbidity and Mortality in the Elderly Population," *Milbank Memorial Fund Quarterly. Health and Society* 60, no. 2 (1982): 183–244).

25 Gaetan Lafortune and Gaëlle Balestat, *Trends in Severe Disability among Elderly People*, vol. 26, OECD Health Working Papers, (Paris: Organisation for Economic Cooperation and Development, 2007). One possibility is that these differences are spurious and result from variations in reporting.

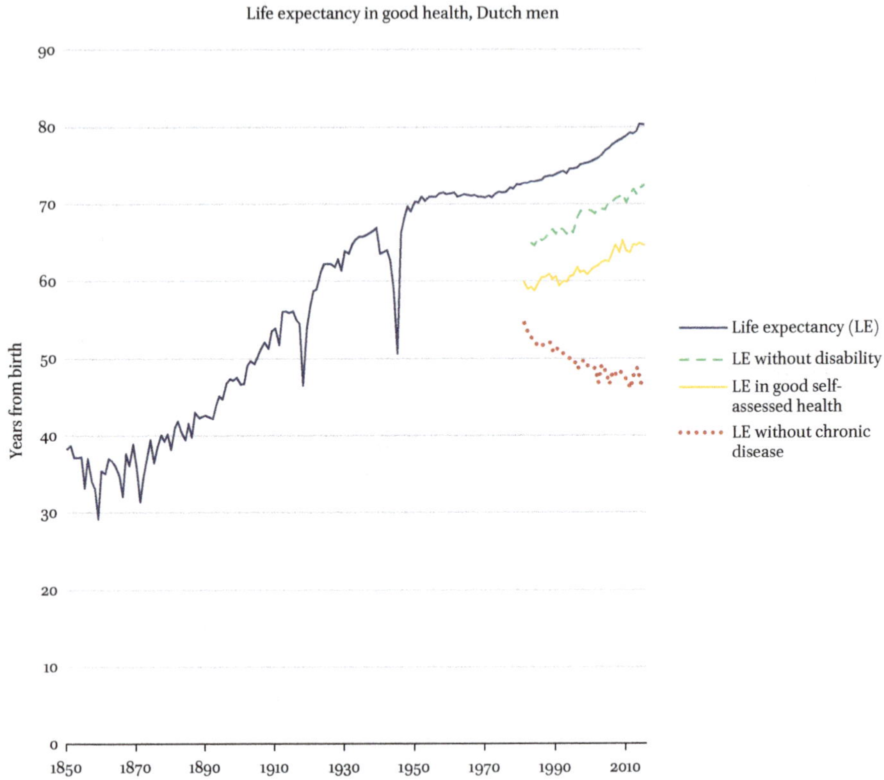

FIGURE 3 Trends in life and health expectancy in the Netherlands, 1850–2010
Notes: Prevalence of disability, self-assessed health and chronic diseases based on self-reports; disability = moderate or severe disability according to GALI *indicator*
SOURCE OF DATA: HUMAN MORTALITY DATABASE (LIFE EXPECTANCY) AND STATISTICS NETHERLANDS (MEASURES OF HEALTHY LIFE EXPECTANCY)

At the same time, life expectancy without chronic disease has declined, and the number of years lived with chronic disease has increased, as a result of earlier detection of chronic diseases. This may have been a necessary condition for the increased benefits of medical care just mentioned – as we will see in later chapters, early detection and treatment of cardiovascular disease and cancer has been an important ingredient of recent advances in medical care.

Nevertheless, when we take a longer time-perspective, it is clear that whatever measure of 'healthy life expectancy' we use, life expectancy in good health is higher in the Netherlands today than total life expectancy 150 years ago, which must mean that the number of years spent in good health has increased enormously. Similar results, but over a shorter period, have been found for other European countries.[26]

That Europeans currently live more years in good health, but at the cost of also living more years in less good health, is confirmed by findings of the Global Burden of Disease study. This study has estimated trends in life expectancy, healthy life-years and years lost to disability since 1990. Of the total number of life-years gained between 1990 and 2017, 26% were spent in poor health, and 74% in good health. Whether the good news in these results outweighs the bad news is difficult to say, even for the specialists who are familiar with these calculations.[27]

Changes in Disease Patterns

Shifting Causes of Death

The remarkable mortality declines that we saw in the previous section were accompanied by profound changes in the share of specific causes of death. Although some countries started to register causes of death before the 20th century, the cause-of-death classifications that were applied at the time differed between countries and are now considered obsolete. Only in a few cases (e.g., tuberculosis and maternal mortality) will it be possible to present pre-20th century cause-of-death data in this book.

Trends in mortality by cause of death show that the increase of life expectancy during the 20th and early 21st centuries was accompanied by important changes in the percentage of deaths attributed to specific diseases. When life expectancy rose from 50 to 70 years, the share of specific infectious diseases (such as tuberculosis and dysentery) and respiratory diseases (such as pneumonia and influenza) declined, whereas that of cardiovascular diseases, cancers and injuries rose (see Suppl. Figure 5).

26 For an European overview for the early 2000s, see Jean-Marie Robine and Emmanuelle Cambois, "Healthy Life Expectancy in Europe," *Population & Sociétés*, no. 499 (2013): 1–4. For the interpretation of trends in total and disability-free life expectancy, see, e.g., Lois M. Verbrugge, "Longer Life but Worsening Health? ," *Milbank Memorial Fund Quarterly. Health and Society* 62, no. 3 (1984): 475–519; Eileen M. Crimmins, Yasuhiko Saito, and Dominique Ingegneri, "Changes in Life Expectancy and Disability-Free Life Expectancy in the United States," *Population and Development Review* 15, no. 2 (1989): 235–67.

27 The figures quoted are for high-income countries; see GBD 2017 Collaborators, "Global, Regional, and National Disability-Adjusted Life-Years (DALYs) for 359 Diseases and Injuries and Healthy Life Expectancy (HALE)," *Lancet* 392, no. 10159 (2018): 1859–922.

After life expectancy had reached a level of 70 years, however, further rises were accompanied by reversals of some of the disease-specific trends. The share of infectious and respiratory diseases started to rise again, instead of continuing to fall, and the share of cardiovascular diseases and injuries started to fall, instead of continuing to rise. Beyond a life expectancy of 70, the share of cancers continued to rise sharply, whereas the share of mental and neurological diseases (including diseases like dementia and Parkinson's disease) also rose sharply.[28]

Most of the earlier changes are well-known, and were already incorporated in Omran's theory of the epidemiologic transition. However, the more recent reversals have not yet fully reached the collective consciousness of demographers and epidemiologists. They point to more radical changes in the health profile of long-lived populations than hitherto recognized.[29]

The rising share of infectious and respiratory diseases that accompanies rises of life expectancy above the level of 70 years, is probably due to the fact that conditions like sepsis and pneumonia are the only remaining gateways to death among very old people, whose lives have been extended by reducing mortality from cardiovascular diseases. Furthermore, the place of cardiovascular diseases appears to have been partly taken by mental and neurological diseases, particularly dementias, which are now more explicitly recognized as a possible cause of death.[30]

The recently declining share of cardiovascular diseases is highly remarkable. Some studies have suggested that recent rises in life expectancy were achieved by shifting the average age-at-death of people suffering from chronic diseases, without changing the distribution of deaths by disease. Yet, this idea is incorrect: the average age-at-death has indeed changed, but so has the

---

28 The cause-specific mortality data from which the shares in Suppl. Figure 5 were calculated, were age-standardized so that the effect of changes in age-distribution of the population, which have occurred in parallel to, and partly as a consequence of, rising life expectancy, do not distort the analysis. Levels of life expectancy cited are for men.

29 An exception must be made for French demographers Jacques Vallin and France Meslé, who have made several studies of recent trends in old-age mortality (France Meslé and Jacques Vallin, "Diverging Trends in Female Old-Age Mortality," *Population and Development Review* 32, no. 1 (2006): 123–45).

30 For the rise of infectious diseases as a cause-of-death among elderly people, see Aline Désesquelles et al., "After the Epidemiologic Transition," *International Journal of Public Health* 60, no. 8 (2015): 961–67. For the rising share of dementias as a cause of death, see Chapter 6 and Johan P. Mackenbach, Marina Karanikolos, and Caspar W.N. Looman, "The Rise of Mortality from Mental and Neurological Diseases in Europe, 1979–2009," *BMC Public Health* 14, no. 1 (2014): 840.

proportion of all deaths attributed to cardiovascular disease, which has declined from around 50% to around 30%.[31]

These changes have occurred throughout Europe, but with important differences in timing. The share of infectious diseases in total mortality was already below 10% in many countries in Northern and Western Europe in the 1930s, whereas countries in Southern, Central-eastern, South-eastern and Eastern Europe often reached that point only in the 1950s. The share of cardiovascular diseases dropped below 40% in the 1990s in many countries in Northern, Western and Southern Europe, but has still not reached that low level in most of Central-eastern, South-eastern and Eastern Europe.

Shifts in the Burden of Disease

Even today, we know much more about mortality and its composition by cause-of-death, than about how the burden of morbidity in a population is built up. The Global Burden of Disease study has recently published the results of a heroic attempt to reconstruct the burden of disease in all countries of the world. Filling up the holes in the data necessitated lots of assumptions and imputations, but the results are of great interest. They do not only give a picture of the present, but may even provide a glimpse of what the historical trends in Europe might have been. This is because the study includes low-income countries in other parts of the world, which give an indication of what the situation in Europe might have been before mortality declined to the very low levels of today.

Taking all diseases together, the total disease burden is only some 10% lower in Europe than in the low-income countries of Sub-Saharan Africa and South Asia. This resembles our earlier conclusion that Europe's increase in life expectancy has not been accompanied by an equally strong rise in 'healthy life expectancy'. The 10% lower disease burden in Europe is entirely due to a lower burden of 'communicable, maternal, neonatal, and nutritional diseases'. By contrast, the burden of 'non-communicable diseases' is somewhat higher in Europe than in low-income countries, as is the burden of 'injuries'.[32]

This suggests that the prevalence of disease has changed much less than one might expect on the basis of the strong declines in mortality. It is the *composition* of morbidity that has changed: communicable diseases and other

31 For the idea that the renewed rise of life expectancy was due to 'delayed degenerative diseases', see S. Jay Olshansky and A. Brian Ault, "The Fourth Stage of the Epidemiologic Transition: The Age of Delayed Degenerative Diseases," *Milbank Quarterly* 64, no. 3 (1986): 355–91.

32 See GBD 2017 Collaborators, "Global, Regional, and National Incidence, Prevalence, and Years Lived", esp. Figure 4.

health problems of the past have declined, but cardiovascular diseases, cancer and other non-communicable diseases, plus the sequelae of injuries, have to a large extent taken their place.

When we stop to think about what exactly happened to these diseases, this is not difficult to understand. The incidence of a disease is the number of new cases arising in the population over a particular period of time, whereas the prevalence of a disease is the number of existing cases present in the population at one point in time. The long-term decline of infectious diseases was mainly a matter of declining incidence, which led to a lower prevalence of disease. On the other hand, the rise of non-communicable diseases was not only due to rising incidence, but also to declining case fatality and thus to a longer duration. The combination of more new cases occurring and longer duration of disease led to a substantially higher prevalence.[33]

Let's look in more detail at some of the underlying trends, starting with infectious diseases. During the 20th century, many European countries have introduced compulsory notification of infectious diseases. This usually included tuberculosis, syphilis, diphtheria, measles and many other diseases. Although notifications were often compulsory for a limited period of time only, the general picture is clear enough: incidence of many infectious diseases has declined enormously.

For example, in England and Wales notifications declined for respiratory tuberculosis (since the early 20th century), scarlet fever (late 1930s), diphtheria (early 1940s), whooping cough (mid-1950s), poliomyelitis (late 1950s), and measles (late 1960s). At the other side of Europe, in the Soviet Union, the incidence of many infectious diseases also declined, albeit often much later than in Western Europe. For example, notifications declined for smallpox (since the early 1920s), malaria (late 1940s), diphtheria (late 1950s), whooping cough (late 1950s), poliomyelitis (late 1950s) and measles (late 1960s). These declines in incidence have dramatically reduced the disease burden from infectious diseases.[34]

33 The relationship between prevalence and incidence is given by the following formula: $P = I \times D$, in which P = prevalence, I = incidence, and D = the duration of disease. This was first noted in Brian MacMahon and Thomas F. Pugh, *Epidemiology: Principles and Methods* (Boston: Little, Brown & Company, 1970), p. 65.

34 The history of infectious disease notification in Britain, which started in the late 19th century already, often against fierce resistance of physicians, employers, teachers and others who had to carry out the necessary procedures, can be found in Graham Mooney, *Intrusive Interventions* (Rochester: Rochester University Press, 2015). Long-term trends in England & Wales are shown in Spence Galbraith and Anna McCormack, "Infection in England and Wales, 1838–1993," in *The Health of Adult Britain 1841–1994. Volume 2*, ed. J. Charlton and M. Murphy (London: The Stationery Office, 1997). Long-term trends in the Soviet Union are shown in S.N. Zatravkin et al., *Заболеваемость Инфекционными*

Let's now look at the data for an important non-communicable disease, cancer. Cancer registries with which trends in incidence can be followed, have only relatively recently been established. In Europe, Denmark was the first country with a cancer registry (1940s), followed by some of the other Nordic countries (1950s). Coverage of more than 10 European countries was only achieved in the 1980s. In most countries, measurement of the average survival rates of cancer patients started even later.

Nevertheless, there can be no doubt that incidence rates of cancer have risen substantially. This can already be inferred from the rise of the mortality rates from cancer since the beginning of the 20th century, but is also clear from the rise of cancer incidence since whenever cancer registrations were first established (Figure 4). Among Danish women, cancer incidence increased continuously since the early 1940s. Rising trends in total cancer (all sites combined) have been found all over Europe, as a result of rising incidence of a majority of specific cancers. Most of these increases have continued until the present day, although some previously rising cancers (such as lung cancer among men) have recently started to fall.[35]

At the same time, cancer survival rates have gradually increased. The Nordic countries were the first to start registering the survival of patients with cancer, and data from Norway and Finland show that between the early 1950s and the early 1970s five-year survival of many cancers already improved a little, and that survival of some cancers improved a lot. For all cancers combined, five-year survival increased from 30% to 40% over this period; cancers for which survival improved most were thyroid cancer, Hodgkin's disease, corpus uteri cancer, malignant melanoma, and testicular cancer, as a result of early advances in cancer treatment.[36]

Болезнями В Ссср. Сообщение 1. 1919–1949 Годы [*The Incidence of Infectious Diseases in the USSR: Myths and Reality. Report 1: 1919–1949*] (Moscow: Semashko National Research Institute of Public Health, n.d.); S.N. Zatravkin et al., *Заболеваемость Инфекционными Болезнями В Ссср: Мифы И Реальность. Сообщение 2. 1950–1990 Годы* [*The Incidence of Infectious Diseases in the USSR: Myths and Reality. Report 2: 1950–1999*] (Moscow: Semashko National Research Institute of Public Health, n.d.).

35 Long-term cancer incidence trends in the Nordic countries from the 1940s (Denmark) or 1950s (other countries) onwards have been documented in T. Hakulinen et al., "Trends in Cancer Incidence in the Nordic Countries," *Acta Pathologica, Microbiologica, et Immunologica Scandinavica* 94 no. S288 (1986): 1–151. For recent trends, see Henrike E. Karim-Kos et al., "Recent Trends of Cancer in Europe," *European Journal of Cancer* 44, no. 10 (2008): 1345–389.

36 On Finland, see Paul W. Dickman et al., "Survival of Cancer Patients in Finland 1955–1994," *Acta Oncologica* 38, no. 12 (1999): 1–103. On Norway, see Cancer Registry of Norway, *Survival of Cancer Patients – Cases Diagnosed in Norway 1968–1975* (Oslo: Cancer Registry of Norway, 1980).

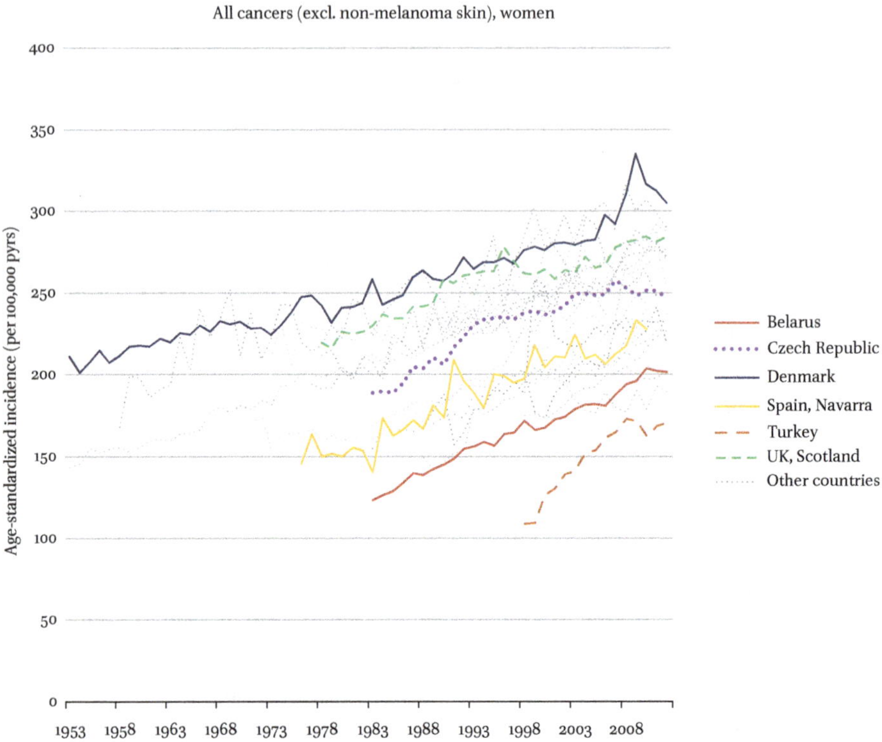

FIGURE 4 Trends in cancer incidence in Europe, 1953–2011
SOURCE OF DATA: NATIONAL OR REGIONAL CANCER REGISTRIES (THROUGH GLOBAL CANCER OBSERVATORY (GCO.IARC.FR; ACCESSED 24/04/2019))

These increases in survival have continued, sometimes accelerated by new advances in treatment. Many more registries now monitor the survival of cancer patients, and European-wide studies show that between the mid-1990s and mid-2000s average five-year survival for all cancers combined increased from 45% to 50%. Survival is, however, considerably better in Northern, Western and Southern Europe than in Central-eastern, South-eastern and Eastern Europe. Progress is slow, and these changes may partly reflect earlier detection of cancer (which artificially increases cancer survival). Nevertheless, the combination of increasing cancer incidence and increasing cancer survival has fuelled a strong rise of cancer prevalence.[37]

---

37 Milena Sant et al., "EUROCARE-4. Survival of Cancer Patients Diagnosed in 1995–1999. Results and Commentary," *European Journal of Cancer* 45, no. 6 (2009): 931–91; Paolo Baili et al., "Age and Case Mix-Standardised Survival for All Cancer Patients in Europe 1999–2007,"

As we will see in Chapter 6, increases in survival have also occurred for ischaemic heart disease and stroke. Although incidence of these diseases has declined much more than the incidence of cancer, the prevalence of cardiovascular diseases has risen as well.

Diseases Rise, Diseases Fall

These changes in the broader composition of mortality and morbidity are the net result of what happened to many specific diseases. Many diseases have manifested themselves in a striking pattern of 'rise-and-fall', but with a total lack of simultaneity. Whereas some 'rises-and-falls' occurred over many millennia, others took only two decades to unfold. Whereas some diseases peaked in the 18th century, others did so in the 19th or 20th century. Yet others are still rising and will hopefully decline in the future.[38]

This will be documented more extensively in Part 2 of this book, of which Table 1 presents a 'sneak preview'. When I started these analyses, I knew that ischaemic heart disease and road traffic injuries had first risen and then declined, because the peak had occurred during my life-time and had been discussed in research papers published in epidemiological journals. Yet, when a sufficiently long time-scale is applied, a pattern of 'rise-and-fall' appears to be the general rule. Ischaemic heart disease and road traffic injuries have risen over more than a half-century before peaking in the second half of the 20th century. Appendicitis and AIDS took a much shorter period to rise to their peak in the 1930s and 1990s, respectively. Tuberculosis and syphilis took several centuries before they reached their peak in the 19th century.

The rise of some other diseases, such as dysentery and other intestinal infections, probably started with the advent of agriculture in the Neolithic period (around 6,500 BCE in Europe). The same applies to famine, which was probably less common among hunter-gatherers than among agriculturalists who

European Journal of Cancer 51, no. 15 (2015): 2120–129. The five-year survival rates cited in the text are age-adjusted, taking background mortality into account.

38 That human diseases tend to occur in a pattern of 'rise-and-fall' was also noted by René Dubos (e.g., René J. Dubos, *Man Adapting* (New Haven and London: Yale University Press, 1965), Chapter 9) whose views we will discuss in more detail in Chapter 3. The notion of 'rise-and-fall' has been used in connection with many specific diseases; see, e.g., Reuel A. Stallones, "The Rise and Fall of Ischemic Heart Disease," *Scientific American* 243, no. 5 (1980): 53–9; David J. Barker, "Rise and Fall of Western Diseases," *Nature* 338, no. 6214 (1989): 371–27). As this book shows it is a truly generalized phenomenon.

were dependent on the growth of a limited number of crops. To my surprise, on a time-scale of millennia even war-related violence has developed in a pattern of 'rise-and-fall': rising until the costs of war finally became prohibitive.[39]

TABLE 1 Rise and fall of diseases in Europe: an overview

Group	Health problem	Rise and fall?	Start of rise[a]	Start of fall[b]
Health problems of pre-industrial societies	War	Rise and fall	(before 4300 BCE)	16th century[c]
	Homicide	Fall only	N/A	16th-17th century
	Famine	Rise and fall	(6500 BCE[d])	18th century
	Plague[e]	Rise and fall	1347	17th century
	Smallpox	Rise and fall	6th century	18th century
	Typhus	Rise and fall	Late 15th century	17th century?
	Malaria	Rise and fall	16th century	18th century
Health problems of industrializing societies	Cholera	Rise and fall	1829-1837	1846-1860
	Intestinal infections[f]	Rise and fall	(6500 BCE[d])	Mid-19th century
	Tuberculosis	Rise and fall	18th century	Mid-19th century
	Syphilis	Rise and fall	Late 15th century	Early 20th century
	Childhood infections[g]	Rise and fall	18th century	Late 19th century
	Pneumonia	Fall only	N/A	Early 20th century
	Influenza	Rise and fall	16th century	1918-1919
	Puerperal fever	Rise and fall	18th century	Mid-19th century
	Infant mortality	Fall only	N/A	Late 18th – late 19th century
	Still-births	Fall only	N/A	1940s
	Pellagra[h]	Rise and fall	18th century	Late 19th century
	Rickets	Rise and fall	17th century	Late 19th century
	Goitre	Fall only	N/A	1920s
	Peptic ulcer	Rise and fall	Late 19th century	1930s-1940s
	Appendicitis	Rise and fall	Late 19th century	1930s-1940s
	Pneumoconiosis	Rise and fall	19th century	Early 20th century
	Mesothelioma	Rise only	1970s	N/A
	Stomach cancer	Rise and fall	19th century?	Early 20th century

39 See Chapters 4–6 for these and many other examples of 'rise-and-fall'. It has not always been possible to capture the complete 'rise-and-fall' trajectory in the figures, because most of these rely on mortality data by cause of death, and because the rise of many diseases occurred before the introduction of national cause-of-death registration. In these cases, the evidence for an earlier 'rise' comes from the literature.

Group	Health problem	Rise and fall?	Start of rise[a]	Start of fall[b]
Health problems of affluent societies	Ischaemic heart disease	Rise and fall	Early 20th century	1970s
	Cerebrovascular disease[i]	Rise and fall	Early 20th century	1970s
	Diabetes mellitus type II	Rise only	Mid-20th century	N/A
	Colorectal cancer	Rise and fall	Early 20th century?	1970s
	Breast cancer	Rise and fall	Late 19th century?	1980s
	Prostate cancer	Rise and fall	First half 20th century?	1980s-1990s
	Lung cancer	Rise and fall	1930s	1970s-1980s[j]
	Liver cirrhosis[k]	Rise and fall	1950s	1970s-2000s
	Dementia[l]	Rise only	1970s	N/A
	Depression	Unknown	N/A	N/A
	Road traffic injuries	Rise and fall	Early 20th century	1970s
	Suicide	Rise and fall	18th century	1920s-1980s
	AIDS	Rise and fall	Early 1980s	Mid-1990s

N/A Not applicable
a Approximate start of documented rise in Europe; between brackets if based on circumstantial evidence re. emergence of health problem
b Approximate start of fall (or peak-year) is for North-western Europe only
c Peak in frequency of war (not in war deaths)
d In Europe, the Neolithic or first Agricultural revolution started in the Aegean c. 6500 BCE
e Second pandemic only
f Dysentery, (para)typhoid fever
g Scarlet fever, measles, whooping cough, diphtheria
h Timing for pellagra is for Southern and South-eastern Europe
i Trend for ischaemic stroke only; for haemorrhagic stroke, see text Chapter 6
j Decline in men only
k There may have been another 'rise-and fall' cycle in the 19th century
l Trend for mortality; no evidence for rise in age-adjusted prevalence

Note: Based on information reviewed in Chapters 4–6

Industrialization and urbanization also went together with a rise of many diseases, ranging from rickets to tuberculosis, and from diphtheria to pneumoconiosis (occupational lung disease). These diseases have since largely disappeared, but have partly been replaced by the health conditions with which we are now familiar, such as ischaemic heart disease, cancer and road traffic injury. This generalized pattern of 'rise-and-fall' is not only fascinating, but also holds important clues for the explanation of long-term trends in population health to which we will come below.

Epidemiologic Transition 2.0

A Theory in Need of Repair

Omran's idea – briefly summarized in Chapter 1 – was that total mortality had declined because, as a result of socioeconomic development, mortality from infectious diseases had declined. After that had occurred, total mortality stabilized because, as a side-effect of the same socioeconomic development, other causes of death had increased and replaced infectious diseases. However, because the new diseases caused death at higher ages (i.e., among the middle-aged and elderly, instead of among babies and children), the exchange led to higher life expectancy. According to Omran, this all happened somewhere between 1870 and 1970, albeit with important differences in timing and pace between countries, e.g., later but faster in Eastern Europe than in Western Europe. At first sight, this may seem a reasonable summary, but upon closer inspection it is far from accurate. There are three important problems.

A first problem concerns Omran's *periodization*. In Northern and Western Europe, the reduction of infectious disease mortality started much earlier than in the last decades of the 19th century. The decline of plague, smallpox and typhus, to mention just a few examples, had already started at least a century earlier. More generally, a clear attenuation of the great fluctuations in mortality, due to devastating epidemics and famine, already occurred in the 18th century, at least in Northern and Western Europe, and represented an important advance in population health that cannot be ignored.

In addition to a problem with the beginning, there is a problem with the end of Omran's epidemiologic transition. Coincidentally, just when Omran published his theory, a renewed decline of mortality started in many high-income countries. A reversal in the trend of ischaemic heart disease was one of its main drivers, but declines in other causes of death such as road traffic injuries also played a role. This renewed decline has sometimes been referred to as a fourth stage of the epidemiologic transition. This has been labelled the "age of delayed degenerative diseases" (because it was mistakenly thought that this did not entail an elimination of mortality from heart disease, but only a delay to older ages) or a "hybristic stage" (because trends were increasingly influenced by individual behaviours and life-styles).[40]

40 Omran defined the end of the epidemiologic transition as the point in time when mortality rates stabilised after their decline. However, when crude mortality rates are analysed,

Another surprise was that it soon appeared that infectious diseases had not been eliminated, but on the contrary seemed to return with a vengeance. After 1970, new infectious diseases emerged (such as legionnaire's disease and AIDS), some old diseases re-emerged as a result of lapses in infectious disease control (such as tuberculosis and whooping cough), and some other infectious diseases became more difficult to control because of antibiotic resistance (such as hospital-acquired staphylococcal infections). Adding to the confusion, it was proposed to either label this a fifth stage of the epidemiologic transition, or to consider this an entirely new epidemiologic transition.[41]

Although a certain rise of mortality from infectious diseases has been noted in many European countries, it is not obvious that this is an important enough phenomenon to warrant the addition of another stage of the epidemiologic transition, let alone to distinguish an entirely new transition. On the other hand, the decline of cardiovascular diseases certainly was important, and qualitatively different from what had happened earlier. This suggests that distinguishing a new stage to accommodate this change may indeed be appropriate.

It does not seem wise, however, to label this a new transition, because by definition a 'transition' is an intermediate stage between two more or less stable states. This can only be accurately identified and defined after the event, and at present we do not yet know where we are heading. Which causes of death will ultimately replace the causes of death that are being pushed back?

---

as in his publications, trends are distorted by changes in the age-composition of the population. In most countries in Western Europe and Northern America, age-standardized mortality rates for women did not stabilise at all, but declined uninterruptedly. The (mistaken) idea that we have entered an "age of delayed degenerative diseases" comes from Olshansky and Ault, "The Fourth Stage of the Epidemiologic Transitio"n, whereas the (gloomy) idea that we have entered a "hybristic stage" comes from Richard G. Rogers and Robert Hackenberg, "Extending Epidemiologic Transition Theory: A New Stage," *Social Biology* 34, no. 3–4 (1987): 234–43.

41 The proposal to label this a 'fifth stage' (of 'emerging and re-emerging infectious diseases') comes from S. Jay Olshansky et al., "Emerging Infectious Diseases: The Fifth Stage of the Epidemiologic Transition? ," *World Health Statistics Quarterly* 51, no. 2–4 (1998): 207–17. The proposal to label this a 'third epidemiologic transition' comes from Ronald Barrett et al., "Emerging and Re-Emerging Infectious Diseases: The Third Epidemiologic Transition," *Annual Review of Anthropology* 27, no. 1 (1998): 247–71. For readers who are losing count: in the latter conception the first epidemiologic transition involved the rise of infectious diseases that accompanied the Neolithic agricultural revolution, while the second one is synonymous with Omran's epidemiologic transition. The idea of a 'second epidemiologic transition' was more fully developed in Molly K. Zuckerman, ed., *Modern Environments and Human Health* (Hoboken: John Wiley & Sons, 2014). In later updates of his 'epidemiologic transition theory' Omran actually embraced some of the extensions (Omran, "Epidemiologic Transition Theory Revisited").

We have seen above that the decreasing share of cardiovascular diseases in total mortality is accompanied by an increasing share of neoplasms and of mental and neurological disorders, but neoplasms have been on the rise for long, and the share of mental and neurological diseases is still very low.[42]

A second problem relates to Omran's *labelling* of groups of diseases. Enormous shifts have occurred in both the absolute rates and relative importance of specific causes of death. But how should these shifts be characterized?

Omran characterized the shift as one from "pandemics" of infectious diseases to "degenerative and man-made diseases." However, although cholera and influenza were pandemic diseases, most of the other infectious diseases that were responsible for declining mortality, such as tuberculosis, pneumonia, and dysentery, were endemic diseases. Furthermore, we now know that some of Omran's 'degenerative' diseases (such as stomach and cervical cancer) have partly infectious origins as well.

Nor is the vaguely moralistic heading of 'degenerative and man-made diseases' an adequate label for the causes of death that have replaced the infectious diseases. Although cardiovascular diseases and neoplasms are diseases of middle and old age, we now know that they are not primarily caused by age-related biological processes of 'degeneration', but are predominantly 'exogenously' caused, just like the infectious diseases that dominated the cause-of-death pattern in previous centuries. Also, while many of these exogenous causes, such as smoking and excessive alcohol consumption and occupational exposures, are 'man-made', so were the living conditions and habits which promoted the transmission of infectious agents.

In theory, it may be possible to solve these terminological problems by finding other umbrella terms, but in practice this has proven to be difficult, and no solution is entirely satisfactory. What this really demonstrates is that the long-term improvement in population health that the epidemiologic transition tries to capture, was a heterogeneous phenomenon. It consisted of sequentially 'falling' diseases, with an emphasis on declines for some infectious diseases in one period, an emphasis on declines for some other infectious diseases in another period, and an emphasis on declines for cardiovascular diseases in still another period, but without clear-cut differences by type of disease, however defined.[43]

---

42 We will see in Chapter 6 that the rise of mortality from Mental and neurological diseases is mainly due to rising mortality from dementia, and that it is uncertain whether this rise of mortality from dementia is real.

43 For some further elaboration, see Johan P. Mackenbach, "The Epidemiologic Transition Theory," *Journal of Epidemiology and Community Health* 48, no. 4 (1994): 329–32.

The third problem is that Omran largely ignored *other health outcomes than mortality*. There is an implicit assumption in many of his interpretations that changes in mortality equal changes in incidence of the underlying diseases. However, some of the changes in mortality, even before the early 1970s, were due to declines in case fatality, as in the case of the treatment of pneumonia and other infectious diseases by antibiotics. Over time, trends in morbidity (and health expectancy) have become at least as important for evaluating population health as trends in mortality (and life expectancy), but they are not captured by the epidemiologic transition theory.

These and related omissions have led to proposals to replace the concept of the 'epidemiologic transition' by that of a 'health transition'. This concept includes changes in morbidity in addition to mortality, but also society's responses to health problems such as the expansion of health care services. While that may risk mixing up the dependent variable (i.e., changes in population health) with the independent variable (i.e., what society does to improve population health), it is certainly important to look beyond life expectancy. As shown above, data on disability-free life expectancy suggest that life expectancy without severe disability has increased in parallel with total life expectancy, implying that years lived with severe disability have remained more or less constant, whereas years lived with any disability and particularly with chronic illness have increased during the last stage of mortality decline.[44]

Taking these problems into account, I propose the following modification of the epidemiologic transition theory: 'epidemiologic transition 2.0'.

How: Characterizing Change

As we have seen above, long-term trends in population health have been the result of many superimposed disease-specific trends, and the latter are more often than not characterized by a distinct pattern of 'rise-and-fall'. One way to understand this endless succession of 'rises-and-falls' is to regard them as an accompaniment of socioeconomic development. As a result of the drive for socioeconomic improvement, and the changes in behaviour associated with this drive, mankind is continuously confronted with new disease risks. However, because higher levels of development also bring higher living standards and a greater desire and capacity to control disease, after some time these disease risks decline again (but often to be replaced by new disease risks).

This suggests that, to the extent that we need a distinction in different stages of population health change, it may be useful to relate disease trends to stages

44 The concept of the 'health transition' was proposed in Julio Frenk et al., "Elements for a Theory of the Health Transition," *Health Transition Review* 1, no. 1 (1991): 21–38.

of socioeconomic development. This is what I have already done, without explicitly mentioning it in the text, in Table 1. In this table I grouped diseases into three large groups, depending on the period in which their mortality rates peaked in North-western Europe: 'health problems of pre-industrial societies', which generally peaked before 1800; 'health problems of industrializing societies', which peaked between 1800 and 1950; and 'health problems of affluent societies', which peaked after 1950. Let me explain.

In the first group I brought together a number of diseases (like smallpox and typhus) and other causes of 'crisis mortality' (war and famine) which caused many of the large peaks in mortality that were mostly gone – at least in North-western Europe – before 1800. These can be regarded as 'health problems of pre-industrial societies', not only because they peaked before most North-western European countries began to seriously industrialize, but also because their causes were linked to the material hardship that was prevalent before modern economic growth took off. (Homicide has been included in this group as well, because it has been in secular decline since the 15th century.)[45]

In the second group I brought together the diseases that were associated with the large-scale industrialization and urbanization of the 19th century. Their rise had often started before the 19th century, but continued or accelerated to reach a peak before the middle of the 20th century, the subsequent decline being partly a result of the success of control efforts. This group includes well-known diseases like tuberculosis and diphtheria, but also infant mortality which, in many countries, had a temporary peak in the late 19th century as a consequence of urbanization. It also includes a few nutrient deficiency diseases, which rose as a result of dependence on a more monotonous diet, as well as occupational lung disease, which increased as a result of the mechanization of grinding, and peaked in the 1920s.[46]

In the third group I brought together the diseases that peaked after 1950, or that have risen but not yet peaked at all. These diseases have been labelled 'diseases of affluence', but this is the trickiest label of the three. During the 20th century, when scientists tried to make sense of the rise of these diseases, various labels have been proposed. In addition to Omran's 'degenerative and man-made diseases', these include 'diseases of affluence', 'diseases of civilization' and 'Western diseases', as well as more neutral terms like 'non-communicable

45 The inclusion of war in this group could be debated, because war-related deaths only peaked in the middle of the 20th century. However, the frequency of war peaked in the 16th century.

46 Stomach cancer and haemorrhagic stroke can also be included in this group, because mortality declined since the early 20th century. However, for practical reasons trends of these diseases will be discussed in Chapter 6.

diseases' and 'chronic diseases'. None of these terms is satisfactory, and all are inaccurate – even a simple distinction between communicable and non-communicable diseases no longer holds.[47]

I have decided to retain the term 'diseases of affluence' because the rise of most of these diseases was facilitated by rising living standards, or by what mankind did to achieve these living standards. This applies to cardiovascular diseases, diabetes mellitus, most cancers, and many causes of injury. I also included dementia and depression in this group, although dementia (and other mental and neurological diseases) may turn out to be characteristic of a future stage of health development, and although it is unclear whether depression is more frequent in affluent societies than it was in the past. Finally, this group includes a 'ghost from the past', i.e., the infectious disease AIDS. This spread as a result of international travel and liberalization of sexual mores, conditioned by the affluence of the second half of the 20th century.

When: Staging Change

This distinction of three categories of diseases also suggests a distinction of three stages of population health change over the past three centuries. This distinction is necessarily somewhat arbitrary, because diseases' peak-years are spread out rather evenly over the three centuries since 1700, without natural dividing-lines. This emerges very clearly from Table 1: the last column of this table shows a virtually continuous succession of diseases starting to fall. Also, the peak-years differed between European regions; for example, whereas typhus may have peaked in the 17th century in Sweden, it probably peaked in the 20th century in Russia. We should thus not assume a universal timing of these changes. Nevertheless, three possible stages would be the following:

---

47 For example, as will be discussed in Chapters 5 and 6, peptic ulcer and stomach cancer are now considered to be essentially infectious diseases. It has been speculated that micro-organisms are also involved in the causation of cardiovascular diseases, which suggests a deeper link between different stages of the epidemiologic transition (Alex Mercer, *Infections, Chronic Disease, and the Epidemiological Transition* (Cambridge: Boydell & Brewer, 2014)). For the term 'diseases of affluence' see Thomas McKeown, *The Origins of Human Disease* (Oxford: Basil Blackwell, 1988), for 'diseases of civilization' see Henry E. Sigerist, *Civilization and Disease* (New York: Cornell University Press, 1943), and for 'Western diseases' see Hubert C. Trowell and Denis P. Burkitt, *Western Diseases, Their Emergence and Prevention* (Cambridge (Mass): Harvard University Press, 1981). All these terms are easy to criticize, but difficult to replace by a satisfactory alternative. Many of the so-called 'diseases of affluence' have fallen in later stages of the rise in living standards; the term 'diseases of civilisation' refers to a Euro-centred view of human civilization; and the idea of 'Western diseases' is obsolete because most of these disease are now global.

In a *first stage* the frequency and amplitude of annual fluctuations in mortality started to diminish, due to a reduction in the frequency and/or severity of famine and epidemics of plague, smallpox, typhus and malaria. In North-western Europe, these declines started before 1800, but some of these problems continued to cause spikes in mortality in the 19th and even 20th century before disappearing completely. This stage thus does not have a natural end, and if an end is necessary it seems best to take the start of the second stage as the end of the first. Before 1800, mortality in non-crisis years may or may not have started to slowly decline as well, but life expectancy at birth remained low at a level not much higher than 30 years.[48]

In a *second stage* a range of health problems characteristic of industrializing societies, and often causally linked to industrialization and urbanization, started to decline. Among the diseases studied in this book, this applies to various infectious diseases (cholera and other diarrheal diseases, tuberculosis, syphilis, childhood infections, pneumonia, ...), maternal and infant mortality, peptic ulcer and appendicitis, nutrient deficiency diseases, and occupational lung disease. This decline was mostly the result of decreasing disease incidence, but during this stage decreasing case fatality also started to play a role, particularly towards the end. Like the first stage, this second stage also does not have a natural end, as declines from these conditions have continued even after the third stage had started.

In North-western Europe the first signs of declining mortality from some infectious diseases (e.g., tuberculosis) could already be noticed in the first half of the 19th century, but declines really got under way in the last decades of the 19th century. At that point, the modest increases in life expectancy that had already occurred, suddenly accelerated, mainly as a result of the start of a rapid decline of infant mortality. In this second stage, the proportion of total mortality due to infectious diseases declined from more than 40% to less than 10%. Life expectancy increased from little more than 30 years in the first half of the 19th century to around 65 years (men) and 70 years (women) in the 1950s.

In a *third stage* a number of diseases that had risen during the second stage, probably as a side-effect of increasing prosperity, started to decline: ischaemic heart disease, stroke, a few cancers, and road traffic injuries and suicide. Like in previous stages, this was still partly the result of declines in incidence, but

48 Perrenoud, "The Attenuation of Mortality Crises" puts the end of the age of large mortality crises in the late 1600s for England, Italy and Geneva, in the early 1700s for France, in the early 1800s for Sweden, Norway and Denmark, and in the late 1800s for Finland. As noted above, however, large mortality fluctuations continued to occur in the 20th century (see Figure 2).

increasingly declines in case fatality also played an important role. In this stage, the share of cardiovascular mortality in total mortality declined from a peak between 40 and 70% to much lower values, whereas the share of cancer continued to increase, and the share of mental/neurological diseases now started to increase.

One other characteristic of this third stage is that mortality decline among the elderly, including the oldest old, accelerated, contributing to a continued increase of life expectancy at birth to levels sometimes exceeding 80 years among men and (more often) women in the first two decades of the 21st century. In this stage, we can also observe what happens to health expectancy: both years-in-good-health and years-in-bad-health go up, but it may well be that years-in-very-bad health have remained stable or even declined somewhat.

Of these three stages, the second more or less corresponds with Omran's epidemiologic transition. There are still good reasons to see this as a very special stage. This was a stage with ultra-rapid increases in life expectancy, in which disease-specific declines strongly dominated disease-specific increases, as a result of unprecedented improvements in living conditions and a series of important breakthroughs in the control of infectious diseases.

Where: Locating Change

In the preceding section we gave an approximate timing of the three stages for North-western Europe. However, there were large differences in timing of these changes between countries (see Suppl. Table 4).

It is challenging to assess differences in timing of the first stage of mortality decline, because so few countries have data going back into the 18th century. It is only at the end of the 19th century that some countries in all European regions were collecting data permitting the calculation of crude mortality rates. At that point in time, annual fluctuations in mortality were still substantial in South-eastern and Eastern Europe, indicating that these countries were late in going through this first stage.

If we take decline of infant mortality as a marker of the second stage, there are again clear differences between European regions. By the beginning of the 20th century, countries in Northern and Western Europe were distinctly ahead of Southern, Central-eastern, South-eastern and Eastern Europe, where levels below 10% would often only be reached after World War II.

In a similar way, when we use the proportion of all deaths due to cardiovascular disease as a marker of progression of the third stage, we find that in the beginning of the 21st century Northern and Western Europe are far ahead of Central-eastern, South-eastern and Eastern Europe. Interestingly, Southern

Europe has now shed off its disadvantage, and has joined the front-runners in Northern and Western Europe.[49]

Although all European regions have experienced a strong increase in life expectancy since the late 19th century, and although some convergence of life expectancy has occurred during the 20th century, it is amazing to see how certain patterns of variation have persisted throughout this period. Broadly speaking, the Nordic countries are still ahead of many other European countries, and South-eastern and Eastern Europe still lag behind. This suggests that some of the causes of these patterns of variation in population health have also persisted over more than a century, and perhaps longer.

At the same time, not all regions have kept their relative position. This applies most clearly to Southern or Mediterranean Europe, which lagged behind North-western Europe until the mid-20th century, but now has some of the longest-lived populations in the world. As we will see in later chapters, this is due, on the one hand, to a process of catching-up with North-western Europe (e.g., in eliminating communicable diseases). On the other hand, these countries have not experienced a similar rise as North-western Europe in cardiovascular disease mortality during the second stage of mortality decline.

49 This pattern is confirmed when we look at differences in the year in which European countries passed certain thresholds for female life expectancy (Suppl. Table 4): 50 years (as a marker of progression of the first stage), 65 years (as a marker of progression of the second stage), and 80 years (as a marker of progression of the third stage). Northern and Western Europe were ahead of the rest in all three stages, but in the third stage they were joined by Southern Europe.

CHAPTER 3

Understanding Trends in Population Health

To understand trends in population health, and to decide between different explanations, it is necessary to have a good theory for what determines population health. In this chapter we therefore review the available theories, and compare some of their predictions with our European data. We end this chapter with an overview of the historical development of public health and medical care, and of its impact on population health in Europe.

Theories of Population Health

Before we can understand long-term trends in population health, we must understand what the causes of disease are. Of course, different specific diseases have different specific causes, but is there no general theory of what causes disease in human beings?

Unfortunately, this general theory is hard to find. Unlike physicists, who spend huge research budgets on finding a 'Theory of Everything' which explains all physical aspects of the universe, health scientists do not seem interested in a unified theory of what causes disease. One will look in vain for such a theory, or even a brief general introduction on the nature and origins of disease, in the textbooks of public health and epidemiology.[1]

What the public health literature offers us is a number of useful, but often shallow, conceptual frameworks. Starting from what we know about the many specific 'determinants' of disease as found in epidemiological studies, these frameworks propose a smaller number of more general categories of determinants of health and disease, plus – sometimes – an idea of how these groups of determinants relate to each other.

A simple example is the 'host-agent-environment' model, which was originally developed for a better understanding of infectious diseases. According to this model, infectious disease occurs when the environment brings an 'agent' (a micro-organism) in contact with a 'host' (a human being). The model

1 And, for that matter, in textbooks of pathology or general medicine. For a critique of the lack of theorizing in epidemiology, and a proposal for an 'ecosocial theory of disease distribution', see Nancy Krieger, *Epidemiology and the People's Health* (Oxford etc.: Oxford University Press, 2011).

suggests that differences in the occurrence of infectious disease can be explained from differences in characteristics of the agent (e.g., the virulence of the micro-organism), the host (e.g., his or her levels of immunity), and the environment (e.g., contamination of drinking water).[2]

After the near-elimination of infectious diseases, epidemiological textbooks adopted a similar conceptual framework for the understanding of chronic diseases, such as cardiovascular disease and cancer. This was done by introducing new types of 'agents', such as 'nutritive excesses' (causing cardiovascular disease and diabetes), allergens (causing asthma and hay fever), and ionizing radiation (causing leukaemia). Although the host-agent-environment model provided no structure for how to understand the interaction between its three components, it did help to emphasize the continuing importance of factors external to the 'host'.

Later, more complex frameworks were proposed, such as that of the 'web of causation' which allows for a larger number of determinants of each disease, some of which may work indirectly through other determinants. This model recognizes that diseases are often caused by a chain of different factors. For example, diabetes may be due to obesity, which may be due to a high-calorie diet, which may be due to high sugar content of food stuffs, which may be due to consumers' preference for both a nice taste and a low price. In addition, it allows for the possibility that different factors may have to come together to produce the outcome. In the diabetes example, the web of causation does not only include consumers' preferences but also producers' profit maximization strategies, which together help to understand why sugar is added to so many foodstuffs.[3]

These frameworks are – to a large extent – empty shells, but other conceptual frameworks have tried to organize environmental and other determinants of disease into a smaller number of groups, and to give labels to each group

---

2 According to Krieger, *Epidemiology*, p. 150, the first explicit mention of 'host', 'agent' and 'environment' as factors determining the occurrence of disease dates to the early 1950s (Gordon JE. Epidemiology – old and new. Journal of the Michigan State Medical Society 1950; 49:194–99).

3 For an elaboration of the 'host-agent-environment' model for non-communicable diseases, see Abraham M. Lilienfeld and David E. Lilienfeld, *Foundations of Epidemiology*, Second ed. (Oxford etc.: Oxford University Press, 1981), pp. 46–47. The 'web of causation' model was proposed in MacMahon and Pugh, *Epidemiology*, pp. 23–24. Incorporating chains of causation often requires multi-level models, which take into account different levels of organization and thus allow for the influence of macro-level factors on micro-level behaviour. For an elaboration, see Mervyn Susser and Ezra Susser, "Choosing a Future for Epidemiology: Ii. From Black Box to Chinese Boxes and Eco-Epidemiology," *American Journal of Public Health* 86, no. 5 (1996): 674–77.

pointing to more general causes of disease. For example, the 'Lalonde model' makes a simple distinction between four groups of factors: 'human biology' (including genetics), the 'environment', 'life style', and 'health care organization'. Another popular model, the so-called 'rainbow model', regards health and disease as the outcome of several layers of influences, graphically depicted as a rainbow. These run from an outer layer of 'general socioeconomic, cultural and environmental conditions', through 'living and working conditions', 'social and community networks', and 'individual lifestyle factors', to an innermost and more immutable part of 'age, sex and constitutional factors'. Recently, a more detailed model of the 'social determinants of health' was proposed by the WHO Commission of the same name. This links the 'socioeconomic and political context' to inequalities in 'social position', and these to inequalities in specific living conditions, and these to inequalities in health and well-being.[4]

All these models usefully emphasize that diseases are often caused by external influences, however defined. This clearly resonates with one of the main findings of this book, which is that diseases tend to rise and fall on a time-scale too short to allow for spontaneous changes in the internal structure and functioning of the human body. Such an 'ecological' view of disease causation has deep historical roots, ultimately going back to Hippocrates' account of the environmental causes of disease in his famous *Airs, Waters and Places*.

In this treatise, Hippocrates (c. 460–377 BCE) described the important effects of climate, diet and other environmental conditions on health and disease in the ancient Greek world. This view of disease causation was revived and further elaborated in the 18th century, and is still relevant and valid today, although the details of the links between the environment and disease have undergone a complete re-think.[5]

4 What came to be known as the 'Lalonde model' was proposed in a report issued in 1974 under the responsibility of the then Canadian Minister of Health Marc Lalonde; see Trevor Hancock, "Lalonde and Beyond: Looking Back at 'a New Perspective on the Health of Canadians,'" *Health Promotion International* 1, no. 1 (1986): 93–100. The 'rainbow model' was proposed in 1991 in Göran Dahlgren and Margaret Whitehead, *Policies and Strategies to Promote Social Equity in Health* (Stockholm: Institute for Future Studies, 1991). The 'social determinants of health' model was first published in Commission on Social Determinants of Health, *Closing the Gap in a Generation* (Geneva: World Health Organization, 2008), p. 43. Later versions also include a 'life-course' perspective, e.g., in Michael Marmot et al., "WHO European Review of Social Determinants of Health and the Health Divide," *Lancet* 380, no. 9846 (2012): 1011–29.

5 For Hippocrates' *Airs, waters and places*, see, e.g., Dona Schneider and David E. Lilienfeld, eds., *Public Health: The Development of a Discipline* (New Brunswick etc.: Rutgers University Press, 2011), Chapter 2. The emergence of 'public hygiene' in the 18th century can be seen as a revival of Hippocratic ideas (James C. Riley, *The Eighteenth Century Campaign to Avoid Disease* (New York: St. Martin's Press, 1987)). This is illustrated by the work of the French

This is illustrated by two more recent attempts to develop a general theory of the origins of disease. The first is by French-American microbiologist René Dubos (1901–1982), who published a couple of profound books on human health and its determinants in the 1950s and 1960s, such as *Mirage of Health* (1959) and *Man Adapting* (1965). The following citation from *Man Adapting* summarizes Dubos' main line of reasoning: "[S]tates of health or disease are the expressions of the success or failure experienced by the organism in its efforts to respond adaptively to environmental challenges" (p. xvii). Dubos underpins this statement by an in-depth analysis of the effects on human health of a wide range of 'environmental challenges', including climate extremes, social competition, malnutrition, microbes, and water and air pollution.

Dubos also discusses the 'rise-and-fall' of diseases, which he relates to the dynamic nature of these environmental challenges. He explains the emergence of 'new' diseases in his own life-time as follows:

> To a surprising extent, modern man has retained unaltered the bodily constitution, physiological responses, and emotional drives which he has inherited from his Paleolithic ancestors. Yet he lives in a mechanized, air-conditioned, and regimented world radically different from the one in which he evolved.
>
> …
>
> The diseases characteristic of highly industrialized and urbanized societies are, to a large extent, the manifestations of the effects of new environmental forces to which man has not had a chance to become adapted.[6]

The second – and somewhat less profound – attempt at a general theory of the causes of disease is by Thomas McKeown, the same person whose work played such an important role in the 'battle of ideas' on the explanation of the increase in life expectancy in the Western world. In the final year of his life, long

proto-hygienist Jean-Noël Hallé (1754–1822) who classified the factors that modify health into *circumfusa* (things that surround us), *applicata* (things that are applied to our bodies), *ingesta* (things that are introduced into our bodies), *excreta* (things that we excrete), *gesta* (our voluntary actions), and *percepta* (our perceptions). See Gérard Jorland, *Une Société à Soigner* (Paris: Gallimard, 2010), Chapter 2.

6 Dubos, *Man Adapting*; citations are from the 13th printing (1977), p. xviii and p. 367. Dubos has criticized the 'utopian' idea that all diseases can be eliminated by environmental control, because man always seeks novelty and thereby exposes himself to new health risks; see René J. Dubos, *Mirage of Health* (New York: Harper & Brothers, 1959), pp. 281–282.

after he published his main work on the historical decline of mortality in England and Wales, he published an interesting book entitled *The Origins of Human Disease*.[7]

In this book, McKeown proposes to classify all diseases in just three categories: 'prenatal diseases' (all diseases manifested before birth), 'diseases of poverty' (diseases manifested after birth that are attributable to deficiencies or hazards related to lack of the essentials for life), and 'diseases of affluence' (diseases manifested after birth that are attributable to maladaptation or hazards related to industrialisation). His category of 'prenatal diseases' includes chromosomal aberrations, single-gene defects, and congenital malformations. Diseases of poverty' include malnutrition and infectious diseases. And 'diseases of affluence' include cardiovascular diseases, most cancers, diabetes, and other so-called 'western' diseases.

In all its simplicity (or simplism?), this classification rests on an explicitly ecological theory of disease causation. After setting aside congenital (and thus potentially genetically caused) diseases, this theory attributes all other diseases to a single etiological factor, of which one can have either too little or too much: prosperity. Of course, McKeown is careful in drawing out the multiple and often indirect links between economic development and the occurrence of disease, and to point out counterexamples and caveats. Yet, this is a parsimonious theory of the fundamental causes of all disease which – if correct – explains why during economic development some diseases fall and others rise.

An 'Ecological-Evolutionary Theory' of the Origins of Disease

After this brief review it is possible – leaning heavily on Dubos – to sketch an 'ecological-evolutionary theory' of the fundamental causes of disease. A summary of this theory in one long sentence is: diseases are caused by 'unfavourable exchanges' between the human organism and its external environment, and/or by 'failures in the structural and functional design' of the organism, which, in the final analysis, are due to the dependence of human organisms on a fundamentally hostile external environment, and to unfortunate evolutionary legacies (Figure 5).[8]

This theory of the 'origins of disease' starts from the recognition that, despite the enormous variety in the diseases that humans suffer from, all manifestations of disease can be understood as resulting from some 'pathologic onset'. This is an unbalancing change in the 'internal milieu' of the organism

7 McKeown, *Origins*.

8 This section has been modified after Johan P. Mackenbach, "The Origins of Human Disease: A Short Story on 'Where Diseases Come From,'" *Journal of Epidemiology & Community Health* 60, no. 1 (2006): 81–86.

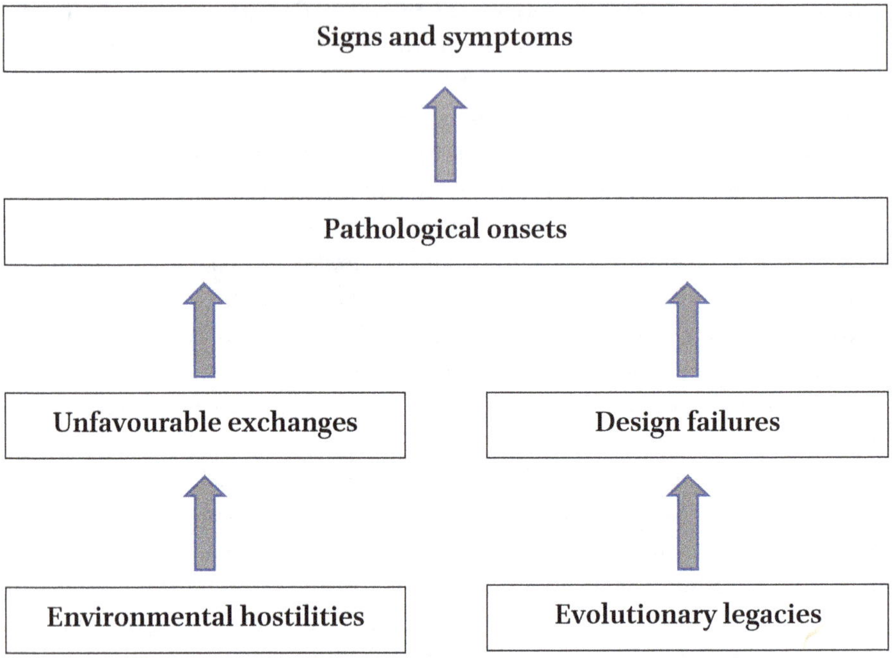

FIGURE 5 The origins of disease
ADAPTED FROM JOHAN P. MACKENBACH, "THE ORIGINS OF HUMAN DISEASE: A SHORT STORY ON 'WHERE DISEASES COME FROM.'" JOURNAL OF EPIDEMIOLOGY & COMMUNITY HEALTH 60, NO. 1 (2006): 81–86

with which it cannot adequately cope, and which sets the whole disease process in motion. Disease processes, i.e., the internal mechanisms that produce the signs and symptoms of disease, are what medical textbooks are keen to describe in detail. However, these mechanisms find their starting-point in a 'pathologic onset', and only this can guide us in our search for the real causes of disease. For example, in the case of infectious diseases this 'pathologic onset' is invasion by micro-organisms, and in the case of cancer it is uncontrolled cell growth resulting from mutations in DNA.[9]

9 Disease processes usually consist of reactions of the organism to 'pathologic onsets'. Further examples of 'pathologic onsets' are: hereditary DNA abnormalities (leading to conditions like Down's syndrome, Huntington's disease), induction of auto-immune reactions (hyperthyroidism, rheumatoid arthritis), induction of allergic reactions (asthma, atopic eczema), nutrient deficiencies (iron-deficiency anaemia, pellagra), derangements of metabolic processes (diabetes), formation of atherosclerotic plaques (ischaemic heart disease, ischaemic stroke), cytogenetic abnormalities (lung cancer, leukaemia), mechanical 'wear-and-tear' to supportive structures (lumbar hernia, osteoarthritis), ingestion of

The next question then is what causes these 'pathologic onsets', and the general answer is that these always result from an unfavourable exchange between the human organism and its external environment, or from a failure in the structural or functional design of the organism, or from a combination of both. Sometimes the unfavourable exchange with the external environment is easier to identify, as in the case of invasion by micro-organisms, or ingestion of noxious chemical substances causing poisoning, or encounters with large kinetic forces causing bone-fractures. In other cases the design failures are easier to recognize, as in the case of hereditary DNA abnormalities causing Huntington's disease, or allergic reactions causing asthma. Yet, as we will see below, deeper reflection often shows that both are necessary for disease to occur.

We can now go one step further, and ask ourselves why human organisms so often have unfavourable exchanges with the environment, and why their design so often has imperfections leading to disease. Let's start with the first question: why are unfavourable exchanges with the environment so common? This can only be understood if we realize that exchanges with the environment are necessary. In order to survive, all living organisms must continuously exchange energy and matter with their external environment, because these exchanges provide the organism with the basic necessities of life (food, oxygen, warmth and water). In addition, human organisms need their environment for material security (housing, income, safety, ...), social interaction (support, intimacy, status, ...), and self-development (knowledge, aesthetics, self-actualisation, ...).[10]

Many of these exchanges are favourable, but some are not. Health problems may arise, when the intake of basic necessities or the fulfilment of more advanced human needs is insufficient, or when, in its necessary exchanges with the environment, the human organism encounters noxious (harmful) influences. These '*noxae*' can be physical in nature (noise, radiation, cold, ...), or chemical (pollutants, tobacco smoke, certain lipids, ...), or biological (parasites, bacteria, viruses, ...), or psychological (bullying, sexual abuse, ...). Almost all diseases can be traced back to one of these unfavourable exchanges, which may range from lack of a basic nutritional factor (causing pellagra) to ingestion of the wrong kind of lipids (ischaemic heart disease), and from encounters with a virus (influenza) to inhalation of tobacco smoke (lung cancer).[11]

---

noxious chemical substances (intoxication, alcoholic liver cirrhosis), and encounters with large kinetic forces (hip fracture, shot wounds).

10 The phrase 'unfavourable exchanges with the external environment' was chosen to include both insufficient intakes from the environment of the necessities of life, and encounters with noxious influences from the environment.

11 These exchanges with the external environment are usually active processes, and are therefore determined as much by the behaviour of the organism as by the environment

But why are these unfavourable exchanges with the environment so common, that mankind is continuously plagued by an enormous variety of diseases? The disheartening answer is: because the external environment on which we depend is more hostile than we like to think. It is hostile in the sense that the basic and more advanced necessities for human flourishing are scarce, and in the sense that this environment contains an abundance of '*noxae*'.

Earth has allowed life to develop, so it must be a relatively life-friendly planet. Yet, it has always been a challenge for mankind to find or grow sufficient food, and human societies have always had difficulty providing for the more advanced needs of all their members. This scarcity is partly natural, and partly man-made in the sense that the increase in human population numbers and human needs has tended to outpace the increase in available resources. And it is not only a matter of scarcity: paradoxically, the same elements in the abiotic, biotic and human environment that we are dependent on, often can make us sick as well.

A simple illustration of this paradox is oxygen: all higher life on earth is dependent on oxygen, but oxygen is a dangerous compound, as one can see from the fact that it destroys iron. During the processing of nutrients in our bodies, oxygen is released, and this causes 'oxidative stress' which is thought to contribute to cardiovascular disease and cancer. Another illustration: all life on earth is dependent on sunlight, but exposure to ultraviolet and other radiation leads to mutations in our DNA and may cause cancer.

There is also a fundamental hostility, in the form of competition, between different life-forms. Bacteria feed on us, and although we have developed sophisticated mechanisms of defence, they are smarter, and continuously succeed in circumventing our countermeasures. Equally important is the fact that, while we need other human beings for survival and flourishing, at all levels of human organization (families, companies, cities, countries, globally) we also compete with each other for resources, causing diseases in those who are less successful.[12]

The active role of mankind in producing its own diseases actually extends much further than the competition just mentioned. Exposure to a hostile

itself. The interaction between organism and environment blurs the distinction between the two; see Richard C. Lewontin, *The Triple Helix* (Boston: Harvard University Press, 2001).

12 For the role of 'oxidative stress' in generating cardiovascular disease and cancer, see Richard G. Cutler and Henry Rodriguez, *Critical Reviews of Oxidative Stress and Aging* (New York: World Scientific Publishing, 2003). Bacteria are not only hostile: we also need them, e.g., for digestion. For the role of human competition in health inequalities, see Johan P. Mackenbach, "Persistence of Social Inequalities in Modern Welfare States," *Scandinavian Journal of Public Health* 45, no. 2 (2017): 113–20.

environment often results from seeking novel environments in which we hope to find a better life, but which contain dangers to which we do not yet have an adequate response. It also sometimes results from human interventions that are intended to improve living conditions, but as a side-effect harm the environment that we depend on. The shift from hunting-and-gathering to agriculture is an example of a change in which human beings have sought to escape one danger (lack of edible wild plants and prey animals), but replaced it with another (dependence on a limited number of cultivated plants and animals). Human development often seems like a forward flight in which frontiers are pushed backwards, but never disappear completely.[13]

While this suggests a purely 'ecological' view of disease causation, it is important to note that some cases of all diseases, and many cases of some diseases, may be entirely attributable to an autonomous derailment of internal mechanisms. This can be seen as a failure in the (genetically determined) structural or functional design of the human organism. Hereditary DNA abnormalities, such as those leading to Huntington's disease, are a clear example of diseases where most cases are probably attributable to such a design failure only, without much influence from the environment. But such examples are uncommon, and the importance of design failures – or perhaps better: design imperfections – in the causation of disease extends much further than their role in rare inherited disorders.

One important design imperfection is that human organisms cannot always cope effectively with unfavourable exchanges with the external environment. Our organism disposes of a large variety of protection and adjustment mechanisms, ranging from protective structures and detoxification mechanisms to immune reactions and behavioural responses. These are supposed to protect us from harm, and some failure of these adjustment mechanisms can therefore usually be identified when disease occurs. For example, invasion of micro-organisms only produces infectious disease when the immune system does not succeed in timely elimination of the invaders – which often happens, indicating that our immune system is imperfect. Similarly, the fact that we sometimes break our bones indicates that our protective structures have not been designed to withstand all the kinetic forces that we encounter.[14]

---

13 Other examples range from the migration out of Africa which opened up new continents for human exploitation but also exposed humans to colder and less sunny climates, to industrialization which massively increased the production of basic necessities but also polluted the environment; see Anthony J. McMichael, *Human Frontiers, Environments and Disease* (Cambridge etc.: Cambridge University Press, 2001). For novelty-seeking, see Dubos, *Mirage of Health*.

14 The distinction between 'unfavourable exchanges with the external environment' and 'design failures' is similar to that between 'nurture' (external environment) and 'nature'

But design failures are not limited to those which interfere with our responses to the external environment. Another design imperfection is that living organisms cannot deal perfectly with 'entropy'. Survival requires constant reproduction – of germ cells (for creating progeny) and of somatic cells (for repair and maintenance of our bodies). However, during cell reproduction small random errors in DNA occur all the time. Although we have highly effective repair and search-and-destroy mechanisms, a small fraction of these errors is not detected in time, leading to congenital disease in our children or to cancer in ourselves. These and other design failures also partly explain why the incidence of many diseases rises with age: the combination of an accumulation of environmental insults with less-than-perfect defence and repair mechanisms ensures that disease risks go up when we age.[15]

Conceivably, due to the very success of improvements of the environment, the balance in the causation of human disease may over time have shifted somewhat from 'exogenous' to 'endogenous' causes, i.e., from a predominant role of unfavourable exchanges with the external environment, to a relatively more important role for design imperfections. The increased importance of neurological diseases like Alzheimer's dementia and Parkinson's disease, for which it has proved difficult to find environmental causes, may be an illustration of this shift.[16]

Purely 'ecological' theories of disease causation may thus be losing some of their explanatory power, but that environmental factors still play an important role is clear from their quantitative contributions to the burden of disease, also in high-income countries.[17]

We may then ask, like we did in the case of unfavourable exchanges with the external environment: why do human organisms have so many design imperfections? This question can best be answered from the perspective of

---

(genes). The distinction can be misleading, because the environment influences living organisms through their genes, and genes influence the way organisms interact with their environment; see Matt Ridley, *Nature Via Nurture. Genes, Experience and What Makes Us Human.* (London: Harper, 2004).

15 A third design failure is that we have limited supplies of vital stocks, such as immune cells that can be directed at specific antigens: after we have exhausted these supplies, we cannot cope with new micro-organisms any more. For the role of 'design failures' in the ageing process, see Robert E. Ricklefs and Caleb E. Finch, *Aging: A Natural History* (New York: Scientific American Books, 1995); Thomas B.L. Kirkwood, *Time of Our Lives* (Oxford etc.: Oxford University Press, 1999).

16 See Chapter 8.

17 For quantitative analyses of the contribution of 'exogenous' determinants to mortality and disability, see, e.g., GBD 2017 Collaborators, "Global, Regional, and National Comparative Risk Assessment of 84 Behavioural, Environmental and Occupational, and Metabolic Risks," *Lancet* 392 (2018): 1923–94.

evolutionary biology. This lack of perfection is partly due to the fact that humans have not evolved to be able to live in good health in our current environment. The structural and functional characteristics of the human organism have been selected for their 'fitness' (i.e., ability for survival and reproduction) in previous hostile environments. Our organism can cope with hunger, and less so with the more recent abundance of food.[18]

Some of these 'imperfections' in our design are due to 'trade-offs' or compromises that were necessary during this long evolutionary trajectory. Sickle cell anaemia is the classic example. People heterozygous for the sickle cell gene, which causes an abnormality in haemoglobin (the oxygen-carrying protein in red blood cells), are protected from malaria, but have difficulty being physically active. On balance, this was advantageous when their ancestors lived in a malaria-infested environment, but has now become a disadvantage. Another example is familial hypercholesterolemia, which increases the risk for cardiovascular disease now, but probably provided protection against famine in the past.

More generally, the ubiquity of design imperfections is due to the fact that during humans' long evolutionary trajectories, achieving perfection was not necessary in the first place. This insight comes from the 'disposable soma' theory, which sees our bodies as nothing more or less than the 'throw-away' vehicles of our genetic material. The successful propagation of our genes does not require a perfect body at all, but only requires that we are able to reproduce before our bodies fall apart, due to the effects of a hostile environment and/or innate imperfections.[19]

Explaining Long-term Change

We are now in a better position to address the question that will concern us in the rest of this book: how to explain long-term trends in population health,

---

18 See, e.g., Randolph M. Nesse and George C. Williams, *Why We Get Sick* (New York: Times Books, 1995). For more extensive analyses, see Stephen C. Stearns, ed., *Evolution in Health and Disease* (Oxford etc.: Oxford University Press, 1999).

19 For the trade-off in familial hypercholesterolemia, see Eric J.G. Sijbrands et al., "Mortality over Two Centuries in Large Pedigree with Familial Hypercholesterolaemia," *British Medical Journal* 322, no. 7293 (2001): 1019–23. Another trade-off follows from the theory of 'antagonistic pleiotropy', which posits that senescence (and disease associated with senescence) is the inevitable by-product of adaptations that increase fitness earlier in life. For example, mechanisms that limit cellular proliferation may protect against cancer in adult life, but will promote degradation of organ function in old-age; see George C. Williams, "Pleiotropy, Natural Selection, and the Evolution of Senescence," *Evolution* 11 (1957): 398–411. For the 'disposable soma' theory, see Thomas B.L. Kirkwood and Steven N. Austad, "Why Do We Age?," *Nature* 408, no. 6809 (2000): 233–38.

in particular the 'rise-and-fall' of so many diseases? At a time-scale of centuries changes in the structural and functional design of the human organism are implausible, and therefore the answer must lie elsewhere. The explanation must lie either in changes in the way mankind has interacted with its environment (which may have either increased or decreased the occurrence of disease) or in changes in the way mankind has handled disease (which may have changed the outcome of the interaction between humans and their environment).

Of course, changes in the occurrence of disease and its consequences has many specific explanations. Many specific exchanges with the external environment are involved, and all of these may have changed, from exposure to famine to working conditions and consumption patterns. Similarly, many specific interventions have been developed, often based on new scientific insights and technological breakthroughs. The latter are the usual stuff of histories of medicine and public health, and their development over time is certainly important for an understanding of the history of population health. Many of these specific changes will therefore be reviewed in the disease-focused chapters in part II of this book.

However, for a deeper understanding of long-term changes in population health we need a second level of explanation which helps us understand why these specific factors changed over time, often simultaneously and in similar directions. For this we need to move from the specific or 'proximal' factors just mentioned, to the more 'distal' factors which have set all the specific changes in motion.

Broadly speaking, the main candidates are *economic* and *sociocultural* change (which may have induced changes in the way mankind interacted with its environment) and the development of *effective systems of health intervention* (which enabled mankind to prevent diseases and their consequences, and to make human health somewhat independent from interactions with the environment). To the extent that these changes relied on collective human action, *political* changes may have played a role as well (both by fostering progress, for example by creating conditions for economic growth and investments in a public health infrastructure, and by causing temporary setbacks).[20]

These are the four groups of factors that we will introduce in the subsequent sections of this chapter. Separating out one of these as the main cause of

20 Omran already wrote that "[t]he determinants of the transition from infectious to degenerative disease predominance are by no means simple," but include "[s]ocioeconomic, political and cultural determinants" and "[m]edical and public health determinants" (Omran, "Epidemiologic Transition", pp. 518–20).

changes in population health is difficult, because they are interdependent and each has specific pathways linking it to long-term changes in European population health. Nevertheless, after reviewing all the evidence we will try to identify the 'prime mover' of these changes, but we delay that to one of the final sections of this book.

Economic, Political and Sociocultural Conditions

Economic History: Improvements in Living Standards

The increase in European life expectancies coincided with a strong increase of countries' living standards. Between 1700 and 1870, North-western European countries went through radical economic changes which started a period of unprecedented economic growth. These changes, usually summarized as the 'Industrial Revolution', started in Britain, spread from there to other parts of Western and Northern Europe, and after 1870 also spread to the South and East. Steam-power, factories, railways and globalization all contributed to the increase in economic productivity, which led to increases in real wages and public expenditure, but also to profound societal changes such as urbanization and secularization.[21]

Long-term trends in national income have been spectacularly upwards. Despite interruptions by two World Wars, the Great Depression of the 1930s, and the economic crises of the 1990s in Central-eastern, South-eastern and Eastern Europe, Europeans now enjoy much higher living standards than their ancestors in the second half of the 19th century. Some countries have changed their relative positions, such as the United Kingdom which lost its top position in the 1940s, and Portugal which moved from the rear-guard to a middle position after World War II. Other countries, such as Albania, retained their positions throughout these three centuries (see Suppl. Figure 6).

21 Economic historians have come to distinguish an 'industrious revolution' preceding the 'industrial revolution', which increased production and consumption by making family labour more efficient (Jan de Vries, "The Industrial Revolution and the Industrious Revolution," *Journal of Economic History* 54, no. 2 (1994): 249–70). For an introduction to European economic history, see Stephen Broadberry and Kevin H. O'Rourke, eds., *Cambridge Economic History of Modern Europe: Volume 1: 1700–1870.* (Cambridge etc.: Cambridge University Press, 2010). Stephen Broadberry and Kevin H. O'Rourke, eds., *Cambridge Economic History of Modern Europe. Volume 2: 1870 to the Present* (Cambridge etc.: Cambridge University Press, 2010); These volumes also contain insightful analyses of the impact of economic growth on population health.

These improvements in living standards led to more and better nutrition, better housing, more leisure time, higher levels of education, and changes in many other aspects of life. Higher living standards are enjoyed throughout Europe – despite continuing and sometimes widening inequalities between countries – and throughout national populations – despite continuing and sometimes widening inequalities in income between social groups. Life is much better now than it used to be, but at the beginning of the 21st century we have become aware of many more "despites" than continuing inequalities.

Let's therefore pause for a moment and acknowledge some of the darker sides of this economic growth. Europe's economic advance would have been less propitious without the exploitation of its colonies in Africa, Asia and the Americas, often involving the use of slaves and brutal repression of indigenous peoples. The industrial revolution and all that followed would have been impossible without the burning of fossil fuels like coal and oil, ultimately leading to planetary climate change. Economic growth was also accompanied by massive environmental degradation and habitat destruction, leading to the extinction of many other living species. These are big issues to which we will need to come back (in Chapter 8).

For the moment, however, let's focus on the human health effects of economic growth. There can be little doubt that the resulting improvement in living conditions has brought many health benefits. The parallel upward movement of national income and life expectancy is striking, and certainly suggestive of a causal relationship between the two. So is the occurrence of simultaneous setbacks, as in the case of the declining life expectancies and average incomes in Central-eastern, South-eastern and Eastern Europe after the collapse of the Soviet Union.

There are several mechanisms that could explain such a causal relationship. Improvements in living standards helped to push back the diseases of the past that were caused by a lack of basic necessities, for example by eliminating famine and improving the quality of nutrition. Furthermore, economic growth allowed countries to invest in research and development, to create an expensive public health infrastructure, and to pay for rising costs of medical care. Through these and other pathways, economic development very likely contributed to long-term improvements in population health.[22]

However, upon closer inspection the relationship is far from straightforward, and the idea that economic growth automatically brings improvements in population health – still popular in public health circles – has been discredited

22 See, e.g., Lant Pritchett and Lawrence H. Summers, "Wealthier Is Healthier," *Journal of Human Resources* 31, no. 4 (1996): 841–68.

by more in-depth studies. As we saw in Chapter 1, Preston's finding of strong upward shifts in the association between national income and life expectancy already fuelled scepticism about a causal link. These upward shifts appeared to be more important for the explanation of the secular increase in life expectancy, than the increase in national incomes *per se*. Later studies have fed this scepticism even further, and have demonstrated that a distinction needs to be made between short-term and long-term effects of economic growth, and between cross-sectional and longitudinal relationships between average income and population health.

Whereas the long-term effect of economic growth on population health must have been positive, the short-term effects have often been negative. This was as true in the 19th century as it is now. In the 19th century, rapid economic growth often reduced population health, because in their early phases industrialization and urbanization had many negative side-effects, such as occupational hazards, air pollution, and infection. Working conditions of labourers were often extremely poor, contaminated by dangerous substances and involving high injury risks. Factories also spewed gigantic amounts of smoke into their immediate surroundings. Living in crowded houses in the rapidly expanding cities multiplied the risks of air- and water-borne infections. These negative side-effects had to be actively counteracted by public health and other measures before the ultimate benefits could get the upper hand.

In the 20th century, the short-term effects also were often negative. Economic expansion and contraction often had 'pro-cyclical' effects, in the sense that mortality usually went up during economic booms (because of an increase in, e.g., road traffic injuries and alcohol-related mortality) and went down again during recessions. Even on the longer time-scale of decades instead of years, economic growth has had many negative health effects, as economic development during the 20th century was accompanied by air pollution and other forms of environmental degradation, and by rises in smoking, obesity and other risk factors implied in the term 'diseases of affluence'.[23]

23 For an analysis of how rapid economic growth in the 19th century often caused "Disruption, Deprivation, Disease, and Death," which needed to be counteracted by public health and other countermeasures, see Simon Szreter, "Economic Growth, Disruption, Deprivation, Disease, and Death," *Population and Development Review* 23, no. 4 (1997): 693–728. Reconstruction of English life expectancy data for the first half of the 19th century clearly shows a deterioration in the first stages of the Industrial Revolution; see Simon Szreter and Graham Mooney, "Urbanization, Mortality, and the Standard of Living Debate," *Economic History Review* 51, no. 1 (1998): 84–112. For the effect of economic recessions on population health, see Christopher J. Ruhm, "Are Recessions Good for Your Health?" *Quarterly Journal of Economics* 115, no. 2 (2000): 617–50. For an analysis linking the rise of

A distinction must also be made between cross-sectional and longitudinal relationships. We almost always find a strong relationship between national income and life expectancy *at one point in time*, as illustrated by the 'Preston-curve'. However, the association between *changes over time* in national income and life expectancy is much weaker. For example, the Great Depression of the 1930s, in which national incomes temporarily declined, coincided with massive increases in life expectancy. More formal studies have also not been able to demonstrate that increases in national income consistently go together with increases in life expectancy. This implies that we cannot assume a causal relationship from rising national income to rising life expectancy, and that the cross-sectional relationship that we observe is probably determined by other mechanisms as well.[24]

One possibility is confounding by third factors. Higher life expectancy may have been produced by other factors that were associated with economic growth, but not caused by economic growth. One possibility is rising levels of literacy and education, which on the one hand helped economic growth, by increasing the productivity of the work-force, and on the other hand promoted population health improvements, by facilitating the diffusion of modern hygienic insights.

Another mechanism which may contribute to a strong cross-sectional association between national income and life expectancy, even in the absence of a strong effect of rising national income on life expectancy, is 'reverse causality'. This occurs if there is an effect of rising life expectancy (or population health improvement more generally) on national income. Studies have found convincing evidence for such 'reverse' effects, which are probably due to the fact that better health leads to higher labour productivity. The mutually reinforcing effects of population health on national income and vice versa can, in this way, give rise to 'virtuous cycles' underpinning longer periods of sustained growth in both.[25]

---

so-called 'diseases of affluence' to economic development, see Majid Ezzati et al., "Rethinking the 'Diseases of Affluence' Paradigm," *PLoS Medicine* 2, no. 5 (2005): e133. As American economist and Nobel laureate Angus Deaton has argued, despite short- and mid-term negative effects, economic growth has in the long run led to better population health; see Angus Deaton, *The Great Escape* (Princeton: Princeton University Press, 2013).

24 For a more rigorous 'longitudinal' analysis relating changes over time in national income to changes over time in life expectancy, see William Easterly, "Life During Growth," *Journal of Economic Growth* 4, no. 3 (1999): 239–76.

25 For an overview of empirical studies of the effects of life expectancy on economic growth, and the mechanisms involved, see David E. Bloom and David Canning, *Population Health and Economic Growth*, vol. 24, Health and Growth, (Washington, DC: World Bank (Commission on Growth and Development), 2009). A recent addition to this literature is

A further complication – loosening a cross-sectional link between national income and life expectancy – is diffusion of knowledge and technology. As we have seen in Chapter 1, Preston's interpretation of the upward shift of the life expectancy curve between the 1930s and 1960s was, that this was due to the diffusion of new technologies, such as malaria control and antibiotics. These spread from the richer countries in which they had been developed, to poorer countries which had not been able to pay for their development, but could now apply them at low cost.

The partial decoupling of technological advances from economic growth may also explain the rapid improvements of life expectancy during the Great Depression in the 1930s. These advances were probably due to innovations (such as sanitation, workers' protection, and better obstetric care) that had been introduced earlier, but had their full population health impact only in the 1930s.[26]

Armed with these insights, we will now have a more detailed look at the European experience, starting with some cross-sectional 'Preston-curves'. The available data cover a very long period, from the 1870s to the 2010s, of which just a few important time-points are shown in Figure 6.

In the 1870s, just before rapid increases in national income and life expectancy began, there was not yet a correlation between the two: European countries with a higher national income, such as Great Britain, did not have a higher life expectancy than poorer countries, such as Sweden or Norway. A positive correlation gradually emerged in the following decades, and is then consistently found from the 1930s onwards. This consistency is surprising, because

---

Matteo Cervellati and Uwe Sunde, *Demographic Change and Long-Run Development* (Cambridge (Mass.) & London: MIT Press, 2017). When health gains are achieved within working ages, population health improvements may produce a 'demographic dividend' (David E. Bloom, David Canning, and Jaypee Sevilla, *Economic Growth and the Demographic Transition*, NBER Working Papers, (Cambridge, Mass: National Bureau of Economic Research, 2001)). Such 'virtuous cycles' are much less plausible for health improvements at higher ages.

26 For how technological advances have contributed to decoupling of life expectancy trends from economic growth, see David E. Bloom and David Canning, "Commentary: The Preston Curve 30 Years On: Still Sparking Fires," *International Journal of Epidemiology* 36, no. 3 (2007): 498–99. For the role of delayed effects in explaining the paradox of increasing life expectancy despite economic turbulence in the interwar period, see Robert Millward and Joerg Baten, "Population and Living Standards, 1914–1945," in *Cambridge Economic History of Europe. Volume 2*, ed. Stephen Broadberry and Kevin H. O'Rourke (Cambridge etc.: Cambridge University Press, 2010). The importance of literacy and education has been demonstrated in studies of rapid mortality declines in Kerala, Sri Lanka and Costa Rica; see John C. Caldwell, "Routes to Low Mortality in Poor Countries," *Population and Development Review* 12, no. 2 (1986): 171–220.

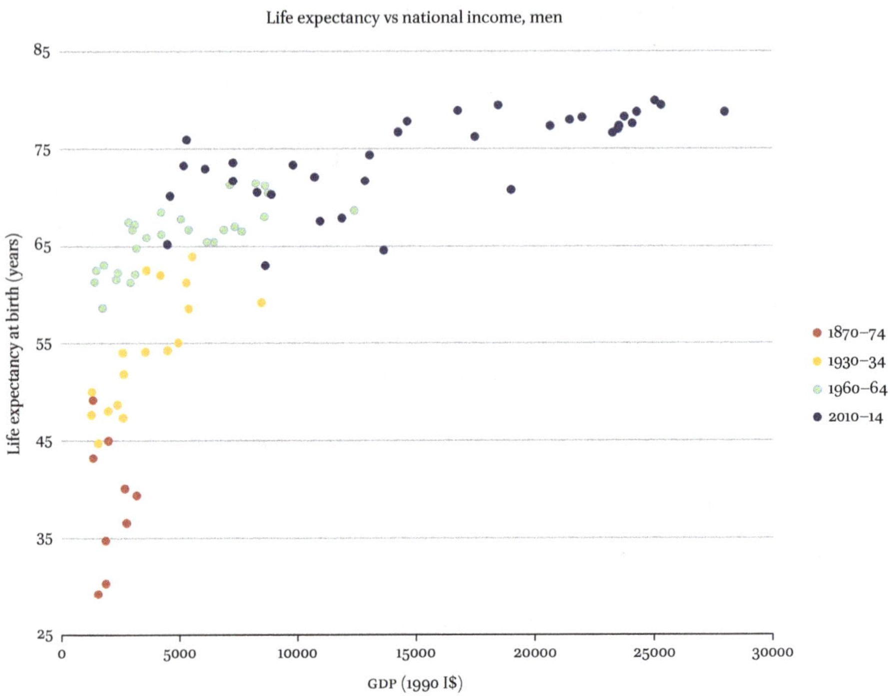

FIGURE 6 National income and life expectancy in Europe, 1870s to 2010s
Notes: Each dot represents one country/period combination
SOURCE OF DATA: WWW.CLIO-INFRA.EU FOR GDP (ACCESSED 28/08/2018), HUMAN MORTALITY DATABASE AND MANY OTHER SOURCES FOR LIFE EXPECTANCY

the cause-of-death composition of mortality changed radically. In the 1930s and 1960s, countries with a higher national income had lower infant mortality and mortality from infectious and respiratory diseases, whereas in the 1990s and 2010s they had lower mortality from cardiovascular diseases.[27]

Figure 6 also shows the large upward shifts in the relation between national income and life expectancy. Because national income has been expressed in

27 For the correlations between national income and life expectancy, see Suppl. Table 3. Simple correlations were statistically significant and positive in 1930–34, 1960–64, 1990–94 and 2010–14, but not in 1870–74 or 1900–04. After adjustment for other determinants (protestant legacy, average education, and level of democracy), statistically significant associations are only found in 1990–94 and 2010–14, suggesting that the effect of national income on life expectancy has become stronger, not weaker, over time. For a more in-depth analysis, see Johan P. Mackenbach and Caspar W.N. Looman, "Life Expectancy and National Income in Europe, 1900–2008," *International Journal of Epidemiology* 42, no. 4 (2013): 1100–10.

1990 international dollars, we can clearly see that at the same level of national income life expectancy was higher in the 2010s than the 1960s, and in the 1960s than the 1930s. This implies that increases in national income provide at most a partial explanation of increases in life expectancy.[28]

Diffusion of new public health and medical technologies from richer to poorer countries in Europe – the mechanism postulated by Preston – has certainly played a role in these upward shifts. In several periods, particularly the 1930–1960 period, countries with a lower national income had larger increases in life expectancy than richer countries, due to stronger declines of infant mortality and mortality from infectious and respiratory diseases. In later sections and chapters, we will repeatedly come back to this remarkable catch-up phenomenon, which was based on rapid implementation in poorer countries of techniques and policies that had already been introduced in richer countries.[29]

As mentioned above, we cannot assume that the cross-sectional relationships seen in Figure 6 are due to a causal effect of national income on life expectancy. The nearest we can get to identifying a causal relationship is by relating changes-over-time in national income to changes-over-time in life expectancy. When we do this in our European dataset, we find positive relationships in the 1900–1930 and 1990–2010 periods only, suggesting that in these two periods, but not in others, rising living standards may have contributed more directly to rising life expectancy.[30]

Over-all, the European experience suggests that improved living conditions did play a role, but may not have been the most important factor in long-term improvements in population health.

Political History: The Rise of the Modern State

One other factor that has played a role is political change. Political conditions, events and actors have often facilitated or hindered population health

28 Although upward shifts occurred in all periods, they were largest in the period 1930–1960, when they accounted for between two-thirds and four-fifths of the increase in life expectancy in Europe as a whole. As shown in Mackenbach and Looman, "Life Expectancy", after 1960 the upward shifts were smaller, and contributed between one-quarter and one-half to the increase in life expectancy in Europe as a whole.

29 For the correlations between national income at the beginning of each period, and changes in life expectancy during each period, see Suppl. Table 3.

30 For the correlations between changes in national income and changes in life expectancy, see Suppl. Table 3. These correlations were statistically significantly negative in 1930–1960, and mostly non-significant in other periods, suggesting that the catch-up in 1930–1960 by poorer countries was independent of improvements in living standards.

improvements, either directly or indirectly. In the few pages that follow, we will focus on two important political developments: the development of the modern state, and changes in the governance of states (particularly the rise of democracy and the adoption of egalitarian ideologies).[31]

The development of the modern state has been given extra emphasis in the title of this section, because it provided the necessary institutions and resources for implementing large-scale measures to improve population health, from sewage systems to old-age pensions and from universal health insurance to road safety. However, without the rise of democracy and of egalitarian ideologies the health benefits would not have been so wide-spread. This increased the leverage of the poorer sections of society, which led to policies and institutions benefiting the health of all, and not only that of the elites. As a result, and as we will see below, differences between European countries in the timing, speed and direction of political change often went together with differences in the timing, speed and direction of population health change.

General histories of Europe agree that the development of the *modern state* was one of the most significant developments of the 18th and 19th centuries. The 18th century saw the emergence of centralized states with uniform taxation, professional bureaucracies, and a gradually expanding scope for national policies. Apart from maintaining an increasingly costly army, these policies came to include the improvement of communications, the promotion of trade, and the containment of epidemics. During the 19th and 20th centuries, European states were further strengthened by promotion of a national consciousness, rising levels of taxation, and a relentless expansion of the responsibilities of the state. These now also came to include the provision of education, social security, mother and child care, health insurance, and many other public policies that most Europeans now take for granted.

These trends were not primarily driven by considerations of public welfare, but by what was perceived to be the national interest. Due to technological developments, warfare became more and more costly, and these costs could only be carried by a centralized state capable of raising taxes. Investments in roads, waterways and (in the 19th century) railways were justified by the necessity of stimulating economic growth. The expansion of the welfare state was not only a means of relieving poverty, but also of containing communism and warding off revolution. Nevertheless, increasing government involvement

31 War – "the mere continuation of politics by other means," according to Prussian general Carl von Clausewitz (1780–1831) – will be dealt with in Chapter 4.

(and effectiveness) was an important pre-condition for many policies that sooner or later improved public welfare, including population health.[32]

The political map of Europe has undergone enormous changes in the course of the centuries covered by this book. In the early 18th century no such thing as Germany or Italy existed yet, Finland was still part of the Kingdom of Sweden, the Ottomans occupied large parts of the Balkans, and the Polish-Lithuanian Commonwealth contained a huge part of Central-eastern and Eastern Europe, until it was partitioned between Russia, Prussia and the Habsburg empire and completely erased from the map at the end of the 18th century.

During the 19th and 20th centuries, Europe's political map was repeatedly changed as a result of the peace settlements after the Napoleonic Wars, World War I and then World War II, and as a result of the collapse of the Soviet Union and Yugoslavia. For example, after World War I, Finland became independent from Russia which had taken it from Sweden in the early 19th century. So did the Baltic countries until they were reconquered by the Soviet Union in 1940. The end of World War I provoked the end of the Habsburg and Ottoman Empires, which resulted in a range of newly independent states in Central-eastern and South-eastern Europe, such as Czechoslovakia, Hungary, Yugoslavia and Albania. After World War II, Germany was first split up and then re-united in 1990. This coincided with the dissolution of the Soviet Union which also saw many new countries in Eastern Europe become independent.

The net effect of these and other changes has been a substantial rise in the number of independent states. Recently, this fragmentation was partly balanced by a slow process of European integration within an expanding European Union that – at the moment of writing (2019) – has 28 member states. Over time, the European Union has played an increasingly important role in population health, for example by regulating the emission of air-pollutants,

---

32 General histories of Europe emphasizing the emergence of the modern state are John M. Roberts, *The Penguin History of Europe* (London etc.: Penguin, 1996), esp. Book 3, and Timothy C.W. Blanning, *The Pursuit of Glory: Europe, 1648–1815* (London: Allen Lane, 2007), Part 2. A distinction can be made between the advent of the modern state (a process starting in the Middle Ages and culminating in the absolutism of the 18th century), the rise of the concept of the 'nation' (i.e., a community founded on national awareness – an idea that gained popularity in the 19th century), and the merging of the two in modern 'nation-states' (which most European countries had achieved by the middle of the 20th century); see Hagen Schulze, *States, Nations and Nationalism* (Oxford: Blackwell, 1996). For a comparative history of the role of the state in dealing with infectious diseases in Britain, France, Germany and Sweden, see Peter Baldwin, *Contagion and the State in Europe, 1830–1930* (Cambridge: Cambridge University Press, 1999). The creation of public health and health care systems reciprocally reinforced the process of state formation; see Abram de Swaan, *In Care of the State* (New York etc. : Oxford University Press, 1988).

harmonizing tobacco control policies, and stimulating road traffic safety programs.[33]

These changes – dissolutions and mergers of political entities – provide interesting opportunities for studying the effect of political conditions on population health. In general, dissolution of a political entity has often increased disparities in life expectancy between its newly independent parts, whereas unification has often reduced such disparities. This strongly supports the idea that states make a difference for the health of their populations.

Here are a few examples, some of which have been illustrated in Figure 7. After independence from Russia, Finland's life expectancy moved away from Russia's, and gradually converged with Sweden's during the 20th century. During the 1920s and 1930s, life expectancy in the newly independent Baltic republics followed a similar upward trend as Finland's, but after World War II their life expectancies followed the unfavourable trends in Russia. It was only after the breaking up of the Soviet Union that their life expectancies diverged again from Russia's. The peaceful splitting up of Czechoslovakia into a Czech and a Slovak Republic in 1993 was followed by a small but measurable divergence of their life expectancies. The merger between the German Democratic Republic and the German Federal Republic in 1991 was followed by a rapid and strong convergence. Also, Slovenia and Croatia have been part of the Habsburg Empire, benefiting from the empire's homogenizing policies in the areas of education and public health. They still have higher life expectancies than parts of former Yugoslavia which have been under Ottoman rule, such as Bosnia, Serbia and North Macedonia.[34]

---

33 From consisting of only six countries (Germany, France, Italy, Netherlands, Belgium, Luxembourg), the European Union has been enlarged in four waves: the 1970s (Denmark and United Kingdom), the 1980s (Spain, Portugal and Greece), the 1990s (Finland, Sweden and Austria) and the 2000s (Malta, Cyprus and many Central and Eastern European countries). The United Kingdom has in a referendum voted to leave, but at the moment of writing (Autumn 2019) it was still unclear when 'Brexit' would occur. For illustrations of the role of the EU in recent health improvements, see Johan P. Mackenbach and Martin McKee, eds., *Successes and Failures of Health Policy in Europe* (Maidenhead: Open University Press, 2013), *passim.*

34 Many of these remarkable patterns of divergence and convergence were documented in Johan P. Mackenbach, "Political Conditions and Life Expectancy in Europe, 1900–2008," *Social Science & Medicine* 82 (2013): 134–46. For an analysis of health convergence between East and West Germany, see Pavel Grigoriev and Markéta Pechholdová, "Health Convergence between East and West Germany as Reflected in Long-Term Cause-Specific Mortality Trends," *European Journal of Population* 33, no. 5 (2017): 701–31. The effect of the dissolution of Yugoslavia has been analysed in Stephen J. Kunitz, "The Making and Breaking of Yugoslavia and Its Impact on Health," *American Journal of Public Health* 94, no. 11 (2004): 1894–904. Although studies of the effect of becoming a member of the European

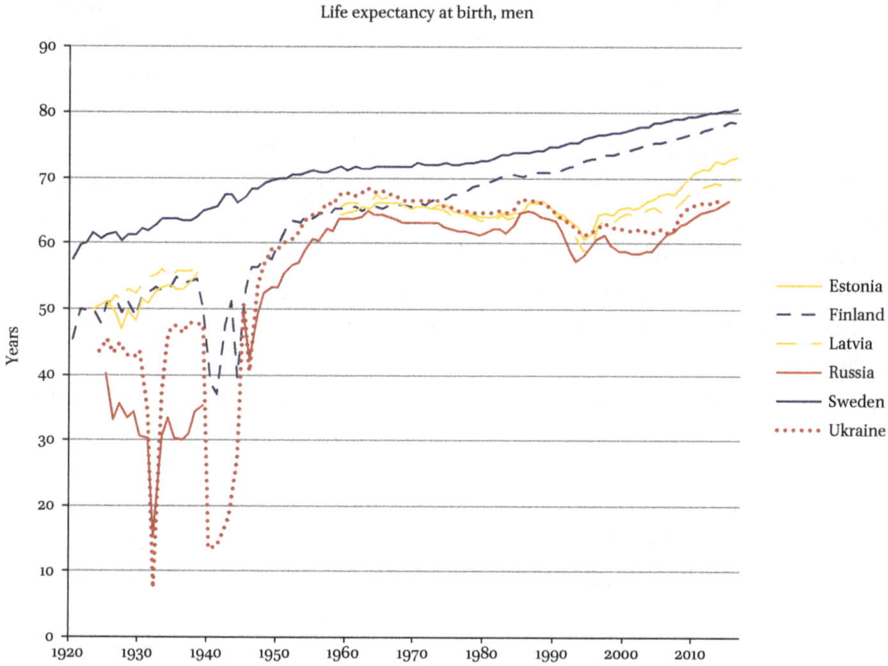

FIGURE 7 Trends in life expectancy in Northern and Eastern Europe, 1920–2015
SOURCE OF DATA: SEE SUPPL. TABLE 1

As in the case of economic growth, and despite being indispensable for population health improvement, the rise of the modern state undoubtedly also had darker sides. The nationalism underpinning the advent of modern 'nation-states' often fuelled mutual enmity, and the state has not merely become more effective in doing good things, but also in doing bad things. This does not only include warfare – already briefly mentioned above – but also colonization and exploitation of other parts of the world, and political oppression and even physical extermination of entire population groups. Sometimes, for example in the Soviet Union in the middle of the 20th century, rapid population health improvements went hand-in-hand with brutal oppression of political opponents of the regime, making a balanced moral judgement nearly impossible (see Chapter 7).

Union have found no clear signs of life expectancy convergence following entry into the EU, as shown in Mackenbach, "Political Conditions and Life Expectancy" some convergence occurred before entry, probably as an effect of preparations for membership.

A second political trend that has contributed to long-term improvements in population health is the *rise of democracy and egalitarian ideologies*. This has changed the way in which European countries govern their internal affairs, to the advantage of the majority of their populations. In the early 18th century, the political systems of European countries varied between republican democracy in Switzerland and full-blown autocratic monarchy in the Ottoman empire. Most European countries, including Russia, the Habsburg Empire, France, Spain and Sweden, still had absolutist monarchies, in which the ruler's will was supreme. Only a few countries, such as the Dutch Republic and Venice, tended towards early forms of democracy, based on a contract with a ruler-elect and rule by code of law (constitutional government). In the United Kingdom, England's Glorious Revolution (1688) had also left a form of constitutional monarchy.[35]

The 19th and 20th centuries witnessed a gradual rise of liberal democracy. This is defined by representative government operating through law, by regular, free and fair elections based on universal suffrage, and by respect for individual rights including freedom of expression and association. Recurring revolts and revolutions often included a demand for more democracy, and because these demands were ultimately effective, many countries in Northwestern Europe developed into liberal democracies during the 19th century, to be followed by many countries in other parts of Europe in the early 20th century. However, during the 20th century many European countries also had shorter or longer periods of autocratic government, either communist or noncommunist (often fascist in inspiration). This happened during the Interbellum and then again after World War II, when many countries in Central-eastern and South-eastern Europe were forced to adopt communist autocratic regimes, and several countries in Southern Europe temporarily had non-communist autocratic regimes.[36]

There is a large literature showing that democracy is good for people's health, although there are also many exceptions to the rule. (Think of Cuba and China, which despite being governed by autocratic regimes have made great advances in population health.) This is not only because democracy is associated with prosperity, but also because democratic governments have more incentives to commit themselves to population health improvement.

35 For an overview of the governance systems of European countries in the 18th century, see Norman Davies, *Europe: A History* (London: Pimlico, 1997), p. 1265.

36 The rise of democracy in Europe can be traced in general histories of Europe (such as Davies, *Europe: A History*,) and has been analysed in more detail in Luciano Canfora, *Democracy in Europe* (Oxford: Blackwell, 2006).

They tend to make decisions in accordance with voters' interests, and thus are usually more actively engaged in promoting the public good than authoritarian governments. This advantage may be strengthened by greater public accountability, greater inclination towards redistributive policies, and greater ability to recruit competent and honest people.[37]

The historical record in Europe shows that, during most of the 20th century, democratically governed countries indeed had higher life expectancies than autocratically governed countries. Despite strong changes in cause-of-death patterns, this positive association has attenuated only slightly over time, and was still clearly present in 2010. In 1930, democratically governed countries had lower infant mortality and mortality from infectious and respiratory diseases, whereas in 1990 democratically governed countries had lower mortality from cardiovascular diseases and injuries.[38]

Although this supports the idea that democracy is good for population health, many other factors may confound this relationship, and longitudinal analyses actually suggest a more complex story, because increases in life expectancy were not always larger in democratically governed countries. On the contrary, the reverse applied in the period 1930–1960, when increases in life expectancy were larger in autocratically governed countries. As we will see later, the catch-up movement of countries in the South and East was actively managed by their autocratic non-communist regimes (as in the case of Spain and Portugal) and by their autocratic communist regimes. No other European country has experienced such a rapid growth of life expectancy as Russia did during the 1940s: 18 years gain in life expectancy in little more than a decade. Large gains in life expectancy were also seen in other Soviet republics, as well

---

37 See, for example, Jeroen Klomp and Jakob de Haan, "Is the Political System Really Related to Health?," *Social Science and Medicine* 69, no. 1 (2009): 36–46; Timothy Besley and Masayuki Kudamatsu, "Health and Democracy," *Political Economy* 96, no. 2 (2006): 313–18; Johan P. Mackenbach, Yannan Hu, and Caspar W.N. Looman, "Democratization and Life Expectancy in Europe, 1960–2008," *Social Science & Medicine* 93 (2013): 166–75. On the counterexamples of Cuba and China, see Vicente Navarro, "Has Socialism Failed? An Analysis of Health Indicators under Socialism," *International Journal of Health Services* 22, no. 4 (1992): 583–601.

38 For the correlations between levels of democracy and life expectancy, see Suppl. Table 3. These correlations were statistically significant and positive in 1930–34, 1960–64, 1990–94, and 2010–14, and non-significant in 1870–74 and 1900–04. After adjustment for other determinants, statistically significant associations are mainly found in 2010–14, suggesting that in earlier periods confounding by other factors probably contributed to the positive association.

as in Central-eastern and South-eastern European countries under Soviet influence.[39]

In the second half of the 20th century, two waves of political reform brought full democracy to Spain, Portugal and Greece in the 1970s, and various degrees of democracy to the countries of Central-Eastern, South-eastern and Eastern Europe in the 1990s. Whereas the first wave was associated with a slight acceleration of the increase in life expectancy in the countries involved, the second wave had mixed effects, probably because too many changes occurred simultaneously. Planned economies were replaced by market economies, and painful economic adaptations were undertaken. As a result of these disruptive changes, life expectancy went down in many countries. However, some countries emerged quickly from this painful phase with a renewed increase of life expectancy, often in tandem with a rapid development towards full democracy. This mainly applies to the Baltic countries and countries in Central-eastern Europe that rapidly linked up with Western Europe.[40]

The rise of democracy would not have occurred without the rise of egalitarian ideologies, emphasizing the equality of all citizens, and this egalitarian ethos has undoubtedly also contributed to long-term improvements in population health. Reducing social inequality in all spheres of life, including income, wealth, access to education, and access to health care, has been a core policy focus for left-wing parties throughout the 20th century. Despite all their failures, when they were in government these parties often at least partly achieved their egalitarian policy goals. When they were not in power the threat of a socialist or communist victory in democratic elections often stimulated other political parties to also embrace redistributive policies, and to support the development of the modern welfare state. This welfare state provided a safety net against poverty, and increased access to education and health care.[41]

39 For the correlations between levels of democracy at the beginning of each period, and changes in life expectancy during each period, see Suppl. Table 3. These correlations were statistically significant and negative in 1930–1960, and mostly non-significant in other periods. On the improvements in population health in Spain under the Franco regime, see Jose A. Tapia Granados, "Politics and Health in Eight European Countries," *Social Science & Medicine* 71, no. 5 (2010): 841–50.

40 The impact of both waves of democratization on life expectancy and cause-specific mortality in Europe has been analysed in Mackenbach et al., "Democratization."

41 On the history and achievements of the welfare state, see, e.g., Evelyne Huber and John D. Stephens, *Development and Crisis of the Welfare State* (Chicago: University of Chicago Press, 2001).

Sociocultural History: the Lights Go On

Over the past three centuries, important sociocultural changes have occurred as well. However, it is more difficult to capture these in quantitative indicators than in the case of economic or even political changes. Thanks to the development of modern survey methods we know quite a lot about current differences between European countries in, e.g., social cohesion, religiousness, and health literacy. Yet, trends in these and other factors can only be measured over relatively short time-periods. Nevertheless, three sociocultural conditions stand out as having had a profound impact on secular changes in population health: long-standing cultural differences between European countries; the 'civilizing process'; and increasing levels of literacy and other indicators of a more 'enlightened' way of life.

Despite a long-term tendency towards convergence, *cultural differences* between European countries have persisted until the present day. Studies have pointed to an important 'cultural fault-line' that runs along a North-South axis through the middle of Europe, and separates Western Christianity from Eastern Orthodox Christianity. In the West, a further distinction can be made between North-western Europe, which became mainly Protestant in the 16th and 17th centuries, and Southern Europe which remained Roman-catholic. These three 'cultural zones' can still clearly be distinguished, partly because their cultures have resulted in different economic, sociocultural and political trajectories. In the West, the historical sequence of medieval Humanism, Renaissance, Reformation/Counter-Reformation and Enlightenment resulted in – to mention a few of the important differences with the Eastern Orthodox zone – individualization, secularization, early advances in science, early industrialization, separation between church and state, and early democratization.[42]

In these developments, which ultimately resulted in the 'rise of the West' as a global power, the Protestant countries in North-western Europe took the lead, and were followed by the Roman-catholic South and later still by the Eastern Orthodox East. Although it is unlikely that religious affiliation is the only cause of these different trajectories, there may be some truth in Max Weber's

42 For 'global cultural zones', see Samuel P. Huntington, *The Clash of Civilizations and the Remaking of World Order* (New York etc.: Simon & Schuster, 1996). Cultural values (such as Ronald Inglehart's post-materialism values, and Welzel's emancipatory values) cluster geographically according to Huntington's cultural zones; see Ronald Inglehart and Wayne E. Baker, "Modernization, Cultural Change, and the Persistence of Traditional Values," *American Sociological Review* 65, no. 1 (2000): 19–51; Christian Welzel, *Freedom Rising* (Cambridge etc.: Cambridge University Press, 2013).

thesis that modern capitalism could thrive in North-western Europe because of the 'protestant ethic' of hard work and savings.[43]

Protestantism is also associated with early improvements in population health. Traditionally-protestant countries always had a higher life expectancy, but the association was strongest in 1870, 1900 and 1930, and has gradually weakened in more recent times. This association is probably due – at least partly – to an effect of average levels of education on life expectancy. Protestantism and education are closely linked: because of the core Protestant idea that every church member should be able to read the Bible, levels of education have for a long time been higher in Protestant than in Roman-catholic and Eastern Orthodox countries.[44]

Religious affiliation is not the only cultural factor with long-standing differences between European countries. 'Cultural values', i.e., broad preferences that the members of a society share, also differ within Europe in rather stable patterns. For example, 'self-expression values' and 'emancipative values' are particularly prevalent in North-western Europe. Although data on long-term trends in these cultural values are not available, it is likely that these have evolved over time, from the more traditional values still prevalent in other parts of Europe. Such cultural changes may have reinforced a shift towards more rational behaviour with a focus on personal well-being, including good health.[45]

---

43 For some further comments on "the rise of the West," see Chapter 7. Max Weber's study of how the Protestant outlook on life may have contributed to the early rise of capitalism in North-western Europe is a classic of sociology (Max Weber, *Die Protestantische Ethik Und Der Geist Des Kapitalismus* (Bd. XX & XXI: Archiv fur Soxialwissenschaft und Sozialpolitik, 1904–05)). However, the empirical evidence for this theory is mixed (Harold B. Jones, "The Protestant Ethic: Weber's Model and the Empirical Literature," *Human Relations* 50, no. 7 (1997): 757–78).

44 For the correlations between Protestantism and life expectancy, see Suppl. Table 3. These correlations were statistically significant and positive in all periods. However, after adjustment for other determinants, statistically significant and positive associations are only found in 1870, 1900 and 1930, suggesting that the effect of Protestantism has become weaker over time. Within countries with mixed populations, such as the Netherlands and Switzerland, Protestants have long had higher life expectancies than Roman-Catholics; see, e.g., Judith H. Wolleswinkel-van den Bosch et al., "Determinants of Infant and Early Childhood Mortality Levels and Their Decline in the Netherlands," *International Journal of Epidemiology* 29, no. 6 (2000): 1031–40. These differences have recently faded; see Johan P. Mackenbach, "Jean Calvin, Calvinism, and Population Health: Impressions from Switzerland," *European Journal of Public Health* 17, no. 1 (2007): 1.

45 European countries' 'cultural values' can be found in, e.g., Welzel, *Freedom Rising*; Ronald Inglehart, *Modernization and Postmodernization* (Princeton: Princeton University Press,

Another sociocultural trend which has probably contributed to long-term changes in population health is the *'civilizing process'*. This is a general change in manners since the Middle Ages that has been described and analysed by German-British sociologist Norbert Elias (1897–1990). Using 'etiquette' books and other historical sources, Elias traced how behavioural norms with regard to violence, sexual behaviour, bodily functions, and table manners were gradually transformed. These changes did not primarily occur for health-related reasons, but because of increasing thresholds of shame and repugnance. For example, eating with one's hands from a common bowl became repulsive and was gradually replaced by eating with a fork from a private plate, long before people became aware of the risks of infection.[46]

This 'civilizing process', with its increasing 'self-restraint', formalization of manners, and repression of emotions, probably had a wide range of effects on population health. Increased sensitivity to bodily contact and to the smells and excretions of the human body may have contributed to the diffusion of hygienic practices, and thus to a decreasing risk of attracting infectious disease. As we will see in Chapter 6, stricter aggression regulation contributed to the decline of homicide. Conceivably, increased sexual restraint facilitated the adoption of fertility control and the decline of syphilis. More generally, increased 'self-restraint' probably facilitated many changes in health-related behaviours.[47]

Although these changes were partly autonomous, they were not completely independent from other societal changes. According to Elias, the requirement of 'self-restraint' originated in the growing interdependency of people, as a result of increasing integration into larger political and economic units. This happened earlier in North-western Europe than elsewhere, so that differences between European countries in this 'civilizing process' can plausibly have contributed to differences in the timing of several population health improvements.

However, the most important sociocultural change underpinning long-term population health improvement probably was a more rational attitude to

1997). For an empirical analysis of their health implications, see Johan P. Mackenbach, "Cultural Values and Population Health," *Health & Place* 28 (2014): 116–32.

46 Norbert Elias, *Uber den Prozess der Zivilisation* (Basel: Verlag Haus zum Falken, 1939).

47 For an analysis of how the 'civilizing process' induced behavioural changes contributing to the decline of leprosy, plague, syphilis and cholera before the contagious nature of these diseases was known, see Johan Goudsblom, "Public Health and the Civilizing Process," *Milbank Quarterly* 64, no. 2 (1986): 161–88. For an application of Elias' theory to the development of public health, poverty relief, education, and social security, see Swaan, *In Care of the State.*

health and disease. This was based on *increased knowledge* and diffused throughout the population by rising levels of literacy and education. These changes started as part of the broader 18th century movement of the 'Enlightenment', and continue until the present day. This is illustrated by the fact that adherence to health guidelines is still better among higher than among lower educated people.[48]

The 'Enlightenment' was the 18th century European movement advancing the idea that 'reason' is the primary basis of all knowledge. It aimed to emancipate human reason from prejudice, superstition and religious dogma, and its ideas and ideals penetrated many areas of life, from agriculture to politics, and from medicine to religion. The 'Enlightenment' started in Britain and the Dutch Republic, and rapidly spread from there to other countries in North-western Europe, including France and Sweden.

Here again, we find an example of where Protestantism (or factors underlying countries' choice for the Reformation) may have made a difference. Repression of Enlightenment ideas was more forceful in Roman-catholic countries, whereas in countries like Great Britain and the Dutch Republic which had adopted Protestantism, governments were more liberal-minded and populations were better educated. Enlightenment ideas were developed in academies, salons, and societies, and were diffused in the first newspapers and other periodicals for which literacy was of course an essential requirement. Consequently, ideals of educating the population led to more emphasis on schooling and, ultimately, compulsory education.[49]

This movement had important consequences for population health, through various pathways. A more rational approach to economic issues helped to start and sustain the agricultural and industrial revolutions. It stimulated the development of physics and other sciences. It led to a movement towards 'enlightened' government and, ultimately, democracy. It led to more rational forms of Christianity and, ultimately, to secularization, which removed some of the barriers to fertility control. It also sparked the rise of a more egalitarian ethos,

---

48 Studies found that rising the age of compulsory education led to better health behaviours (and lower mortality) in adulthood. For a review, see Mackenbach, *Health Inequalities*, Chapter 3.

49 For a general overview of the Enlightenment and its spread in Europe, see Ulrich Im Hof, *The Enlightenment: An Historical Introduction* (Oxford: Blackwell, 1994). The development of the Enlightenment in Britain, and its impact on all aspects of life, have been detailed in Roy Porter, *Enlightenment: Britain and the Creation of the Modern World* (London: Allen Lane, 2000). For an enthusiastic review of the many contributions of the Enlightenment to human well-being, see Steven Pinker, *Enlightenment Now* (London: Allen Lane, 2018).

which underlay the humanitarian reforms of the 18th and 19th centuries that were necessary for population-wide health improvement.

By fostering science and a more rational approach to disease it also stimulated medical science and the adoption of new scientific insights by medical practitioners. In the general population, starting with the elites, new attitudes with regard to the care of the body emerged, with more attention to preventing disease. As part of this medical revolution, it also stimulated the development of personal and public hygiene. Even among the elites, regular washing of body and clothes only became habitual in the late 18th and early 19th centuries, partly because previous generations had mistakenly believed that contact with water increased the risk of illness. The sanitary reforms of the second half of the 19th and first half the 20th century were accompanied by health education campaigns which contributed importantly to further changes in popular conceptions of disease and acceptance of modern hygienic insights. Pushed to the extremes, 'Enlightenment' thinking led to the previously unthinkable idea that perhaps, in the future,

> the improvement of medical practice [...] will mean the end of infectious and hereditary diseases and illnesses brought on by climate, food or working conditions. It is reasonable to hope that all other diseases will likewise disappear as their distant causes are discovered.[50]

As a result of this movement, and the schooling program to which it led, levels of literacy and education rose tremendously in all European countries, but with important differences in timing between countries. Trends in levels of literacy are pictured in Figure 8. Literacy can be measured by the proportion of brides and bridegrooms (or other people who had to sign documents) who were able to sign their names. This can be traced over a much longer period than trends in levels of education.[51]

---

50 For a general overview of the changes in medical science and medical practice stimulated by the Enlightenment, see Roy Porter, *The Greatest Benefit to Mankind* (London: HarperCollins, 1997), Chapter x. The emergence of 'enlightened' attitudes towards the care of the body in France were traced in G. Vigarello, *Histoire des Pratiques de Santé: Le Sain et le Malsain depuis le Moyen Âge* (Paris: Éd. du Seuil, 1999). A study of changes in attitudes towards common infectious diseases in late 19th century London has documented the rise of modern hygienic practices under the influence of prevention campaigns; see Anne Hardy, *The Epidemic Streets: Infectious Disease and the Rise of Preventive Medicine, 1856–1900* (Oxford etc.: Oxford University Press, 1993). The quote is from the Marquis de Condorcet (1743–1794), and is reproduced here from Porter, *Greatest Benefit*, pp. 245–46.

51 More recently other measures for literacy have been proposed, such as 'numeracy', indicated by the ability to give your exact age (Brian A'Hearn, Jörg Baten, and Dorothee

Around 1800, countries in North-western Europe, such as Britain, Sweden and the Netherlands, had much higher levels of literacy than countries in Southern or Eastern Europe. This was the result of differences between countries in the promotion of literacy in previous centuries. The Swedish example is particularly striking: during the 17th and 18th centuries, massive campaigns were held to enforce a national law that required all parishioners to be able to read the Bible. The campaigns were based on home schooling, and included yearly examinations. A central register of parishioners' reading ability was kept, and shows a strong rise of reading ability in response to the campaigns.

During the 19th century, many other North-western European countries also achieved a rise in literacy, with countries in Southern and Eastern Europe often only catching up during the 20th century. The steepest rises ever were seen in the Soviet Union and Albania, where intensive literacy campaigns in the 1930s, 1940s and 1950s succeeded in rapidly eradicating illiteracy. Portugal stands out as a laggard in Southern Europe, with a proportion of literate people of only 80% as late as in 1975. Largely similar trends are seen for average levels of education (see Suppl. Figure 7).[52]

Rising levels of literacy and education made important contributions to long-term population health improvements. This worked not only indirectly, e.g., via promoting economic development, but also more directly via promoting the adoption of health-conducive behaviours in the population. Individual-level evidence of the effects of literacy and levels of education on mortality in historical times indicates, that in the last decades of the 19th century infant mortality declined earlier among the babies of literate mothers. These were probably more able or willing than illiterate mothers to apply modern hygienic insights and to restrict fertility. As mentioned above, level of education has remained an important determinant of health until the present day, partly because of the greater 'health literacy' of higher educated people.[53]

Crayen, "Quantifying Quantitative Literacy: Age Heaping and the History of Human Capital," *Journal of Economic History* 69, no. 3 (2009): 783–808). Trends in numeracy generally mirror those for conventional measures of literacy (Dorothee Crayen and Joerg Baten, "Global Trends in Numeracy 1820–1949 and Its Implications for Long-Term Growth," *Explorations in Economic History* 47, no. 1 (2010): 82–99).

52 For the rise of schooling in Europe, see Robert A. Houston, *Literacy in Early Modern Europe* (Edinburgh etc.: Pearson Education Limited, 2002). For the Swedish experience, see Egil Johansson, *The History of Literacy in Sweden: In Comparison with Some Other Countries*, vol. 12, Educational Reports Umeå, (Umeå: Umeå universitet, 1977). The rise in literacy during the 19th century was largely due to voluntary schooling, and often preceded the introduction of compulsory schooling.

53 Protective effects of mothers' literacy on infant mortality in the later 19th century have been found in the Netherlands (O.W.A. Boonstra, *De Waardij van eene Vroege Opleiding*

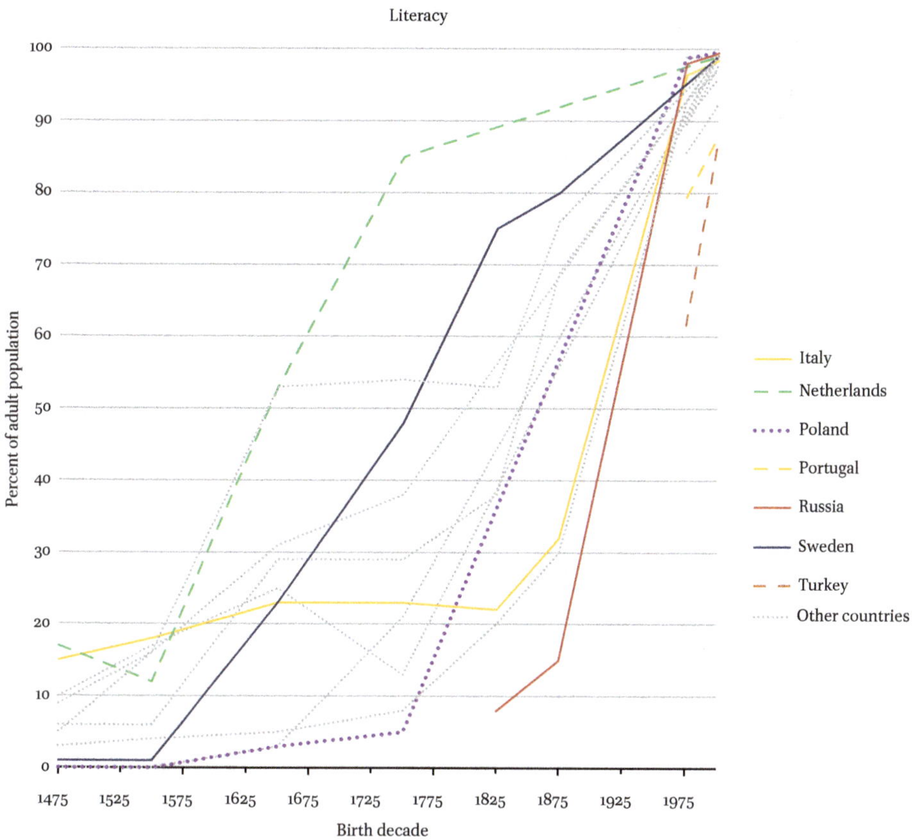

FIGURE 8 Trends in literacy in Europe, 1475–2000
SOURCE OF DATA: WWW.OURWORLDINDATA.ORG (ACCESSED 01/08/2019)

Before national income became an important determinant of life expectancy, a country's average level of education was strongly positively associated with life expectancy. This was the case in 1870, 1900 and 1930, and was due to the fact that countries with a higher average level of education had lower infant mortality and lower mortality from infectious and respiratory diseases. However,

(Wageningen: Wageningen University, 1993), Chapter 9), England and Wales (Woods, *Demography*, Chapter 7), and the US (Samuel H. Preston and Michael R. Haines, *Fatal Years* (Princeton: Princeton University Press, 1991), Chapter 4). For a recent study of 'health literacy', see Kristine Sørensen et al., "Health Literacy in Europe: Comparative Results of the European Health Literacy Survey (HLS-EU)," *European Journal of Public Health* 25, no. 6 (2015): 1053–58.

the strength of this association gradually diminished over time, perhaps because of converging levels of education between countries.[54]

Having come at the end of this rather optimistic account of the many benefits of the Enlightenment, it is time to ask ourselves – like we did in the case of economic and political change – whether there was (or is) a darker side as well. This is a difficult question that – if addressed seriously – would bring us into deep philosophical waters. Let me just mention, therefore, that the 'Enlightenment project' has been criticized on several grounds. One is its emphasis on the autonomy of the individual, which may have contributed to a loosening of social cohesion and mutual responsibility. Another is that the use of reason for instrumental purposes, i.e., as a means to whatever end we choose to pursue, may have fuelled our will to domination over others and the natural world, thereby contributing to the rise of totalitarian regimes and environmental destruction. We will briefly come back to this 'dialectic of the Enlightenment' in Chapter 8.[55]

Public Health and Medical Care

A Short History of Public Health

Tracing the history of 'public health' over three centuries, during which its name has changed several times, is not easy. The problem is aggravated by differences in national language which make it difficult to recognize 'public health' (or the concepts, professions and institutions hiding behind other English terms) in other European countries. It is only recently that the un-translated term 'public health' has come into use throughout Europe – indicating a certain degree of European convergence.[56]

---

54 For the correlations between average years of education and life expectancy, see Suppl. Table 3. These correlations were statistically significant and positive in 1870–74, 1900–1904, 1930–34, and 1960–64, and non-significant in 1990–94 and 2010–14. The correlations between changes-over-time in education and changes-over-time in life expectancy can be found in the same table.

55 For a summary of the most common critiques of the Enlightenment, see James Schmidt, "What Enlightenment Project?," *Political Theory* 28, no. 6 (2000): 734–57. "*Dialektik der Aufklärung*" is the title of a famous book by German philosophers Horkheimer and Adorno, who saw the seeds of Nazi totalitarianism in the 'instrumental reason' promoted by the Enlightenment (Max Horkheimer and Theodor W. Adorno, *Dialektik der Aufklärung* (Amsterdam: Querido, 1947)).

56 For a comparison of current terminology in eight European languages, see Sanja Kaiser and Johan P. Mackenbach, "Public Health in Eight European Countries: An International Comparison of Terminology," *Public Health* 122, no. 2 (2008): 211–16. The European Public

A common definition of 'public health' is: "the art and science of preventing disease, prolonging life and promoting health through the organized efforts of society." This emphasizes the collective nature of public health interventions, as distinct from the individualized nature of medical interventions. If we take this as our definition, we can roughly divide the history of the field in four phases. These are each characterized by a different name: 'medical police' (18th century), 'public hygiene' (19th century), 'social hygiene' (first half of 20th century), and 'new public health' (second half of the 20th century).[57]

'Social medicine' is another frequently used term, both in the past and today, but it has developed too many different meanings to be useful for this overview. These range from an almost-synonym with 'public health' (in continental Europe in the 19th century), to the branch of medicine involved in 'state medicine' (e.g., medical assessments for social insurance benefits, in continental Europe in the 20th century), to a socially critical approach to population health issues (in Britain in the middle of the 20th century, and in Latin America until the present day).[58]

The field of 'public health' did of course not come out of the blue. It built on earlier approaches, such as the precepts for individual hygiene that had been practiced in Greek and Roman times. It also built on the idea that governments had a certain responsibility for the health of their citizens which already came up in the Middle Ages, e.g. with respect to quarantine measures against epidemic diseases. However, after 1700 it gradually developed an identity, widened its scope to cover all population health issues, and built a growing body of empirically based knowledge as well as dedicated institutions and a dedicated profession.[59]

Health Association, founded in 1992, brings together 41 national associations of public health.

57 The definition of 'public health' given in the text is from Acheson (Department of Health, *Public Health in England (the Acheson Report)* (London: Her Majesty's Stationery Office, 1988)). The proposed division in four phases is schematic, and in reality many other terms have been used as well, both in Britain and in other European countries. For example, the term 'public hygiene' has not been regularly used in Britain (where, in the 19th century, the term 'public health' was coined instead), and for some time in the 1970s Britain referred to the field as 'community medicine' before returning to the classical term 'public health'.

58 See, e.g., Porter, *Health Citizenship*; George Rosen, "What Is Social Medicine?," *Bulletin of the History of Medicine* 21, no. 5 (1947): 674–733.

59 Rosen, *History*. A comparative history of public health in Europe is not available; closest comes Porter, *The History of Public Health and the Modern State* which contains essays on France, Germany, Great Britain, Sweden and Russia. Porter, *Health, Civilization and the State* has a deeper analysis of the connections between the rise of the modern state and the development of public health, as does Baldwin, *Contagion and the State in Europe*.

This started in the 18th century which saw the emergence of an approach called '*medical police*'. This term often confuses modern readers, but it refers to the creation of a systematic 'medical policy' by governments, and to its implementation through administrative regulations such as laws, taxes and inspections. It fitted in a more general movement to increase the role of the state in economic and demographic affairs in order to maximize its power ('mercantilism'), which was important in these times of inter-European competition. The development of 'medical police' culminated in the work of Johann Peter Frank (1745–1821), a German physician who held positions throughout Europe (Saxony, Lombardy, Austria, Russia) and who published his *System einer Vollständigen Medicinischen Polizey* between 1779 and 1819.

This was a work in six parts that became highly influential, as illustrated by the fact that it was translated into many languages. It described in detail how the state could promote the health of its inhabitants and the size of its population, systematizing the available arsenal of collective measures to improve population health. This arsenal was – of course – based on contemporary insights into the causes of disease. In the 18th century, many new insights had been gathered thanks to the revival of Hippocratic or 'ecological' theories of disease, for example by the extensive use of geographical comparisons ('medical geography'). Frank's six-volume compendium contained detailed guidance with regard to the care of pregnant women, infants and children, accident prevention, the hygiene of food and housing, sanitation, and many other topics.[60]

Frank's thinking fitted better in the autocratic political regimes of the German states and the Habsburg Empire than in the more liberal regimes of Britain and the Dutch Republic, and even in the German-speaking parts of Europe his ideas were not widely implemented. Together with the political ideal of 'enlightened despotism', the concept of 'medical police' generally went out-of-fashion in the first decades of the 19th century. Nevertheless, the insights

60 Medical historian George Rosen (1910–1977) published several papers on Frank's life and works (George Rosen, "Biography of Dr. Johann Peter Frank Written by Himself," *Journal of the History of Medicine and Allied Sciences* 3, no. 2 (1948): 279–314), the origins of his ideas (George Rosen, "Cameralism and the Concept of Medical Police," *Bulletin of the History of Medicine* 27 (1953): 21–42), and the reception of the concept of 'medical police' in Europe (George Rosen, "The Fate of the Concept of Medical Police 1780–1890," *Centaurus* 5, no. 2 (1957): 97–113). Frank also authored "The People's Misery: Mother of Diseases," probably the first systematic exposition of the relationship between poverty and disease (1790); see Henry E. Sigerist, "Frank, Johann Peter. The People's Misery: Mother of Diseases," *Bulletin of the History of Medicine* 9 (1941): 81–100.

and interventions systematized by Frank were, to varying degrees, applied in many European countries.

In what has been called "the eighteenth century campaign to avoid disease," many environmental measures were taken which may have reduced disease. Measures were taken to drain low-lying, swampy areas, because standing water had been recognized as a source of disease. Measures were taken to flush away the filth from urban areas, because filth did not only stink, but was also suspected to cause disease. Measures were taken to improve the ventilation of closed areas such as houses, ships and prisons, because odours were another suspected cause of disease. Measures were taken to re-inter corpses from inside churches and built-up areas to cemeteries and places outside cities, where they could no longer spread disease. Measures that had already proven their effectiveness in earlier centuries, such as *cordons sanitaires* and quarantine of ships, were also strengthened in this period of 'medical police'. Although these ideas spread throughout Europe, we can safely assume that there were huge differences between European countries in the adoption of these measures.[61]

The *'public hygiene'* that emerged at the beginning of the 19th century represented a new twist in the collective approach to health problems. It was, on the one hand, encouraged by the emergence of new health problems, and, on the other hand, inspired by an increased understanding of the causes of disease. Industrialization and urbanization were accompanied by a worrying rise of infectious disease mortality. The arrival of cholera epidemics in the 1830s and 1840s, in particular, acted as a strong catalyst for developing a more effective approach to avoid disease. At the same time, scientific advances made it possible to more precisely pin-point the environmental conditions causing disease, and – equally importantly – increased people's confidence that disease and mortality could be fought with rationally designed measures.[62]

Initially this was no more than an intuition, as is evident from the *Encyclopédie ou Dictionnaire Raisonné des Sciences, des Arts et des Métiers* by Diderot and d'Alembert, published in the last decades of the 18th century (Plate 4). This

61 "The eighteenth century campaign to avoid disease" is the title of a book by James Riley (Riley, *Campaign*). That such a campaign did really exist is also clear from 18th century attempts to make London a healthier place (Roy Porter, "Cleaning up the Great Wen: Public Health in Eighteenth-Century London," *Medical History* 35, no. S11 (1991): 61–75).

62 For an analysis of the treatment of hygiene in the *Encyclopédie*, see William Coleman, "Health and Hygiene in the Encyclopédie: A Medical Doctrine for the Bourgeoisie," *Journal of the History of Medicine and Allied Sciences* 29, no. 4 (1974): 399–421. Condorcet's statement, cited above, is another example of the naïve optimism about the possibilities to eliminate disease, which would, however, at least partly be justified by the developments in the following two centuries.

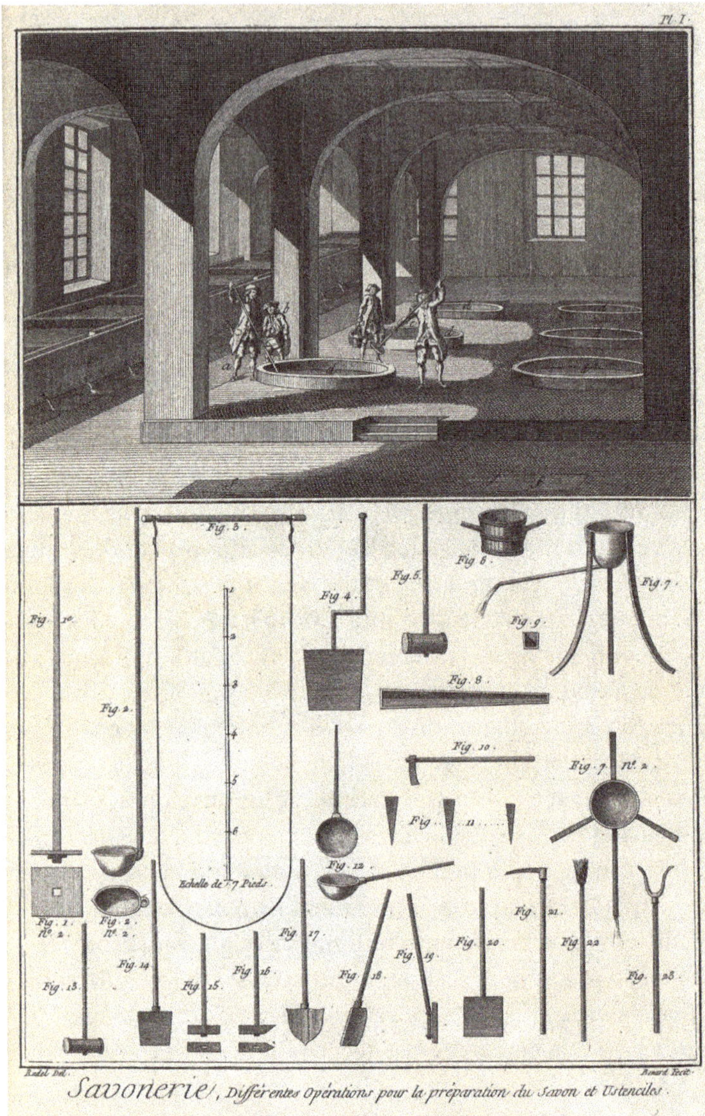

PLATE 4 *Savonerie* [Soap factory] as explained in the *Encyclopédie*, 1771
Detailed plates in Volume IX of the Encyclopédie ou dictionnaire raisonné des sciences, des arts et des métiers by Diderot and d'Alembert, which appeared in 1771, explain how soap can be made. In the 18th century, soap production was still artisanal and small-scale, and soap was expensive, partly because of a tax on soap levied by governments. Soap was not generally used for bathing until it was produced on an industrial scale in the second half of the 19th century.
COLLECTION KONINKLIJKE BIBLIOTHEEK, THE HAGUE. REPRODUCED WITH PERMISSION

has an optimistic lemma on *Hygiène* arguing that prevention is more useful than treatment, and that for the maintenance of health 'only' three things are necessary: to keep the individual in a healthy situation, to remove all causes of disease, and to comply with all health precepts.

This 'public hygiene' movement originated in France after the Revolution of 1789, which created room for reforms of the health system that had been in debate for decades, and that now suddenly seemed practicable. For the first time in history, a 'right to health' of all citizens was agreed on in the *Assemblée Constituante* in 1790. Committees were installed to prepare a national program of medical assistance for the poor and a new public health system. However, before most of these proposals could be carried through, the revolution ended in chaos, dictatorship, the Napoleonic Wars, and lack of funds.[63]

Despite these negative immediate results, several of the ideas developed during the French revolution were revived in the following decades. For example, the proposal for a multidisciplinary health council (*Conseil de Salubrité*) was already implemented in Paris in 1802, and in other French cities and *départements* in the following decades. In the 1820s and 1830s, the science of public hygiene developed in France under the intellectual leadership of people like Alexandre Parent-Duchâtelet (1790–1836) and Louis-René Villermé (1782–1863). In practical applications, however, France soon lagged behind other European countries, perhaps because of the conservative backlash after the violence of the Revolution and Napoleonic Wars.[64]

From France the 'public hygiene' movement spread to other European countries, and most importantly to England where it inspired Edwin Chadwick (1800–1890) to his 'sanitary idea' which would ultimately be adopted everywhere. This idea implied that the major health problems of the time had to be combated by a combination of safe disposal of faeces and provision of safe

63 The French revolution of 1789 was one of three European revolutions that acted as a catalyst for important changes in public health policy, the other two being the European revolutions of 1848, and the Russian revolution of 1917. The practical results were mixed, and only the Russian revolution resulted in rapid and radical changes to the health system, but at a very high price in personal freedom and human lives (see Chapter 7).

64 The leading role for France in the initial phase of 'public hygiene' is illustrated by the fact that the first ever professor in hygiene, Jean-Noël Hallé (1754–1822), was appointed at the *Ecole de santé* in Paris in 1794, that the first scientific journal in the field of public health, the *Annales d'hygiène publique et de médecine légale* was founded in France in 1829, and that the first scientific handbook on public hygiene was published in Paris in 1836; see Matthew Ramsey, "Public Health in France," in *The History of Public Health and the Modern State*, ed. D. Porter (Amsterdam: Editions Rodopi, 1994); Ann E.F. La Berge, *Mission and Method* (Cambridge etc.: Cambridge University Press, 2002).

drinking water, and thus by connecting houses to sewerage systems and piped drinking water.[65]

With England as an intermediate station, public hygiene and the 'sanitary movement' then spread to many other European countries. There it was given similar names (sometimes retrospectively), such as *Hygiénistes* in France and *Hygiënisten* in the Netherlands. During the 19th century this movement gradually succeeded in implementing a range of sanitary reforms, not only in the area of faeces disposal and drinking water, but also in areas like housing conditions, working conditions, infant care, and child labour. Here again, there were huge differences between European countries in the speed of adoption of these measures, with North-western Europe being distinctly ahead of Southern and Eastern Europe.[66]

Some of the delays were due to political opposition from conservative and liberal circles, for example when taxes had to be raised to pay for investments in sanitation infrastructures, or when the need for government interventions in trade and industry clashed with *laissez-faire* economic policies. It is no surprise, therefore, that political conditions remained important for the development of 'public hygiene'. This is illustrated by the catalytic role of the widespread political unrest in 1848, partly sparked by bad harvests and famine, of which the revolutions in Paris and Berlin are the most widely known.[67]

Most of the 1848 revolts and revolutions were repressed by military force, often with the backing of conservative sections of society, but they often did lead to some constitutional changes (e.g., to increase the number of people who had the right to vote in elections). They can also be seen as the birth-place of public health in many continental-European countries. For example, on 8 March 1848, in the middle of the revolution in Paris, orthopaedic surgeon and editor of the *Gazette Médicale de Paris* Jules Guérin (1801–1886) was the first to use the term *médecine sociale* in an editorial celebrating the revolution.

---

65 For the spread of ideas from France to England, see Erwin H. Ackerknecht, "Hygiene in France, 1815–1848," *Bulletin of the History of Medicine* 22 (1948): 117–55. For the early development of public health in Britain, see Christopher Hamlin, "Public Health in Great Britain," in *The History of Public Health and the Modern State*, ed. D. Porter (Amsterdam: Editions Rodopi, 1994).

66 Several national histories of 'public hygiene' are available, e.g. for Britain (Anthony S. Wohl, *Endangered Lives* (London etc.: Dent and Sons, 1983)), France (Jorland, *Société*), and the Netherlands (Eduard S. Houwaart, *De Hygiënisten* (Groningen: Historische Uitgeverij Groningen, 1991)). For the history of public hygiene in some other European countries, see Chapter 7.

67 For political opposition to public health reforms, see, e.g., Christopher Hamlin and Pat Sidley, "Revolutions in Public Health: 1848, and 1998?," *British Medical Journal* 317, no. 7158 (1998): 587–91.

Equally emblematic is the role of German pathologist Rudolf Virchow (1821–1902) during the revolution in Berlin. Earlier in 1848, Virchow had been sent on a mission to Upper Silesia to study the causes of a typhus epidemic. In his report, Virchow not only established the medical diagnosis of the disease, but related the epidemic to a famine resulting from crop failure in the previous years, whose effects were concentrated among poor Polish peasants. Virchow blamed the epidemic on the oppression of these peasants by the local German aristocracy, and his conclusion was that elimination of social inequality was the only way to prevent further typhus epidemics in the future.

On 19 March 1848, just after returning from his trip, and inflamed by the conclusions of his investigations, Virchow joined the revolution. He even defended a barricade using an old pistol borrowed from a medical colleague. During the rest of the year Virchow actively participated in the democratic, republican and socialist movements, and created a weekly journal called *Die Medicinische Reform*, in which he published many of his famous one-liners, including "Medicine is a social science, and politics nothing else than medicine at a larger scale."[68]

During most of the 19th century, there was no consensus on whether or not some of the most prevalent diseases were contagious or not, and if so how diseases exactly spread from person to person. This did not always prevent the implementation of effective countermeasures – the non-contagionist 'miasma theory' prescribed the removal of rotting organic material, which accidentally also helped in reducing risks of infection. Nevertheless, lack of more precise knowledge certainly reduced their precision. It was only towards the very end of the 19th century that the role of micro-organisms in the causation of many diseases was definitively shown.[69]

This 'bacteriological revolution' did not only help to more precisely target sanitation measures, but also opened up a whole arsenal of other interventions. These included antitoxins (which reduced mortality from diphtheria), antisepsis and asepsis (which made surgery and childbirth safer), and isolation of patients known to be infective (which reduced transmission of tuberculosis

68 Literally: "*Die Medizin ist eine soziale Wissenschaft, und die Politik ist weiter nichts als Medizin im Großen.*" For a more extensive analysis of the link between the revolutions of 1848 and the development of public health, see Johan P. Mackenbach, "Politics Is Nothing but Medicine at a Larger Scale: Reflections on Public Health's Biggest Idea," *Journal of Epidemiology & Community Health* 63, no. 3 (2009): 181–84.

69 The difficulty of getting contagionist ideas accepted was partly due to opposition from economic interests, which feared that trade would be harmed by quarantine and other measures to stop contagion; see Erwin H. Ackerknecht, "Anticontagionism between 1821 and 1867," *Bulletin of the History of Medicine* 22 (1948): 562–93.

and other contagious diseases). Due to the triumphs of bacteriology, traditional 'public hygiene' suddenly seemed to be based on false premises. However, the application of bacteriological insights to the solution of many population health problems still required collective interventions, such as pasteurization of milk, inspection of food products, and screening for tuberculosis.[70]

Although the collectivist approach of 'public hygiene' could easily be adapted to carry out some of these new measures, other measures required a new, more personal approach. In the first decades of the 20th century, this new approach emerged in the form of '*social hygiene*'. This involved the development of preventive programs for vulnerable groups: pregnant women and newborns (antenatal and perinatal care), children (consultation clinics for infants and toddlers, school health care), workers (occupational health care), and sufferers from certain infectious diseases and their contacts (consultation clinics for tuberculosis and venereal diseases).

For all these groups, effective prevention depended on the successful merging of bacteriological and other scientific insights with an understanding of the social determinants of disease. Social hygiene also became involved with another rapidly growing area of collective interference with population health, namely social security, as many European countries developed their first schemes of protection against loss of income in the event of accident, illness, and unemployment.

In the development of social hygiene, which went hand in hand with the first steps towards a welfare state, Germany took the lead, as illustrated by the international influence of Alfred Grotjahn (1869–1931). In Grotjahn's conception, social hygiene should focus on influencing social conditions in order to combat contagion, poor nutrition and other specific risk factors of disease. Consultation clinics, in which clients were called up for regular visits with a doctor or nurse, and district nurses, who brought modern hygienic and dietary practices into many people's homes, were the characteristic way of working in this new approach. These ideas diffused throughout continental Europe, including the early Soviet Union where Nicolai Semashko (1874–1949) established a system of primary care based on the principles of social hygiene.[71]

---

70 See Rosen, *History*, Chapter VII. For how the 'bacteriological revolution' changed the practice of public health, see David S. Barnes, *The Great Stink of Paris and the Nineteenth-Century Struggle against Filth and Germs* (Baltimore: Johns Hopkins University Press, 2006).

71 For an analysis of the rise of social hygiene within wider concerns with the "quality of population," see Porter, *Health, Civilization and the State*, Chapter 10. On the role of Grotjahn in developing social hygiene, see S. Milton Rabson, "Alfred Grotjahn, Founder of Social Hygiene," *Bulletin of the New York Academy of Medicine* 12, no. 2 (1936): 43–58.

The Interbellum, the period in which social hygiene blossomed all over Europe, also witnessed two new phenomena which both had a profound impact on the development of public health: eugenics and international health action. After World War I, health was a central concern of many European nations. This was not only because it was important to recover from heavy population losses, but also because collective actions for health were a natural way to unite their populations. Some of these had been brought together in newly formed countries, whereas other populations were sharply divided between left-wing and right-wing political ideologies.[72]

Whereas one important strand of social hygiene stressed the importance of environmental factors, another strand emphasized the role of genetics. This competing strand, 'eugenics', believed that improvements in environmental conditions could only lead to degeneration of the population, because they would promote the survival of genetically weaker individuals. It propagated selective reproduction instead – an idea that came in many gradations, ranging from relatively benign to outright malicious. When it combined with feelings of national or racial superiority, eugenics could derail into 'racial hygiene', as in the case of Nazi Germany where these ideas were taken to the extremes and led to the genocide of 6 million Jews. Because of these and other criminal applications, we tend to forget that 'eugenics' in milder forms was popular throughout Europe.[73]

A second important development of the interwar period is the rise of international organizations in public health. International cooperation in public health had started in the 19th century, with international sanitary conferences in which European countries tried to reach an agreement on stemming the spread of infectious diseases across national borders. However, after World War I, a step-change occurred with the creation in 1920 of the League of

72 This was a fascinating period beset with contradictions and ambivalences. For the connections between state building and social hygiene in newly formed states such as Czechoslovakia and Yugoslavia, see Iris Borowy and Wolf Gruner, eds., *Facing Illness in Troubled Times* (Frankfurt am Main: Peter Lang, 2005), various chapters.

73 Eugenics built on the growing understanding of genetics, for which the basis had been laid by Gregor Mendel (1822–1884). For an in-depth analysis of Nazi health policies, and the connections between German social hygiene and genocide, see Paul Weindling, *Health, Race and German Politics between National Unification and Nazism, 1870–1945* (Cambridge etc.: Cambridge University Press, 1993); Paul Weindling, *Epidemics and Genocide in Eastern Europe, 1890–1945* (Oxford etc.: Oxford University Press, 2000). Sweden had a program of compulsory sterilization of people with mental illness or an antisocial lifestyle. These and more benign applications of 'eugenics' were all part of the same 'social hygiene' movement which easily combined with authoritarianism; see Mark Mazower, *Dark Continent* (London: Allen Lane, 1998), Chapter 3.

Nations Health Organization (LNHO), the precursor of the current World Health Organization (WHO). Apart from producing statistical overviews and acting as a platform for exchanging information and expertise, the LNHO also engaged in several field studies of post-war outbreaks of infectious diseases in Europe, such as typhus and malaria, with keen attention to the social determinants of disease.[74]

In these activities the LNHO was supported by the International Health Division of the Rockefeller Foundation, a philanthropic organization that became strongly engaged in public health work in the interwar period in Europe (and elsewhere in the world). Whereas the LHNO was a (politically and financially) weak organization, the Rockefeller Foundation was rich and competent, and made important contributions to population health improvement, particularly in Southern Europe. By providing expertise and financial support, the Rockefeller Foundation helped in tackling tuberculosis in France and malaria in many Southern European countries. It also helped to bring local expertise up-to-date by supporting the foundation of national schools of public health. Although politically independent, the Rockefeller Foundation worked within the foreign affairs policy goals of the United States. These included strengthening newly formed nations in Southern, Central-eastern and South-eastern Europe, and opposing the perceived threats of the communist Soviet Union.[75]

In the meantime, the arsenal of effective public health interventions had greatly expanded beyond what was available in the beginning of the 20th century. Vaccinations had been developed against several infectious diseases, as had chemical methods for vector control, such as delousing by fumigation to prevent typhus, and destruction of larvae or mosquitoes by insecticide spraying to prevent malaria. Workplaces could be made safer by new methods of accident prevention and worker protection, and by the introduction of safer production methods. Nutrient-deficiency diseases like rickets, goitre and pellagra could be prevented by making sure that essential micro-nutrients were present in people's food.

---

74 On international sanitary conferences, see Mark Harrison, "Disease, Diplomacy and International Commerce," *Journal of Global History* 1, no. 2 (2006): 197–217. On the League of Nations Health Organization, see Patricia A. Sealey, "The League of Nations Health Organisation" (Doctor of Philosophy Ohio State University, 2011); Paul Weindling, ed., *International Health Organisations and Movements, 1918–1939* (Cambridge etc.: Cambridge University Press, 1995).

75 For a history of the International Health Division of the Rockefeller Foundation, see John Farley, *To Cast out Disease* (Oxford etc.: Oxford University Press, 2004). Aspects of its history are also described in various chapters of Weindling, *International Health Organizations*.

After World War II it soon became clear that old health problems were being replaced by new ones. Mortality and morbidity patterns had become dominated by diseases that – at first sight – had little to do with poverty or other forms of misery. They seemed to be caused by an affluent lifestyle, and were mainly chronic in character and thus led to a great demand for health care. Tackling cardiovascular disease and cancer required a new approach that ultimately – in the 1990s – came to be labelled '*new public health*'. The philosophy of 'public hygiene' was refreshed and applied to the health problems of the second half of the 20th century.

Like in the 19th century, the challenge was to find collective approaches that would reach sufficient numbers of people to ensure a population-wide impact. This had to involve massive behaviour change, for which the directive and sometimes authoritarian approach of social hygiene was no longer suitable. The new public health therefore incorporated the insights that had been developed within the field of 'health promotion', which used psychological and sociological insights to develop interventions and policies to change health-related behaviour. This implied, among other things, that health education had to be supported by changes in the environment, e.g., by changing food composition or regulating the sales of tobacco.[76]

The term 'new public health' has been retained for this overview to emphasize some of its innovative aspects, but in reality most professionals now use the term 'public health' *tout court*. Since World War II, the field has gone through considerable terminological confusion. This is due to the fact that collective approaches to population health problems have come to include such a wide variety of methods, and to involve such a wide range of disciplines, that it is often difficult to recognize public health's boundaries.[77]

The incorporation of health promotion is not the only important development of the field of public health of the last half-century. In addition to new methods of behaviour change many other new methods for improving population health became available, and are now seen as core components of public health. For example, screening has become a powerful tool in public health's

---

76 The term 'new public health' was elaborated in Frances Baum, *The New Public Health: An Australian Perspective* (Melbourne etc.: Oxford University Press, 1998). For the genesis of the concept, and its relationship with previous approaches to public health, see Niyi Awofeso, "What's New About the 'New Public Health'?," *American Journal of Public Health* 94, no. 5 (2004): 705–09.

77 This terminological confusion is reflected in frequent name-changes. For example, the United Kingdom adopted the term 'community medicine' in the 1970s, changed this into 'public health medicine' in the 1980s, and since then settled on 'public health' again, now conceived as a multidisciplinary field.

toolbox. This includes screening for risk factors of disease, as in the case of detection of hypertension and high serum cholesterol, followed by dietary advice and/or drug treatment, as well as screening for early stages of disease, as in the case of mass screening for cervical and breast cancer, followed by further diagnosis and treatment. Another example of a new intervention option is accident prevention. Road traffic safety and prevention of drowning, poisoning, and falls have not only become highly effective, but also much needed in the face of the rising death toll from various causes of injuries.[78]

The Impact of Public Health

What has been the contribution of this expanding arsenal of public health interventions to long-term improvements in population health? As mentioned in Chapter 1, this has been the object of an important debate. This debate has, however, largely focused on a single country (the United Kingdom) and a somewhat limited period of time (mainly the second half of the 19th, and first decades of the 20th century).

McKeown, in his interpretation of the mortality decline in England and Wales, not only concluded that medical care had made a negligible contribution, but also that public health measures (sanitation and other improvements in hygiene) had contributed very little. This was because they arrived long after mortality decline had set in, and could only have been responsible for the decline of mortality from diarrheal diseases. It could not have been responsible for the decline of respiratory tuberculosis which accounted for a much larger part of total mortality decline.

However, both McKeown's timing of mortality decline and his rejection of the role of public health measures in explaining the decline of tuberculosis mortality have become under serious attack. Due to fluctuations in mortality it is difficult to pin-point the exact year in which mortality definitely started to decline, and public health measures like isolation of tuberculosis patients and improvements of housing and working conditions may well have contributed to the decline of respiratory tuberculosis.[79]

78 The expanded scope of public health, and the widened arsenal of effective interventions, can easily be recognized in modern textbooks of public health, such as the (massive) Oxford Textbook of Public Health (Roger Detels et al., *Oxford Textbook of Global Public Health*, 5 ed. (Oxford etc.: Oxford University Press, 2015)).

79 These and several other criticisms of McKeown's analysis of mortality decline in England and Wales were published in 1988 by British historian Simon Szreter (Szreter, "Social Intervention"), and have since been widely accepted (see, e.g., Woods, *Demography*, Chapter 8).

Extending our scope over the whole period of three centuries covered by this book, and over the whole of Europe, as we do in the following chapters when we discuss this issue disease-by-disease, it becomes obvious that public health interventions have made substantial contributions to mortality decline. Britain was a special case, because it had relatively high tuberculosis mortality and like some other North-western European countries experienced an early mortality decline. The impact of public health measures is easier to discern in other European countries with a later mortality decline. Also, over the last decades many more studies have been done, providing convincing empirical evidence that specific public health interventions have had significant impacts on a range of health outcomes.[80]

Starting with '*medical police*', it is difficult to say whether this contributed to the main achievement of the 18th century, i.e., the reduction of the frequency and amplitude of mortality crises. German-speaking countries, where these ideas originated, were not among the most advanced in terms of population health in this period. However, as we will see in Chapter 5, the *cordon sanitaire* of the Habsburg Empire against the introduction of plague from the Ottoman Empire was a successful form of 'medical police'. The good performance of Sweden has also been attributed to the popularity in this country of ideas closely related to the concept of 'medical police'. Sweden was not only one of the first countries to create a national system of vital statistics (1748), but in response to the appalling mortality figures that this system revealed, it also created a tax-financed system of medical officers, midwives and hospitals throughout the country.[81]

More generally, the "eighteenth century campaign to avoid disease" has been credited with some first declines of mortality, for example from malaria due to the draining of swamps, although quantitative data are difficult to find. Furthermore, the introduction of smallpox inoculation in the 1720s, and of

80 Tuberculosis was more important as a cause of death in England than in some other European countries, such as Italy. Whereas the contribution of the broader group of infectious diseases to mortality decline was similar in both countries, the percentage contribution of respiratory tuberculosis was one-and-a-half times larger in England & Wales; see Graziella Caselli, "Health Transition and Cause-Specific Mortality," in *The Decline of Mortality in Europe*, ed. Roger S. Schofield, David S. Reher, and Alain Bideau (Oxford: Clarendon Press, 1991).

81 For the effectiveness of the *cordon sanitaire* of the Habsburg empire, see Gunther E Rothenberg, "The Austrian Sanitary Cordon and the Control of the Bubonic Plague: 1710–1871," *Journal of the History of Medicine and Allied Sciences* 28, no. 1 (1973): 15–23. For Sweden's adoption of the principles of 'medical police', see Jan Sundin and Sam Willner, *Social Change and Health in Sweden: 250 Years of Politics and Practice* (Stockholm: Swedish National Institute of Public Health, 2007).

smallpox vaccination in the early 1800s, often with strong government backing, has certainly made important contributions to mortality decline long before the 1840s (the starting-point of McKeown's mortality analyses).[82]

The impact of '*public hygiene*' is somewhat easier to discern. McKeown acknowledged the role of sanitation in bringing down mortality from diarrheal diseases, but could only point to the correspondence of national mortality trends with the timing of introduction of Chadwick's 'sanitary idea'. Since then, many more detailed studies have been done, and have provided more robust evidence that introduction of sewage systems and/or piped drinking caused mortality to decline in many countries.[83]

When we lump together the period of '*social hygiene*' with that of '*new public health*', and assess the contribution of public health interventions developed during the 20th century, the picture is very clear. Around the year 2000, the US Centers for Disease Control (CDC) celebrated the public health achievements of the 20th century in a number of important overviews, of which most of the conclusions also apply to European countries. Improvements in work safety, mother and child care, vaccination and other forms of infectious disease control, quality and safety of food, and quality of housing undoubtedly contributed to mortality decline, particularly in the first half of the century.

Similarly, some of the newer approaches have had an important impact on population health in Europe during the second half of the 20th century. The success of the decline of ischaemic heart disease mortality has many fathers, but one of them is health promotion, e.g., systematic efforts to reduce smoking and make diets healthier. Tobacco control has contributed to stopping the rise

---

82 For the mortality effects, see Riley, *Campaign*, Chapter 6. The effects of smallpox inoculation and vaccination will be discussed in more detail in Chapter 4.

83 A review by Dutch demographer Frans van Poppel, published in 1997, found that the evidence for an effect of improved drinking water supply on infant and childhood mortality was rather mixed (Frans van Poppel and Cor van der Heijden, "The Effects of Water Supply on Infant and Childhood Mortality," *Health Transition Review* 7, no. 2 (1997): 113–48). Since then, several more rigorous studies have been published, finding more convincing effects of either improved drinking water supply (David Cutler and Grant Miller, "The Role of Public Health Improvements in Health Advances," *Demography* 42, no. 1 (2005): 1–22), or sewage systems (Lionel Kesztenbaum and Jean-Laurent Rosenthal, "Sewers' Diffusion and the Decline of Mortality: The Case of Paris, 1880–1914," *Journal of Urban Economics* 98 (2017): 174–86), or investments in sanitation more generally (Frances Bell and Robert Millward, "Public Health Expenditures and Mortality in England and Wales, 1870–1914," *Continuity and Change* 13, no. 2 (1998): 221–49). The implementation of sanitary reform often gained speed only towards the end of the 19th century.

of lung cancer, at least among men, and accident prevention has contributed to sometimes spectacular declines in injury mortality.[84]

Some European countries, such as the former Soviet Union and its satellites in Central-eastern and South-eastern Europe, have been unable or slow to make the switch from the 'old public health', with its emphasis on infectious diseases and paternalistic methods, to the 'new public health'. These countries have also been unable or slow to reduce ischaemic heart disease mortality. Also, differences between countries in trends for cervical and breast cancer mortality are partly due to differences in implementation of population-based screening programs for these diseases.[85]

Plate 5 has miniature portraits of a few figureheads of European public health mentioned in this Chapter or elsewhere in this book.

A Short History of Medical Care

Writing a "short history of medical care," as this section's title suggests, is much more difficult than writing a "short history of public health." Medical care, with its huge knowledge base, multiple specializations and complex organization, is a much larger field than public health. We will therefore have to reduce the scope of this "short history" to make the exercise manageable. We will do this by focusing on what mattered for improving population health.

Scientific breakthroughs have, of course, been important but are only one of the factors that have increased the impact of medical care on population health. Surprisingly, the role of scientific medicine is still disputed. Writing in 1997, historian Roy Porter in his *The Greatest Benefit to Mankind: a Medical History of Humanity from Antiquity to the Present* notes that "medicine's historical balance sheet [is] hard to assess. [...] Its standing is now highly contested. Never has it achieved so much or attracted so much suspicion." Echoing McKeown, he writes that

> the facts indicate how little medicine weighs in the balance of health. [...] We have invested disproportionately in a form of medicine ('Band Aid'

84 For the CDC study, see Centers for Disease Control and Prevention, "Ten Great Public Health Achievements – United States, 1900–1999," MMWR. *Morbidity and mortality weekly report* 48, no. 12 (1999): 241; John W. Ward and Christian Warren, *Silent Victories* (New York etc.: Oxford University Press, 2006). For an update, see Centers for Disease Control and Prevention, "Ten Great Public Health Achievements – United States, 2001–2010," MMWR. *Morbidity and mortality weekly report* 60, no. 19 (2011): 619.

85 See, e.g., Ahti Anttila and José M. Martin-Moreno, "Cancer Screening," in *Successes and Failures of Health Policy in Europe*, ed. Johan P. Mackenbach and Martin McKee (Maidenhead: Open University Press, 2013).

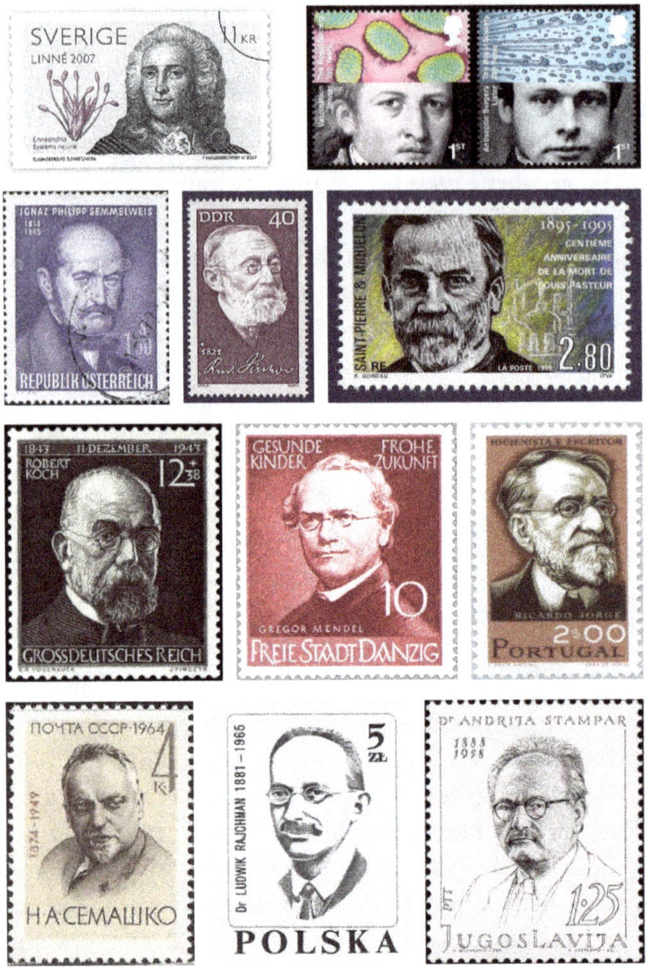

PLATE 5 European public health history on 20th century postage stamps

Many 'standard bearers' of public health have been immortalized on postage stamps. From left to right: Top row: Carl von Linné (one of the earliest disease classifications, Sweden, 18th century), Edward Jenner (smallpox vaccination, Britain, 19th century), Joseph Lister (antiseptic surgery, Britain, 19th century). Second row: Ignaz Semmelweis (cause of puerperal fever, Austria-Hungary, 19th century), Rudolf Virchow (pathology and public health, Germany, 19th century), Louis Pasteur (bacteriology, France, 19th century). Third row: Robert Koch (bacteriology, Germany, 19th century), Gregor Mendel (genetics, Austria-Hungary, 19th century), Ricardo Jorge (public health, Portugal, early 20th century). Bottom row: Nicolai Semashko (public health, Soviet Union, 20th century), Ludwik Rajchman (public health, Poland, 20th century), Andrija Stampar (public health, Yugoslavia, 20th century)

> salvage) whose benefits often come late, which buy a little time, and which are easily nullified by external, countervailing factors.[86]

Is this a fair assessment? In the next section I will show that it is not, but first it needs to be understood that the population health impact of medical care is determined by three, equally important factors. The first is availability of effective treatments, as resulting from the scientific breakthroughs and other advances that form the core of the usual histories of medicine. The second is coverage of the relevant patient groups, as determined by diffusion of the innovation among medical professionals and by access of patients to the health care system. The third is quality of application, which is dependent on, among others, training, experience and guideline adherence of professionals and on patient compliance. Over time, each of these three factors has changed, mostly in a favourable direction albeit with large differences in tempo between countries.[87]

There can be little doubt that the availability of *effective treatments* has increased enormously. It is not necessary to go into the details of Porter's 700+ pages of medical history to identify the main advances in medical treatment over the last three centuries, at least if we restrict ourselves to the advances that have demonstrably improved patient outcomes. Until the late 1930s, advances in specific treatments numbered less than ten, and included a few traditional remedies derived from plants (digoxin against heart failure, aspirin against various pains, and quinine against malaria), antitoxins against diphtheria and tetanus and salvarsan against syphilis, some hormone replacements (insulin against diabetes and thyroxin against hypothyroidism), and sulphonamides (against pneumonia and a few other infections). In addition, there had been some generic advances in fields like obstetrics, surgery, trauma, and nursing care.[88]

Starting around World War II, however, progress accelerated and a whole range of new, specific therapeutics became available. British general practitioner and author James Le Fanu has listed the breakthroughs that brought several important diseases under medical control. These include penicillin

86 Cited from Porter, *Greatest Benefit*, Chapter XXII.

87 This idea that the population health impact of medical care is dependent on 'innovation', 'coverage' and 'quality' was developed by British public health scientist and advocate Martin McKee; see Johan P. Mackenbach et al., "Using 'Amenable Mortality' as Indicator of Healthcare Effectiveness in International Comparisons," *Journal of Epidemiology and Community Health* 67, no. 2 (2013): 139–46.

88 Henry H. Dale, "Advances in Medicinal Therapeutics," *British Medical Journal*, no. 4644 (1950): 1–7.

(against various infectious diseases, 1941), cortisone (against immunological and many other diseases, 1949), streptomycin (against tuberculosis, 1950), chlorpromazine (against depression, 1952), artificial ventilation and intensive care (against poliomyelitis and other life-threatening conditions, 1952), open heart surgery (to replace rheumatic heart valves or lay bypasses around clotted coronary arteries, 1955), hip replacement (against hip fractures and arthrosis, 1961), kidney transplantation (against chronic kidney diseases, 1963), antihypertensive drugs (against stroke and other cardiovascular diseases, 1964), and chemotherapy (against childhood cancer, 1971).[89]

Although Le Fanu, writing in the 1990s, thought that the era of progress had ended due to a slowing down of the development of new effective drugs, it is not difficult to see continued progress in a number of fields. In addition to life support and bypass surgery, the treatment of acute myocardial infarction now includes thrombolysis and percutaneous coronary interventions (both introduced in the 1980s), as well as drug treatment to prevent re-thrombosis, as a result of which survival has increased remarkably. Statins were developed to lower serum cholesterol (1980s), which helped to reduce incidence as well. The management of acute stroke has also improved considerably due to the introduction of comprehensive stroke centres (1990s), as has the management of injury. After the development of effective chemotherapy against acute lymphoblastic leukaemia and other childhood cancers, remarkably effective therapies were developed against other forms of cancer, such as Hodgkin's disease and testicular cancer (1970s). More modest improvements in the treatment of breast cancer (1980s) and colorectal cancer (1990s) – to mention two important examples – have also contributed to a gradual increase in cancer survival.[90]

These are just the specific therapeutics which are relatively easy to pinpoint, but in addition to these, many more general advances were made. For example, due to the introduction of asepsis, blood transfusion and antibiotics surgery became safer, and improvements in surgical techniques then made it possible to treat a wide range of diseases, from appendicitis and cholecystitis to cancers and eye cataracts. While the examples given mostly relate to potentially fatal diseases, important advances have also been made in pain relief and treatment or rehabilitation of sensory and motor disabilities.[91]

---

89 James Le Fanu, *The Rise and Fall of Modern Medicine* (London: Little Brown & Co, 1999).

90 See, for example, Ellen Nolte and Martin McKee, *Does Health Care Save Lives? Avoidable Mortality Revisited* (London: The Nuffield Trust, 2004); Mackenbach et al., "Using 'Amenable Mortality' as Indicator of Healthcare Effectiveness."

91 All these advances should be weighed against the increase in 'iatrogenic disease' resulting from the widening scope and expanding use of medical care, but seen over a longer

These innovations can only affect population health if they achieve sufficient *coverage*, and are applied to all patients whose health problems can be alleviated by the new treatment. Whereas the history of medical innovation can be written from a universal standpoint – streptomycin, blood transfusion and stroke units were invented only once – the history of treatment coverage is much more locally specific. New treatments diffuse like all innovations, with early and late adopters, both among countries and within countries among population groups and professionals. Studies show that even in the last decades of the 20th century, and even in North-western Europe, this diffusion was often a lengthy process taking a decade or more before the last country had introduced the innovation. Between introduction and full use of the innovation, often another decade or more had to pass.[92]

When Europe as a whole is considered, differences in uptake of new medical treatments are even larger. Southern European countries used to be late adopters as compared to North-western European countries, and so were Central-Eastern, South-eastern and Eastern Europe under communism. The latter did not, or only with much delay, adopt the advances in medical treatment which were developed in the West. Although antibiotics such as penicillin and streptomycin diffused rapidly towards Central-Eastern European countries and the Soviet Union in the 1940s, modern drugs developed from the 1960s onwards, such as anti-hypertensive drugs, cancer chemotherapy, and cimetidine (against peptic ulcer), did not. This was due to international isolation (e.g., inability to read the English-language literature) as well as to a different scientific paradigm.[93]

---

period the benefits have almost always outweighed the harms; see John P. Bunker, "The Role of Medical Care in Contributing to Health Improvements within Societies," *International Journal of Epidemiology* 30, no. 6 (2001): 1260–63.

92 See, e.g., Ragnar Westerling et al., "The Timing of Introduction of Pharmaceutical Innovations in Seven E Uropean Countries," *Journal of Evaluation in Clinical Practice* 20, no. 4 (2014): 301–10, for a study of six European countries between the 1970s and 1990s. The delay in introduction varied between 8 years for antiretroviral drugs (against AIDS) and 22 years for cisplatin (against testicular cancer), and the subsequent delay between introduction and peak use varied between a few years and more than 20 years.

93 The study by Westerling et al., "Timing of Introduction" found that, whereas Spain still lagged behind North-western European countries in the 1970s, it no longer did so in the 1980s and 1990s. In Estonia most modern drugs were only introduced after independence in the early 1990s. On the isolation of Soviet medicine, and the role of a scientific paradigm based on communist orthodoxy instead of empirical evidence, see Martin McKee, "Cochrane on Communism," *International Journal of Epidemiology* 36, no. 2 (2007): 269–73.

Achieving sufficient coverage is not only a matter of diffusion of the innovation among medical professionals, but also of patient access. Over time, patient access to medical care has increased considerably. This was due to a combination of increased supply (e.g., rising numbers of doctors, hospital beds, pharmaceutical drugs, equipment) and reduced financial barriers to care utilisation. The expansion of health care into an economic sector absorbing more than 10% of national income has created an enormous machinery to deliver medical treatment. This happened mostly in the second half of the 20th century: health care still accounted for less than 1% of national income in the 1930s, but after World War II health expenditure exploded and now often accounts for more than 10%.[94]

This was facilitated by another factor crucial to coverage: the introduction and expansion of social insurance schemes and (in some countries) a tax-based national health service. The origins of health insurance go back to the Middle Ages, when guilds created mutual assistance associations which – because of their restriction to guild members – covered less than 5% of the population. When the guilds were abolished, voluntary health insurance continued ('sick funds') to exist in various forms, but participation was usually highly restricted.

Germany, under its chancellor Otto von Bismarck (1815–1898), was the first European country to place these sick funds under the authority of the state, and to create a legal framework making health insurance compulsory for all workers in 1883. Most other countries in North-western Europe followed the German example, with coverage often rising to around 20% of the population just before World War I, and to around 40% just before World War II.

It was only in the aftermath of this war, that governments decided to expand coverage to all workers, their dependants, the unemployed and pensioners. Most countries in North-western Europe achieved this without abandoning a social insurance system, by creating a complex regulatory framework and adding heavy state subsidies. However, a few countries chose to switch to a simpler tax-based 'national health service': the United Kingdom did this in 1946 and the Nordic countries followed in the 1960s and 1970s. This ultimately raised coverage to more than 90% of the population in the 1970s.[95]

94 For a long-term history of spending on health care, see Vito Tanzi and Ludger Schuknecht, *Public Spending in the 20th Century* (Cambridge etc.: Cambridge University Press, 2000).

95 A good introduction to the history of social health insurance in Europe is Richard B. Saltman and Hans F.W. Dubois, "The Historical and Social Base of Social Health Insurance Systems," in *Social Health Insurance Systems in Western Europe*, ed. Richard B Saltman, R. Busse, and J. Figueres (Maidenhead: Open University Press, 2004), from which the figures cited in the text have been taken. Some studies have found that stronger expansion

Countries in other European regions often lagged behind considerably. In Southern Europe, coverage rates remained low until the 1960s, but climbed rapidly in the following decades, often coinciding with the switch from dictatorship to democracy, and often based on the introduction of a tax-based national health system. In Central-eastern, South-eastern and Eastern Europe, coverage was raised to nominally 100% with the advent of communism. Under communism, everyone was theoretically entitled to free medical care, but quality of services was usually low, and informal 'under-the-table' payments were often required to obtain better quality care. After the collapse of the Soviet Union, most formerly communist countries rapidly transitioned to some kind of social health insurance system, but with vastly reduced government funding and high user fees.[96]

Finally, *quality of delivery* is the third essential ingredient of the success of medical care in improving population health. Quality of care delivery can change over time, and vary between countries, independent of the diffusion of innovations and independent of access to care. For example, the Soviet Union, as part of its modernization efforts and ambition to provide universal access to health care, succeeded in a 20-fold rise of its number of medical doctors between 1913 and 1963. This must have made a contribution to improving population health, but standards of medical training were low, doctors were badly paid, and incentives were mainly to raise quantity of production, not quality. Russia and other former Soviet republics are still suffering from this legacy.[97]

More generally, however, quality of delivery has probably increased over the 20th century, as a result of better training of medical personnel, increased access of medical professionals to the international literature, and the rise of evidence-based medicine which – at least in some European countries – has

of health insurance coverage was associated with stronger mortality decline; see Calman R. Winegarden and John E. Murray, "The Contributions of Early Health-Insurance Programs to Mortality Declines in Pre-World War I Europe," *Explorations in Economic History* 35, no. 4 (1998): 431–46.

96 On the historical increase in population health coverage, see Khalid Malik, *Human Development Report 2014* (New York: United Nations Development Programme, 2014), Fig. 4.2. On the transition to social health insurance in Eastern Europe, see Hugh R. Waters et al., "Health Insurance Coverage in Central and Eastern Europe: Trends and Challenges," *Health Affairs* 27, no. 2 (2008): 478–86; Bernd Rechel and Martin McKee, "Health Reform in Central and Eastern Europe and the Former Soviet Union," *Lancet* 374, no. 9696 (2009): 1186–95.

97 On the successes and failures of the Soviet health care system, see Mark G. Field, *Soviet Socialized Medicine: An Introduction* (New York: Free Press, 1967). For the persistence of this legacy, see, e.g., Bernd Rechel et al., "Health and Health Systems in the Commonwealth of Independent States," *Lancet* 381, no. 9872 (2013): 1145–55.

increased homogeneity of medical practice through the use of clinical practice guidelines.

The Role of Medicine

McKeown, echoed by Porter and many others, has argued that medical care made only a small contribution to the historical decline of mortality, because most of the decline of infectious diseases antedated the introduction of specific medical interventions, such as antibiotics. In his view, therefore, the "role of medicine" should be modest: "to assist us to come safely into the world and comfortably out of it, and during life protect the well and care for the sick and disabled."[98]

In the 40 years that have passed since his work was published, it has become clear that medical care did have some impact before the introduction of antibiotics, and that, although these and other effective medical technologies arrived late in the historical decline of mortality, they did contribute to a further lowering of mortality. However, it is less clear how important exactly the contributions of medical care have been.[99]

When addressing this question from a European perspective it is again important to note that the British experience is unlikely to be generalizable. As mentioned above, not only was the cause-of-death composition of mortality in England different from that in many other European countries, but like other countries in North-western Europe, England had also experienced an early mortality decline. This left less scope for medical care to contribute than in other parts of Europe, where mortality from infectious diseases was still high in the middle of the 20th century.

A simple look at Figure 1 shows that at the end of the 1930s life expectancy at birth in Europe varied between less than 40 and more than 60 years, with the United Kingdom at the upper end of the distribution (60 years for men, 64 years for women). For countries at the lower end of the distribution, the scope for antibiotics and other medical innovations to contribute to increases in life expectancy was therefore much larger. Also, since the early 1970s, where

98 McKeown's *The Role of Medicine – Dream, Mirage or Nemesis* was published in 1976, 30 years into the post-World War II period of expanding medical care (McKeown, *Role*). The quote is from p. 173. McKeown's attack on the idea that modern medicine had made important contributions to life extension was part of his agenda to re-direct emphasis towards softer goals; see, e.g., Stephen J. Kunitz, "Explanations and Ideologies of Mortality Patterns," *Population and Development Review* 13, no. 3 (1987): 379–408.

99 Mackenbach, "Contribution" reviews these critiques. See also some disease-specific chapters in Part II.

McKeown's analyses ended, life expectancy has increased by another 10 years in many countries, raising the possibility of new contributions of medical care.

Three pieces of evidence suggest that medical care did not only have a measurable impact, but that this impact was substantial, both in absolute and relative terms. These include more detailed analyses of the impact of medical innovations on cause-specific mortality; empirical analyses of the contributions of declines in 'amenable' mortality to total mortality decline; and model-based assessments of the contribution of medical care to total mortality decline.

Sometimes, the impact of medical innovations can be observed in the form of an immediate change in cause-specific mortality. This occurs when a new treatment has a large effect, when it rapidly reaches patients with the relevant conditions, and when quality issues do not dilute the effect. This is rather exceptional – mostly, the expectation should be for more gradual changes – but it does sometimes happen.

The prime example is the introduction of sulphonamides (1935) and antibiotics (1944)(Plate 6). Studies from several countries in North-western Europe have found that, after the introduction of these drugs, the rate of decline for many infectious diseases accelerated. For many infectious diseases there was also an instantaneous, stepwise decrease in mortality coinciding with the introduction of antibiotics. These effects – already substantial in North-western Europe – were considerably larger in other European countries, where mortality from infectious diseases was still very high in the 1940s.[100]

Instantaneous effects have also been found for a few other innovations. The introduction of integrated chemo- and radiotherapy against Hodgkin's disease in the early 1960s was almost immediately followed by rapid mortality decline in many countries in North-western and Southern Europe, but only much later in Central-eastern, South-eastern and Eastern Europe. Similarly, the introduction of platinum-based chemotherapy against testicular cancer in the 1970s was followed by a reversal from rising to declining mortality from this disease

100 For example, in the Netherlands mortality from all infectious diseases together declined by 4% per year before the introduction of antibiotics, and by 10% per year after the introduction; see Johan P. Mackenbach and C.W.N. Looman, "Secular Trends of Infectious Disease Mortality in the Netherlands, 1911–1978," *International Journal of Epidemiology* 17, no. 3 (1988): 618–24, and Chapter 5. Similar findings were reported from Sweden and Finland (Elina Hemminki and Anneli Paakkulainen, "The Effect of Antibiotics on Mortality from Infectious Diseases in Sweden and Finland," *American Journal of Public Health* 66, no. 12 (1976): 1180–84) and from England & Wales (Galbraith and McCormack, "Infection in England and Wales", *passim*).

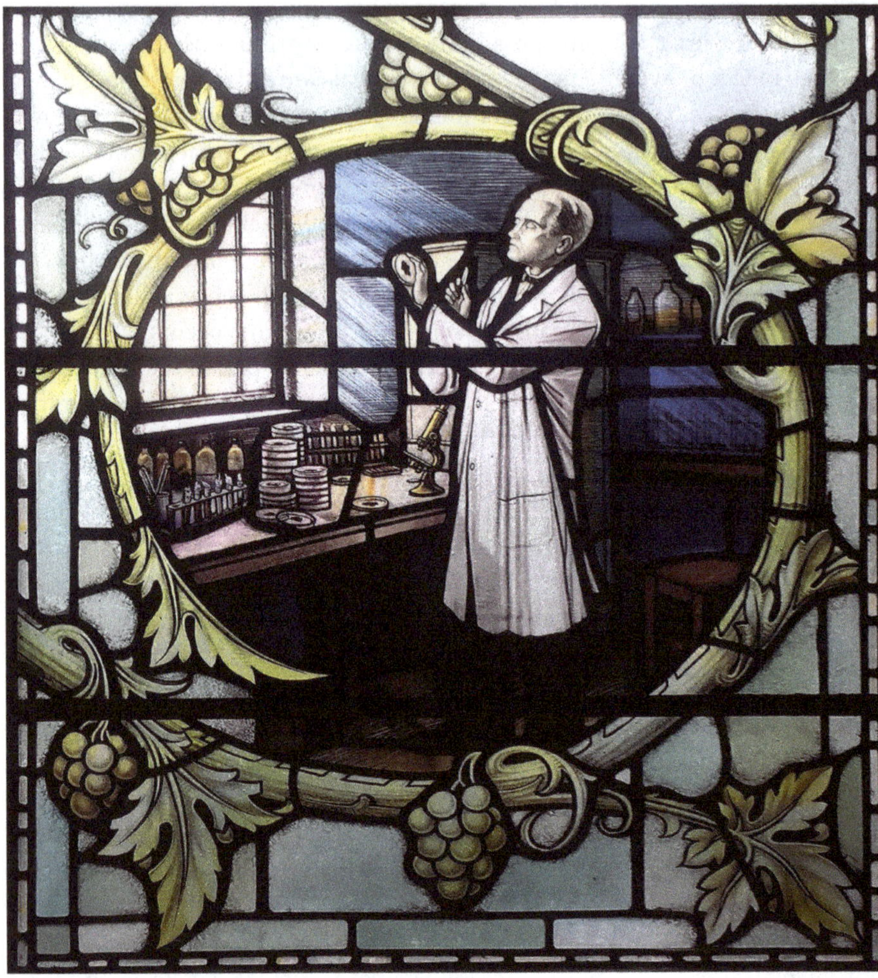

PLATE 6 Alexander Fleming on a stained glass window in St. James's Church (London), 1952
Sir Alexander Fleming (1881–1955) accidentally discovered the bactericidal properties of penicillin in 1928. This stained glass window shows Fleming at work in his laboratory, which was located in the vicinity of this church. Inadvertently, it illustrates the almost religious worship of modern medicine in a secularized society
HTTPS://COMMONS.WIKIMEDIA.ORG/WIKI/FILE:ALEXANDER_FLEMING_STAINED_GLASS_WINDOW.JPG (CC0 1.0; ACCESSED 18/10/2019)

in North-western and Southern Europe, only to be followed much later in the rest of Europe.[101]

Less clear-cut changes have been found for breast, colorectal and other cancers, as well as for innovations in treatment of cardiovascular diseases. This can be explained by the reasons mentioned in the previous section, and by the fact that many improvements in treatment (and sometimes prevention) occurred simultaneously, so that it is impossible to disentangle their effects. Other approaches must therefore be used to estimate the effect of medical care on population health.[102]

One, frequently used approach is to simply take the trends in mortality from conditions which have become amenable to medical intervention, and to compare these to the trends in mortality from non-amenable conditions or total mortality. Examples of causes of death usually included in selections of 'amenable' causes are tuberculosis, pneumonia, Hodgkin's disease, appendicitis, and maternal and perinatal deaths.[103]

Trends in mortality from these conditions have indeed often been rapidly downward over the past half-century, and more so than trends in mortality from non-amenable conditions. This suggests that general improvements in living conditions or behavioural risk factors cannot fully explain their decline, and that medical care also made a contribution. Within Europe, there have been important differences in decline of these conditions, along expected lines. For example, during the communist period declines of mortality from amenable conditions have been much less in Central-eastern, South-eastern and Eastern Europe, and it is only recently that some of this disadvantage has been recovered. Higher mortality from 'amenable' conditions in these parts of

101 For trends in mortality from a range of cancers in many European countries, including Hodgkin's disease and testicular cancer, see Fabio Levi et al., "Cancer Mortality in Europe, 1990–1994, and an Overview of Trends from 1955 to 1994," *European Journal of Cancer* 35, no. 10 (1999): 1477–516. See also Fabio Levi et al., "Trends in Mortality from Hodgkin's Disease in Western and Eastern Europe," *British Journal of Cancer* 87, no. 3 (2002): 291–93; Peter Boyle, Patrick Maisonneuve, and Stanley B. Kaye, "Therapy for Testicular Cancer in Central and Eastern Europe," *Lancet* 335, no. 8696 (1990): 1033.

102 For two attempts to measure the impact of innovations in treatment of cancer and cardiovascular disease in European countries, see Rasmus Hoffmann et al., "Innovations in Health Care and Mortality Trends from Five Cancers," *International Journal of Public Health* 59, no. 2 (2014): 341–50; Rasmus Hoffmann et al., "Innovations in Medical Care and Mortality Trends from Four Circulatory Diseases," *European Journal of Public Health* 23, no. 5 (2013): 852–57.

103 For the origins of this approach, see David D. Rutstein et al., "Measuring the Quality of Medical Care: A Clinical Method," *New England Journal of Medicine* 294, no. 11 (1976): 582–88; Walter W. Holland, "The 'Avoidable Death' Guide to Europe," *Health Policy* 6, no. 6 (1986): 115–17.

Europe, even after risk factor standardization, persists until the present day, and accounts for a substantial part of the differences in life expectancy with North-western and Southern Europe.[104]

The results of these studies can be used for a rough estimate of the contribution of improvements in medical care to total mortality decline. For example, between the early 1950s and early 1980s declines of mortality from 'amenable' conditions added 3 and 4 years, respectively, to life expectancy at birth of men and women in the Netherlands. Because life expectancy actually increased by only 2 and 6 years, improvements in medical care more than compensated for unfavourable trends for other causes of death among men (such as ischaemic heart disease and road traffic injury), and accounted for two-thirds of the total increase in life expectancy among women.[105]

That improvements in medical care have probably made a substantial contribution to recent declines in mortality (and increases in life expectancy) has also been shown in model-based calculations. One study from the United States combined results from Randomized Controlled Trials, in which the effect of specific interventions on mortality among study participants had been measured, with data on the coverage of these interventions in the population. It concluded that between 1950 and 1989, medical treatments had increased average life expectancy by 4.5 years.[106]

A somewhat similar approach was applied in the Netherlands. In this case, the conclusion was that, between the early 1950s and early 2000s, improvements

104 For analyses showing a more rapid decline of 'amenable' mortality, see Nolte and McKee, *Does Health Care Save Lives*; John Charlton and Ramon Velez, "Some International Comparisons of Mortality Amenable to Medical Intervention," *British Medical Journal* 292, no. 6516 (1986): 295–301. Less rapid decline in Central-eastern Europe between the 1950s and late 1980s was documented in Richard J. Boys, Donald P. Forster, and Peter Jozan, "Mortality from Causes Amenable and Non-Amenable to Medical Care: The Experience of Eastern Europe," *British Medical Journal* 303, no. 6807 (1991): 879–83. In Russia, 'amenable' mortality decline stagnated between the 1960s and 1980s, reversed into increasing mortality in the 1990s, and then started to decline again (Evgueni M. Andreev et al., "The Evolving Pattern of Avoidable Mortality in Russia," *International Journal of Epidemiology* 32, no. 3 (2003): 437–46).

105 As estimated in Johan P. Mackenbach et al., "Post-1950 Mortality Trends and Medical Care," *Social Science & Medicine* 27, no. 9 (1988): 889–94. In Mackenbach, "Contribution", which reported on another study for the Netherlands spanning the period between 1875 and 1970, and therefore included some earlier innovations as well, improvements in medical care accounted for between 5 and 20% of total mortality decline.

106 This study also estimated the effect of improvements in medical care on quality of life in non-fatal conditions (John P. Bunker, Howard S. Frazier, and Frederick Mosteller, "Improving Health: Measuring Effects of Medical Care," *Milbank Quarterly* 72, no. 2 (1994): 225–58).

in medical care for infectious diseases, cardiovascular diseases and cancer contributed around 4 years to life expectancy at birth among men and women. This is about half of the total increase in life expectancy over that period.[107]

---

107 Willem J. Meerding et al., *Hoe Gezond Zijn De Zorguitgaven?*, vol. 6, Zorg Voor Euro's, (Bilthoven: Rijksinstituut voor Volksgezondheid en Milieu, 2007).

PART 2

Zooming in: The Rise and Fall of Diseases

CHAPTER 4

Health Problems of Pre-industrial Societies

In this chapter we review some of the main health problems of the *Ancien Régime* – a term originally referring to the old political order which came to an end in the French revolution of 1789, but here referring more generally to the pre-industrial period. We will start with war, homicide and famine, and then deal with plague, smallpox, typhus and malaria. Three other diseases involved in mortality crises, cholera, influenza and AIDS, will be dealt with later. The main question that will concern us is: how did Europeans rid themselves of these 'health problems of pre-industrial societies'?[1]

Violence and Hunger

War

Europe has often been a theatre of war, and wars have caused innumerable numbers of deaths throughout the three centuries covered by this book. Like homicide – with which we will deal in the following section – war and war-related deaths are not a 'disease', so readers may wonder why they are discussed on a par with smallpox, tuberculosis and ischaemic heart disease. The answer is, first, that apart from their direct effects wars have indirect effects on population health, e.g., by precipitating epidemics (Plate 7), and, second, that in the end it does not matter whether a person dies from war (or homicide) or from disease. We would be less enthusiastic about progress in the prevention or treatment of disease if this is accompanied by an increase in the risk of death from war – and isn't that what seems to have happened in the 20th century?

---

1 Leprosy, which declined even earlier than plague, and had largely disappeared from most European countries before the year 1700, will not be dealt with in this book. Neither will yellow fever, although epidemics of this tropical disease, arriving by ship from the Americas and the West coast of Africa, heavily struck Spain and Portugal in the 18th and first half of the 19th centuries (see August Hirsch, *Handbook of Geographical and Historical Pathology*, trans. Charles Creighton (London: New Sydenham Society, 1883), Vol. I, pp. 335–37). Please note that this Chapter mainly focuses on causes of crisis mortality, and not on the causes of mortality in pre-industrial societies in 'normal' years. These included many of the causes dealt with in Chapter 5; see, e.g., Alex Mercer, *Disease, Mortality, and Population in Transition* (Leicester etc.: Leicester University Press, 1990).

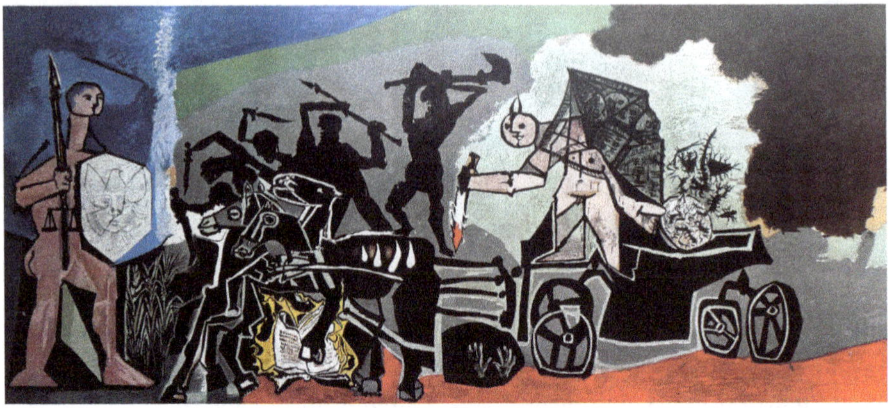

PLATE 7 *La Guerre* [War]. Painting by Pablo Picasso, 1951
The link between war and disease is illustrated in this lithograph, based on a wall painting with the same title by Pablo Picasso (1881–1973). Picasso executed this wall painting, together with another one illustrating 'La Paix' *[Peace], in 1951 in a small chapel in Vallauris (Southern France). Less well-known than his* 'Guernica', *which illustrates the atrocities of the Spanish Civil War, this painting was inspired by the ravages of World War II. It shows how armed conflict is often accompanied by the spread of infectious diseases, symbolized by the black creatures escaping from the cart on the right-hand side.*

What long-term trends in the occurrence of war look like, strongly depends on how we count wars: as events, with each single war counting as one, or as the number of war-related deaths. Military historians have identified a long-term trend since the Middle Ages of decreasing frequency but increasing severity of war: since 1500, war between the great European powers gradually became less frequent, but at the same time more devastating, until the death toll peaked in the 1940s and interstate war almost stopped completely.

Let's first look at the number of war-related deaths. Counting these numbers is far from straightforward, not only because vital registration systems are often interrupted in war-time, but also because wars cause many more deaths than the military casualties that can readily be identified, and because it is difficult to draw a line between more and less strictly war-related deaths. Nevertheless, the trends are pretty clear (see Suppl. Table 5).[2]

2 Because famines and epidemics are treated separately in this chapter, deaths from famine and epidemics 'indirectly' caused by war are not included in the estimates of Suppl. Table 5. If war deaths are expressed per 100,000 of the European population, we see a peak in the early 1800s, a trough in the rest of the 19th century, another much larger peak in the first half

The 18th century started with the War of the Spanish Succession (1701–1714, involving Britain, the Dutch Republic, Austria, Spain, Portugal, France and Savoy) and the Great Northern War (1700–1721, mainly between Sweden and Russia, but also involving Denmark, Poland-Lithuania, various German states and the Ottoman empire). Both caused hundreds of thousands of deaths – substantially less than the great war of the 17th century, i.e., the Thirty-Years War which caused an estimated 6 million deaths – but disastrous nonetheless.

Between the early 18th century and the early 20th century several more wars occurred, of which the most devastating were the combined French Revolutionary Wars (1792–1802) and the Napoleonic Wars (1803–1815), in which France stood opposed to many other European states, and which together caused 2 million deaths. At that time, the population of Europe counted around 200 million people, which implies that a staggering 1% of the entire European population perished in this war.

Clearly, however, the 20th century was the most deadly of the three. Estimates of deaths caused by World War I vary enormously, depending on the source and on whether indirectly caused deaths have been included, between 10 and 40 million. The conservative estimate of 10 million deaths includes 8.5 million military deaths plus 1.5 million civilians killed in hostilities on the Eastern front or dying as a result of food blockades. With a population of around 400 million people, this implies a 2.5% death rate for Europe as a whole.[3]

These numbers almost dwindle, however, when compared to the numbers of deaths caused by World War II. Here again estimates differ wildly, but if we again take a conservative estimate, leaving out indirectly war-related deaths, we find some 14 million military killed in action or dead of wounds, plus some 27 million European civilians killed by states, including Jews killed in the Holocaust. With a 1940 population of 550 million people, this implies a 7.5% death rate for Europe as a whole.[4]

of the 20th century, and then a trough again (see Steven Pinker, *The Better Angels of Our Nature* (London: Allen Lane, 2011), Fig. 5–18).

3 This estimate excludes many millions of deaths caused by war-related epidemics, by the influenza pandemic of 1918–19, by the Armenian genocide, and by the Russian Civil War, and it excludes deaths occurring outside Europe.

4 The estimates of numbers of deaths have been taken from Davies, *Europe: A History*, pp. 1328–329. In the Holocaust (1941–1945), Nazi Germany killed around 6 million Jews, or two-thirds of Europe's Jewish population. On top of that, the Nazis systematically killed many others, including hundreds of thousands of Roma and disabled people.

In addition, the 20th century also counted huge numbers of deaths due to state-based violence against civilians that was not or less directly war-related. These include the victims of the Armenian genocide in Turkey (1915, around 1 million killed), the victims of Stalin's Great Purge (1937–1938, around 1 million killed), and the victims of Franco's regime in Spain and of communist regimes in Yugoslavia, Romania and other communist countries in Central-eastern Europe (between 100,000 and 200,000 each).

The causes of all these wars and atrocities have been heavily disputed between historians, and impartiality is often difficult to find. Whereas historians agree that the blame for World War II lies squarely with Nazi Germany, opinions are more divided about the blame for World War I, but the majority opinion seems to be that here too most of the blame lies with Germany. One of the underlying factors in both wars was the expansionist drive of Germany, which as a result of rapid industrialization had become Europe's most powerful country at the beginning of the 20th century. This expansionist drive was directed towards the East, where the Germans easily could overrun several weaker states but then collided with a mighty and ruthless competitor, Russia/Soviet Union. This explains why most of the civilian deaths in both World Wars, and most of the military deaths counted in World War II, fell in the East.[5]

Similarly, Russia's expansionist drives underlay several of the most bloody wars of the 19th century. These were mainly directed against the crumbling Ottoman Empire, partly in an attempt to get access to the Mediterranean. Already in the 18th century there were four Russo-Turkish Wars, and several more followed in the 19th century. The Russo-Turkish War of 1828–1829 started after Russia had helped to defeat the Ottoman fleet in the war for Greek independence. The Crimean War (1853–1856) started when Russia occupied parts of modern Romania which then were still under Ottoman sovereignty. The Ottomans had to be helped by the British and the French to – temporarily – defeat the Russians. The Russo-Turkish War of 1877–1878 was fought by the Russians to help Bulgarians, Romanians and Serbs gain independence from the Ottomans, and to gain territory for itself in the Caucasus.[6]

5 The historical literature on both World Wars is too vast to oversee, and still expanding. This section was inspired by Davies, *Europe: A History*, Chapter XI. For the impact of the struggle between Nazi Germany and the Soviet Union on the "bloodlands" of Central-eastern and Eastern Europe, see Timothy Snyder, *Bloodlands: Europe between Hitler and Stalin* (London: Bodley Head, 2010).

6 Between 1683 and 1914, Russia's expansion continued at an average rate of 55 square miles per day (Davies, *Europe: A History*, p. 869). The expansionist drives of Germany and Russia can be seen as the collective expression of a desire for better living standards – another dark side of the quest for a better life underlying population health improvements.

After the 1940s Europe has experienced almost no further wars, with the exception of the Yugoslav Wars of the 1990s. This brings us back to the long-term trend in the number of wars, which is radically different from the trend in the number of war-related deaths. Since the early 1500s, the number of European wars (counted as events per decade) has gradually declined, whereas their severity (counted in number of deaths) has increased.

This increasing severity was, to some extent, an unfavourable side-effect of the formation of the modern state. This made European countries more and more effective in waging war, by enabling them to raise the financial means for increasingly expensive, but also increasingly effective, military technologies, and by giving them the bureaucratic means to raise massive conscription armies. This has gradually raised the European death toll of war until it reached an all-time high in the middle of the 20th century, with the carnage of World War II.[7]

For the decreasing frequency of war several explanations have been offered. One is that the increasing expensiveness of military technologies – which increased the severity of war – have also become an almost unsurmountable-barrier to waging war. Another is that the potential benefits of territorial conquest – which was often an important war aim in the past – have become less tempting because of the declining importance of agriculture. A third is nuclear deterrence: the almost-certainty that full-out European war would lead to even more massive destruction than the last conventional war, must also have played a role in preventing any further wars.

However, another explanation – on a more optimistic note – is that over time European countries have become inherently less belligerent. Generalized prosperity has taken away some of the economic pressures for war, and economic and political integration within an expanding European Union has increased mutual dependence and fostered better mutual understanding. War has also been 'denormalized': whereas on the eve of the World War I many Europeans looked forward to a good fight, war has since then been more or less outlawed by international treaties, and many people now feel convulsion at the thought of killing other people. This may be another, belated effect of the Enlightenment during which the first philosophical treaties denunciating

7 For trends in the frequency and severity of wars, see Jack S. Levy and William R. Thompson, *The Arc of War* (Chicago: University of Chicago Press, 2011). The earliest evidence for warfare in Western Europe dates from 4300 BCE, implying that the rise of warfare in Europe must have started (long) before that. Several accelerations in the frequency and/or severity of war have occurred, followed by a recent fall in the number of war-related deaths, producing an over-all pattern of rise-and-fall ("The Arc of War"), not unlike that seen for many other (health) problems of humanity.

war saw the light. Whereas the 19th century saw the 'balance of powers' as the best way to prevent further war after the destruction of the Napoleonic Wars, countries now increasingly rely on the enforcement of international law by the United Nations, if necessary with internationally funded peace-keeping forces.[8]

It is paradoxical that the century in which European population health improved the most, was also the century in which wars caused more deaths than ever before. How are the two connected? Upon reflection, the connections are actually many. The main reason why wars caused more deaths in the 20th than in the 18th or 19th century is that wars were fought with different means and with a different concept of war. Warfare had become industrialized, permitting a vastly larger scale of destruction, and were fought as 'total wars', in which civilians and civilian infrastructures were considered legitimate targets. Both changes were products of 'modernization' – more destructive weaponry was a side effect of industrialization, and the adoption of the concept of 'total war' was a product of the 'rationalization' of military-strategic thinking.

While this suggests that large-scale warfare and population health improvement have overlapping causes, we should also consider the possibility that the European wars of the 20th century have indirectly accelerated population health improvements. They destroyed old infrastructures, such as houses and factories, which had to be replaced by new and more healthy facilities after the wars. Precisely because these were mass wars, they catalysed state involvement in public health and in social security, in order to keep the population healthy and motivated. And they increased investments in medical technology and accelerated medical innovation, which have in peace-time continued to benefit the population. Think of delousing techniques, vaccines, emergency departments and triage, surgical techniques, antibiotics, ... The best known – but far from only – example is penicillin, whose development was accelerated immensely by World War II.[9]

---

8 For an analysis of the origins of war, see Jack S. Levy and William R. Thompson, *Causes of War* (Chichester: Wiley-Blackwell, 2011). Some down-to-earth explanations for the decline of interstate war are offered in Levy and Thompson, *The Arc of War*, whereas Pinker, *Enlightenment Now* emphasizes the role of the Enlightenment, changing attitudes and improving international diplomacy.

9 On the interrelationships between 'war, medicine and modernity', see Peter Neushul, "Fighting Research," in *War, Medicine and Modernity*, ed. Roger Cooter, Mark Harrison, and Steve Sturdy (Phoenix Mill: Sutton Publishing Limited, 1998). Penicillin went from a laboratory phenomenon in 1942 to mass production in 1946, thanks to a rapid transfer of knowledge and scaling up of production which would have been unthinkable without the war effort.

Homicide

Nowadays, homicide – the act of one or more private persons killing another – is a much less frequent cause of death than suicide. In most European countries the rate of death from homicide is around 1 per 100,000 per year, whereas the rate of death from suicide is around between 10 and 20 per 100,000 per year. Long ago, however, it was completely the reverse: in the Middle Ages and the early modern period, homicide was much more frequent than suicide – as if since then the aggression against other people has been internalized.[10]

Studies have shown that in the 1300s and 1400s the homicide rates in England, the Low Countries, Germany, Sweden and Italy still lay between 25 and 75 per 100,000 per year. The secular decline of homicide started in England and the Low Countries in the early 1500s, with Germany and Sweden following in the 1600s, and Italy following much later in the 1800s.[11]

This decline has been attributed to a combination of cultural and political changes that mutually reinforced each other. On the one hand, the 'civilizing process' (Chapter 3) has increased the individual sensitivity to violence. Changing notions of 'masculinity' and 'honour', propagated by the church and reinforced by the Enlightenment, gradually led to a more peaceful lifestyle, first of the upper social classes and later trickling down to the lower social classes. In this process, medieval 'feuds' were first replaced by strictly regulated 'duels', and then the idea of male 'honour' disappeared almost completely, to be replaced by an ideal of 'inner virtue'.

On the other hand, the creation of the state monopoly on violence also increasingly restricted the use of physical violence in interpersonal conflicts. In the 16th and 17th centuries homicide was criminalized, and the judiciary started to prosecute the perpetrators. In the late 18th century, a shift in punishment occurred from fines to imprisonment, and in the 19th century many European cities established a police force which could, among other things and

10 A negative association between suicide and homicide has not only been found over time, but also comparing countries or population groups; see Jean-Claude Chesnais, *Histoire de la Violence en Occident de 1800 à Nos Jours* (Paris: Robert Laffont, 1981), Chapter 8. This has fuelled speculations that the suppression of aggression towards others has led to more depression and an increased tendency to self-harm; see Marzio Barbagli, *Farewell to the World* (Cambridge & Malden: Polity Press, 2015), Chapter 3.

11 For systematic analyses of long-term trends in homicide, see Manuel P. Eisner, "Modernization, Self-Control and Lethal Violence," *British Journal of Criminology* 41 (2001): 618–38; Manuel P. Eisner, "From Swords to Words," *Crime and Justice* 43, no. 1 (2014): 65–134.

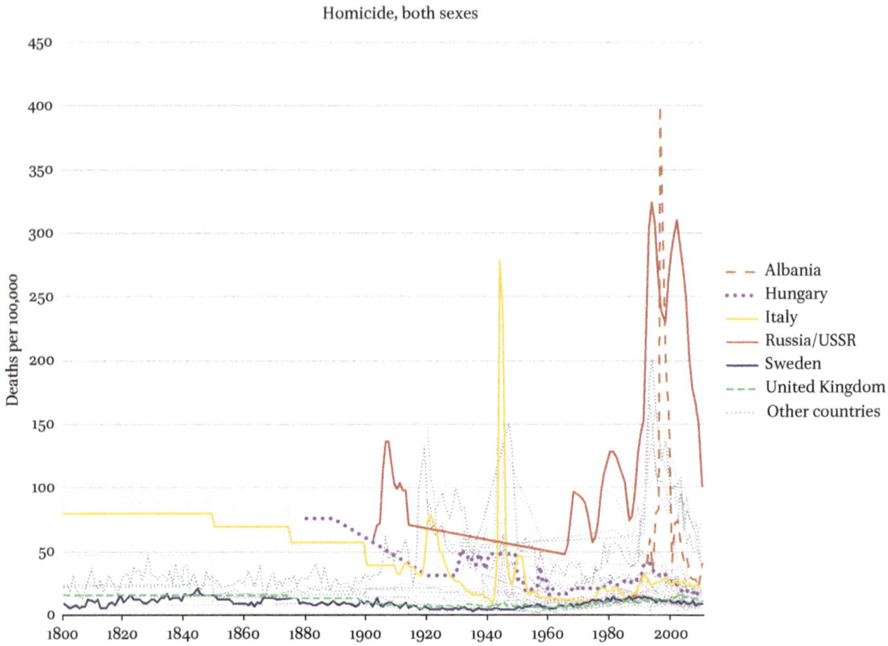

FIGURE 9 Trends in homicide in Europe, 1800–2010
SOURCE OF DATA: WWW.CLIO-INFRA.EU (ACCESSED 28/08/2018)

sometimes against the protests of the local population, investigate crimes and try to apprehend suspects.[12]

Figure 9 shows trends in homicide in European countries since 1800. In view of what has just been said, it is important to keep in mind that this figure does not capture the secular decline of homicide rates that occurred in Western and Northern Europe in the preceding period. For example, in the year 1800 the homicide rates in England, Belgium and Sweden were already down to 1 or 2 per 100,000 per year. We do, however, see that Southern European countries such as Italy (and Spain, not highlighted in the graph) were still in the process of reducing their homicide rates from the much higher pre-modern levels.

When we take 1800 as our starting-point, what strikes us most in Figure 9 is, first, the absence of a general decline in homicide and, second, the enormous 'spikes' in homicide mortality that keep returning throughout the 19th and 20th centuries. It is thus not immediately clear from the graph that

12 On comprehensive explanations of long-term trends in homicide, see Chesnais, *Histoire*; Pieter Spierenburg, *A History of Murder* (Cambridge: Polity Press, 2008). An attempt to relate the decline in homicide to the increase in 'social disciplining' and 'self-control' can be found in Eisner, "Swords."

Europe-as-a-whole has made much progress in eliminating homicide mortality. It is important, therefore, to look in more detail at what has happened. What we see in Figure 9 is the result of at least four superimposed processes.

First, homicide rates in the Western European countries in which homicide rates were already very low in the early 1800s, have followed a pattern of slow, and sometimes multiple, but always modest 'rises-and-falls'. For example, in Sweden homicide rates rose somewhat during the first half of the 19th century, then declined for a very long period, rose again in the second half of the 20th century, and then started to decline again. In many European countries – also in the South and East – homicide rates reached their lowest point ever in the 1940s and 1950s, and have since risen again.

The minimum values obtained in the middle of the 20th century have been interpreted as the result of the long-term 'civilisation process' mentioned above. The increase since then has been interpreted by some as a temporary 'reversal of direction' of this process, i.e., a 'de-civilising process' resulting from the loosening of norms in the 1960s. However, because homicides within the family did not increase at all, others have suggested other explanations. These point to violence between non-European immigrants among whom male 'honour' is still important, proliferation of organized crime leading to violent conflicts between drug dealers and other criminals, and increased night-time recreation with alcohol intoxication.[13]

Second, homicide rates in many less advanced countries have converged, to a greater or lesser degree, towards the low values already obtained in a number of Western European countries in the early 1800s. This is what happened in, for example, Italy and Spain during most of the 19th century, and in Hungary during a large part of the 20th century (Figure 9). Because this process of convergence was slow, it resulted in starkly contrasting homicide rates within Europe during most of the period observed.

In the 19th century, Europe became divided in an inner and an outer zone, with the outer zone consisting of Ireland, the Mediterranean, the Balkans, Eastern Europe, and Finland, where homicide rates remained high. Within their respective countries, the islands of Corsica, Sardinia and Sicily also long kept their higher homicide rates. This has been attributed to cultural delays (e.g., extended family ties and honour remaining important for longer) combined with

13 See Manuel P. Eisner, "Modernity Strikes Back?," *International Journal of Conflict and Violence* 2, no. 2 (2008): 288 – 316 and Spierenburg, *History* for an analysis of these recent trends. Pinker, *The Better Angels of Our Nature*, Chapter 3, has argued for the role of a 'de-civilising process', due to the rise of anti-authoritarian attitudes in the 1960s. A similar explanation has been suggested for the rise of sexually transmitted diseases (see Chapter 5, Syphilis).

delays in the creation or imposition of the state monopoly on violence (e.g., persistence of knife fighting, feuding, and banditry). It was only after World War II that these contrasts in homicide rates between North and West on the one hand, and South and East on the other hand, more or less disappeared.[14]

Third, superimposed on these longer-term processes are several massive increases in homicide rates coinciding with episodes of political disruption. For example, homicide rates in Finland spiked in the early 1900s in connection with the 1905 Russian revolution, and then again around 1920 in the aftermath of the civil war that resulted in Finland's independence from Russia. Homicide rates in Russia itself spiked in the early 1900s as well, as they did in the late 1990s and early 2000s, in connection with the political and economic disruption after the collapse of the Soviet Union. Homicide rates in Italy spiked in the last years of World War II, as they did in many other European countries. The largest spike of all occurred in 1997 in Albania, when the 'pyramid crisis' resulted in massive civil unrest and violence between armed gangs, the police and civilians.[15]

Clearly, this is a different type of homicide as compared to the interpersonal violence seen in normal times. In war-time, the normal restrictions on the use of violence, both psychological and judicial, partly disappear. Conflicts between opposing parties are not only fought by armies, but also, and usually on a smaller scale, by civilians, as in resistance movements or retaliations for actions of the other party. Nevertheless, these massive spikes, in which homicide rates briefly rise to medieval levels, illustrate the fragility of the social fabric that protects us from wide-spread violence in normal times.

Fourth and finally, some of the homicide trends and variations seen in Figure 9 reflect changes and variations in one of the most important risk factors for homicide: excessive alcohol consumption. Both in the past and nowadays, many acts of homicide are committed during a fight between two persons, usually young or middle-aged men, who are both under the influence of alcohol.

---

14 See Chesnais, *Histoire,* Chapter 2, and Spierenburg, *History,* Chapter 6, for an analysis of these contrasts in homicide rates within Europe.

15 In 1905 Finland was still part of the Russian empire. On trends in Finland's homicide rates, see Jukka Savolainen, Martti Lehti, and Janne Kivivuori, "Historical Origins of a Cross-National Puzzle: Homicide in Finland, 1750 to 2000," *Homicide Studies* 12, no. 1 (2008): 67–89. Although data on homicide in Russia/Soviet Union are not available between the start of World War I and the mid-1960s, we know that the Civil War following the October 1917 revolution was accompanied by a massive rise in homicide; see Chesnais, *Histoire,* Chapter 14. On the Albanian 'pyramid crisis', see Chapter 7.

Finland's high rates of homicide arose in the early 19th century, when, due to ample availability of alcohol, binge drinking became common in newly established forest-industrial towns and lumber-producing rural communities. During the 20th century, Finland's rates converged somewhat with Sweden's, but a new rise in homicide started in the late 1960s after the relaxation of alcohol control measures. To a large extent, the connection between excessive alcohol consumption and homicide also 'explains' the levels and variations in homicide in Russia and other countries of the former Soviet Union.[16]

Famine

As we saw in Figure 2, until quite recently large-scale famine was a very important cause of mortality crises in Europe. The origins of these famines were often complex. In early modern Europe a single crop failure due to bad weather was no longer enough to produce starvation, because public stores of grain and commercial trade with other, non-afflicted areas could compensate for temporary shortages of food.

Famines were therefore usually due to a combination of factors, such as rapidly rising population numbers plus a succession of harvest failures. Disastrous human intervention could also produce a famine, for example in World War II during the infamous German siege of Leningrad in 1941–44 (Plate 8) and during the '*Hongerwinter*' in the Netherlands in 1944.[17]

Famines must have accompanied humans since at least the Neolithic period. This is because agriculture allowed them to increase their numbers, but also made them dependent on a limited number of self-grown foods, whose growth was subject to weather and other conditions beyond their control. Over time, however, the severity of famines declined: so-called super-famines in which many millions of Europeans perished, all occurred before the 18th century. The last of these super-famines occurred in the 1690s. On a very long

16 See Savolainen et al., "Historical Origins of a Cross-National Puzzle" for the history of homicide in Finland. Many studies have shown an association between excessive alcohol consumption and homicide in Russia, e.g. Yury Razvodovsky, "Homicide and Alcohol Intoxication in Russia, 1956–2005," *Alcoholism* 43, no. 1 (2007): 36–50.

17 See Guido Alfani and Cormac Ó Gráda, "Famines in Europe: An Overview," in *Famine in European History*, ed. Guido Alfani and Cormac Ó Gráda (Cambridge etc.: Cambridge University Press, 2017) for a general overview of the factors causing European famines. The Dutch '*Hongerwinter*' had a complex explanation, including a strike by Dutch railway personnel (in response to a call from the exiled Dutch government to help the advance of the allied troops) and a German blockade of inland shipping; see Ingrid de Zwarte, *De Hongerwinter* (Amsterdam: Prometheus, 2019).

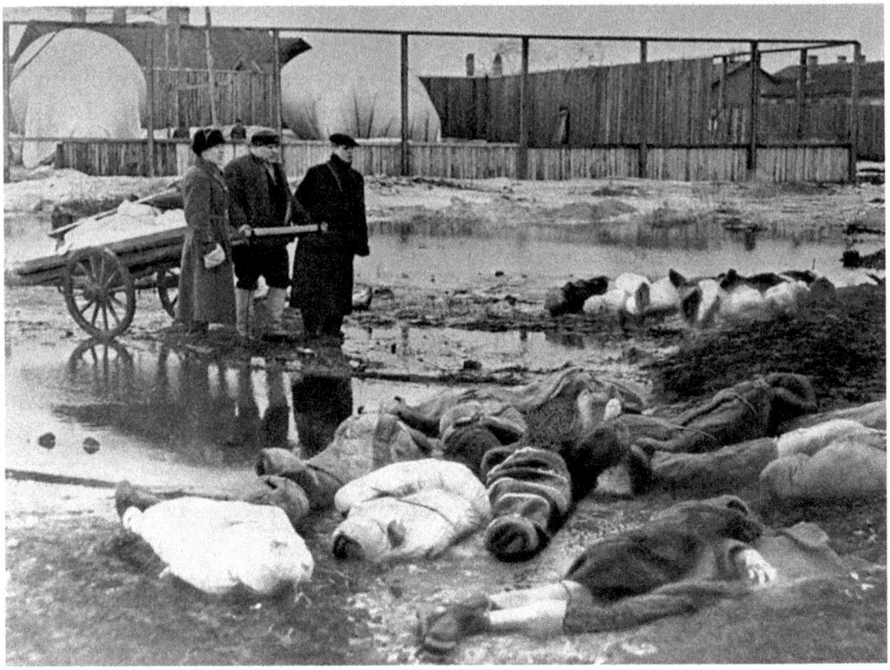

PLATE 8 Three men burying famine victims during Leningrad's siege, 1942
During European history, wars have often caused famines. The siege of Leningrad by the German army during World War II started in 1941 and lasted for two-and-a-half years, causing 1.5 million deaths, mostly by starvation. Many people died on the streets. Photograph by Boris Kudoyarov
HTTPS://COMMONS.WIKIMEDIA.ORG/WIKI/CATEGORY:VOLKOVSKOE_CEMETERY#/MEDIA/FILE:RIAN_ARCHIVE_216_THE_VOLKOVO_CEMETERY.JPG (CC BY SA 3.0; ACCESSED 18/10/2019)

time-scale, famine's secular trend is therefore characterized by a pattern of 'rise-and-fall', just like many other health conditions.[18]

The gradual decline of the risk of famine was due to favourable changes in its structural determinants. Extreme meteorological events became less severe or frequent when the Little Ice Age came to an end, which may have contributed to a lower frequency of crop failures. More importantly, the availability of food increased at a faster rate than population numbers increased, due to an 'agricultural revolution'. (Not to be confused with the Neolithic or first

18 According to Alfani and Ó Gráda, "Famines in Europe" table 1.1, three super-famines that struck large parts of the European subcontinent and killed many millions of people occurred in 1315–17, 1590–98, and 1793–97.

agricultural revolution.) This (second) revolution started in the 17th and 18th centuries in England and the Low Countries, and later spread to the rest of the European continent. It is not a coincidence that England was the first European country to remain free of famine.[19]

This agricultural revolution had two main components: an increase in agricultural output, and a change from subsistence farming to production for national and international markets. Agricultural productivity was increased by new systems of crop rotation, introduction of new foods like the potato, and expansion of arable land by drainage of lakes and marshes. Breakdown of regulations on marketing and improvements in transport allowed farmers to specialize and produce for the market, which would in the 19th century lead to the globalization of food trade networks and increased availability of non-locally grown food.[20]

However, although these changes gradually reduced the risk of famine, two counter-forces ensured that famines continued to occur into the 19th and 20th centuries (for some of the largest famines occurring after 1700, see Suppl. Table 6). Some countries became strongly dependent on a single crop, such as potatoes or maize, which increased their vulnerability to crop failures. And as warfare became more large-scale, hostilities more often led to wide-spread famine.

Famines in the 18th century were less severe than those in earlier centuries, but several major famines still occurred, including the 'Great Frost' of the 1740s which caused a visible spike in mortality in the Nordic countries (Figure 2). The most notorious among the 19th century famines are those of 1816–17, 1845–50, and 1866–68. The first followed the eruption of Mount Tambora in present-day Indonesia, whose dust clouds caused a European 'Year without a Summer' in 1816. The third was due to an exceptionally rainy and cold summer in 1866

19 The Little Ice Age (ca. 1400 – 1800) reached its minimum temperatures around 1650. European fine art museums still exhibit the romantic skating scenes that this period of severe winters produced, but this was also a period in which harvests suffered and epidemics raged; see Brian Fagan, *The Little Ice Age* (New York: Basic Books, 2000); Alfani and Ó Gráda, "Famines in Europe" . However, for a different view-point see Morgan Kelly and Cormac Ó Gráda, "The Waning of the Little Ice Age: Climate Change in Early Modern Europe," *Journal of Interdisciplinary History* 44, no. 3 (2013): 301–25. England suffered famines until the mid-17th century but remained free since then, in contrast to other European countries; see Richard Hoyle, "Britain," in *Famine in European History*, ed. Guido Alfani and Cormac Ó Gráda (Cambridge etc.: Cambridge University Press, 2017).

20 See Mark Overton, *Agricultural Revolution in England* (Cambridge etc.: Cambridge University Press, 1996) for an analysis of the agricultural revolution in England.

and a succession of crop failures in Northern and Eastern Europe, and is also clearly visible in Figure 2.[21]

The second, the 'Potato Famine' of the 1840s, is one of the best documented. This is because it occurred at a time when a keen interest in quantification was already present in many European countries, and some countries already kept death registers. Although several countries in North-western Europe were struck, Ireland was struck the most severely. The best estimate for the total number of deaths caused by the 'Great Irish Famine' is 1 million, or around 12% of the Irish population.[22]

As was so often the case, the causes of this famine were complex. A mold disease, 'Potato Blight', partially destroyed several potato crops in a row, and as the Irish people were highly dependent on this staple food large-scale starvation ensued. Yet, other factors also played a role, such as the rapid increase in population numbers of the preceding decades, suggesting that the rise of mortality also represented a 'Malthusian crisis'. Furthermore, the response of local and national government (Ireland was still part of the United Kingdom and governed from London) was callous. Poor farmers were evicted from their lands without regard to their livelihood, and famine relief was grossly insufficient.[23]

In the 20th century, large famines continued to occur, but now mainly as an accompaniment of international or civil war. The main famines of the 20th century occurred in the Soviet Union. The civil war following the Bolshevik revolution led to a famine in 1917–22; a combination of drought and disastrous policies led to famine in Ukraine and parts of Russia in 1927–33; and a combination of crop failures and the destruction of World War II led to a severe famine in Moldova in 1946–47.

Each of these famines caused at least 1 million deaths, but the 1933 famine was the worst of all, with a death count amounting to 2.5 million in Ukraine alone. This famine was different from the other two 20th century famines in

---

21 The 'Great Frost' famine, and the way it influenced mortality rates in Europe, has been analysed in John D. Post, *Food Shortage, Climatic Variability, and Epidemic Disease in Preindustrial Europe* (New York: Cornell University Press, 1985). Post argues that social disarray, including the failure of famine relief measures, was as important as undernutrition in causing excess mortality.

22 Although these deaths occurred over several years, the Irish spike in mortality in the late 1840s would have been one of the highest in Figure 2, if only national mortality rates for Ireland would have been available for plotting.

23 The causes of this famine, and particularly the role of the British government, has been fiercely debated. A monument to the famine in Belfast even speaks of 'genocide' on the Irish people. See Ó Gráda, "Ireland" for a balanced discussion.

the Soviet Union because it occurred in plain peace-time. It has therefore given rise to accusations of 'genocide' on the Ukrainian people by Joseph Stalin. This idea is also captured in the name given to this famine, 'Holodomor', which literally means 'killing by starvation'. Although there is no convincing proof that there was an intent to kill on the part of the Soviet authorities, the forced collectivization of agriculture that Stalin pursued in these years, the redirection of food from grain-producing areas to urbanized regions in the North of Russia, and lack of adequate famine relief certainly played a role.[24]

Great Epidemics

Plague

Plague, the disease which we now know to be caused by infection with *Yersinia pestis*, has produced some of the most devastating epidemics which mankind has ever encountered. Before the modern era, 'plague' used to be a general name for all diseases with high mortality, but some stories about 'plagues' in the Bible and Herodotus contain details about symptoms suggesting that plague in its current sense already occasionally raged in the Middle East before the Common Era.[25]

Plague is a disease that can manifest itself in several forms: 'bubonic plague' (infection of the lymph nodes), 'septicemic plague' (infection in the bloodstream), and 'pneumonic plague' (infection of the lungs). It is spread through the bites of infected rat-fleas, but in the case of 'pneumonic plague', the most lethal version, also from person to person through air-droplets. The responsible micro-organism, *Yersinia pestis*, circulates in animal reservoirs, particularly in rodents, and plague pandemics which reached Europe probably originated in reservoirs in remote Asian regions. The disease had a short incubation period and very high case fatality, causing great panic in affected populations.[26]

---

24 The estimate for Ukraine is from Jacques Vallin et al., "A New Estimate of Ukrainian Population Losses During the Crises of the 1930s and 1940s," *Population Studies* 56, no. 3 (2002): 249–64. This famine also caused at least 1 million deaths in Russia; on the causes of this famine, see Stephen G. Wheatcroft, "Eastern Europe (Russia and the USSR)," in *Famine in European History*, ed. Guido Alfani and Cormac Ó Gráda (Cambridge etc.: Cambridge University Press, 2017).

25 For the ancient history of plague, see, e.g., Hirsch, *Handbook* vol. 1, pp. 494–96.

26 This paragraph is a short summary of the current consensus on the aetiology of plague, and ignores several scientific controversies, such as whether or not the human flea can transmit the disease. For an overview of unexplained aspects of plague epidemics, see Paul Slack, "The Black Death Past and Present. 2. Some Historical Problems," *Transactions of the Royal Society of Tropical Medicine and Hygiene* 83, no. 4 (1989): 461–63. DNA testing

Plague struck Europe long before national or even municipal statistical data were collected, so reconstructing the timing and diffusion of plague epidemics has been a matter of studying archival sources. Like other diseases, plague is characterized by a clear pattern of 'rise-and-fall', in this case in several waves stretching over some 1500 years. The decline of plague started before the 18th century, but because several epidemics still occurred in Europe after the year 1700 we will briefly discuss its history and the reasons for its decline.[27]

The first documented plague epidemic in Europe was the 'Justinian plague', which arrived in Constantinople from the Middle East in 542. It spread along the coasts of the Mediterranean and into Southern Europe along seafaring routes and along rivers, causing huge numbers of casualties in the 540s. After this first wave, the plague returned in cyclical patterns throughout the 6th, 7th and 8th centuries, always arriving from the East. It mysteriously disappeared after a last epidemic in the 760s, perhaps due to an interruption of long-distance trade with Asia as a result of the Islamic conquests of the Mediterranean.

The second plague pandemic reaching Europe from Asia was the 'Black Death', which arrived in Constantinople in 1347 on board a Genoese ship coming from the Crimea, where during a siege the Tartars had catapulted the bodies of plague victims into the Genoese trading post of Caffa. The disease spread along the coasts of the Mediterranean, the Atlantic, the North Sea and the Baltic into most of Europe, always arriving in port cities and travelling along trading routes. It caused huge numbers of casualties in the late 1340s, perhaps up to 25 million in Europe as a whole, and its massive mortality probably caused profound changes in European culture.[28]

---

of victims of the plague in London (1348) and Marseille (1722) has confirmed the presence of *Yersinia pestis* in their dental pulp; see Michel Drancourt et al., "Detection of 400-Year-Old Yersinia Pestis DNA in Human Dental Pulp," *Proceedings of the National Academy of Sciences* 95, no. 21 (1998): 12637–40; Kirsten I. Bos et al., "A Draft Genome of Yersinia Pestis from Victims of the Black Death," *Nature* 478, no. 7370 (2011): 506–10.

27 For a recent overview of the world-wide epidemiology of plague, including an analysis of some unexplained aspects of its spread in Europe, see Samuel K. Cohn, "Epidemiology of the Black Death and Successive Waves of Plague," *Medical History* 52, no. S27 (2008): 74–100.

28 For example, the emergence of new art forms like Dances of Death suggest profound changes in attitudes in the 14th century. Effects on the economy were also huge: during and immediately after the Black Death economies collapsed, but in later years the reduction in population numbers and the resulting shortage of man-power led to wage increases and a rise of living standards; see Norman F. Cantor, *In the Wake of the Plague* (New York: Free Press, 2001).

After this first wave, the plague retreated and returned in cyclical patterns, but until much later never disappeared entirely. Devastating epidemics in North-western Europe occurred as late as the 1620s and 1660s, ravaging even capital cities like London and Amsterdam. Southern and Eastern Europe still experienced some plague epidemics in the 18th century, including an epidemic in the early 1720s in Marseille (Southern France), one in the early 1740s in Messina (Sicily), and one in the early 1770s in Moscow (Russia). In the 19th century, however, epidemics of plague were almost completely limited to South-eastern Europe. The decline of plague, including the last spikes in the 18th and 19th centuries, can clearly be seen in Figure 10.[29]

The gradual disappearance of plague from Europe has never been completely explained. Factors that have been considered – without much direct evidence – are a change in rat populations, a change from wooden to stone-built houses, increased immunity of rats or fleas, and decreased virulence of *Yersinia pestis*. While it is difficult to rule out such 'spontaneous' changes, there is also a lot to be said for an impact of intentional 'human agency', particularly public health measures. Plague was recognized as contagious early on, and in North-western and Southern Europe this resulted in the development and implementation of increasingly effective measures to prevent contagion.[30]

This included isolation of patients and disinfection of the houses of the deceased, forced quarantine of ships suspected of carrying infected persons, and military cordons to prevent infected persons and/or goods to leave or enter cities and countries. The first quarantine station was established in the Republic of Ragusa (modern-day Dubrovnik on the coast of Croatia) in 1377, and from the early 1400s onwards the principalities of Italy established a sophisticated system of defence against plague and other infectious diseases that was kept in place for several centuries. This included an outer ring of armed sailing boats in the Mediterranean and the Adriatic, a middle ring of forts and observation towers on the Italian coast, and an inner ring of land-based cavalry to stop anyone and anything that had penetrated the first two rings. This system was

29 Figure 10 is based on counting the number of localities afflicted by plague, and not on counting numbers of people infected with or dying from plague. The gradual increase seen between the early 14th and mid-17th centuries is probably an artefact of the increasing availability of archival sources, or simply of the increasing numbers of inhabited localities. Most of the information in this section about the diffusion of plague through Europe comes from Jean Noël Biraben, *Les Hommes et la Peste en France et dans les Pays Européens et Méditerranéens* (Paris: Mouton, 1975) and Hirsch, *Handbook* vol. 1, pp. 494–96.

30 See, e.g., Slack, "Black Death" and Cohn, "Epidemiology" for a balanced account of the factors involved in the decline of plague.

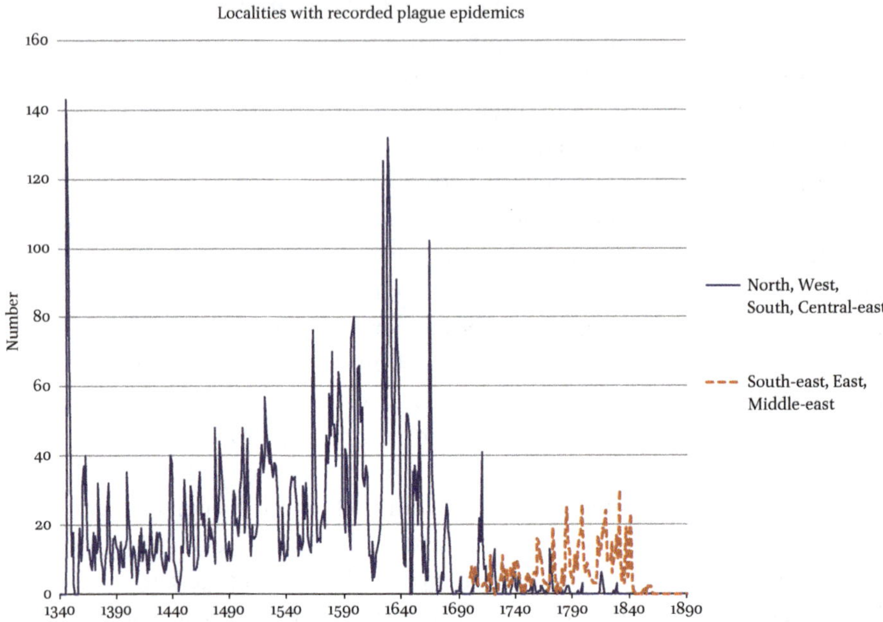

FIGURE 10 Plague epidemics in Europe and the Mediterranean, 1340–1890
Notes: Central-east includes North-western Russia; Middle-east includes Turkey and North Africa
SOURCE OF DATA: JEAN-NOËL BIRABEN. *LES HOMMES ET LA PESTE EN FRANCE ET DANS LES PAYS EUROPÉENS ET MÉDITERRANÉENS*. PARIS: MOUTON, 1975, ANNEXE III

not 100% water-tight, as illustrated by the 1743 epidemic in Messina, but has likely prevented many epidemics from entering the country.[31]

Another important countermeasure was the *cordon sanitaire* on the border – more than 1000 kilometres long – between the Habsburg and Ottoman Empires. This was created by the Habsburg Empire during the 18th century, in order to prevent introduction of plague from the Ottoman Empire where the disease was still endemic. It was completed in 1770 and kept in place until the

31 On the Italian system of defence against plague, see Andrew D. Cliff, Matthew R. Smallman-Raynor, and Peta M. Stevens, "Controlling the Geographical Spread of Infectious Disease: Plague in Italy, 1347–1851," *Acta Medico-Historica Adriatica* 7, no. 2 (2009): 197–236. Evidence for an effect of *cordons sanitaires* also includes the experience with the last great plague epidemics in France. In contrast to London, Paris could avoid the plague epidemic of the 1660s, by a *cordon sanitaire* in the North of France, shielding it off from the Low Countries where Amsterdam was already struck by plague. France also stopped the plague epidemic of the 1720s by a *cordon sanitaire* in Provence and Languedoc; see P. Bourdelais, *Les Épidémies Terrassées. Une Histoire de Pays Riches* (Paris: Éditions de la Martinière, 2003), Chapter 1.

1860s. It included a chain of military look-out posts, guarded frontier crossings, regulations for who and what could enter the Empire, and quarantine stations to isolate and disinfect suspicious people and goods. It also included a plague intelligence service in the Ottoman empire which could send timely warnings to step-up protection measures. Even though occasional lapses occurred, the implementation of this system coincided with the disappearance of plague from the Habsburg Empire.[32]

Plague did not disappear from all parts of Europe in the same pace, and the fact that it persisted longer in the South-east, as illustrated in Figure 10, supports the idea that preventive measures were at least partly responsible for the decline of plague. In the Ottoman Empire, both the largely illiterate public and the governing bodies were reluctant to implement the measures recommended by Western experts. During the first decades of the 19th century, yearly epidemics still occurred in the Balkans, then still part of the Ottoman Empire. It was not until the 1830s that the Ottoman authorities, pressed by Western governments, adopted stricter measures to prevent the spread of plague, after which plague also disappeared from the South-east.[33]

Smallpox

In contrast to what its innocuous name suggests, smallpox was a big killer during Europe's Middle Ages and early modern period. This disease, which is caused by infection with the *Variola* virus, was probably already known to Galen (third century CE), and received its first clear description from Persian physician Rhazes (854–925). It is likely that smallpox was already common in Southern Europe in the sixth century, and penetrated into Northern Europe during the Middle Ages, reaching Iceland in the 13th century.[34]

Since then, regularly returning smallpox epidemics with a periodicity of between 5 and 15 years, depending on the size of populations, have been a constant feature of the European mortality pattern. It was mainly a disease of children, which not only caused skin vesicles and pustules, but in its malignant form also caused a high fever, septicaemia and extensive bleeding, leading to a

32 See Rothenberg, "Austrian sanitary cordon."

33 Due to international sanitary cooperation, the third pandemic of plague, which started in China in the 1850s, and reached Hong Kong, Bombay and Alexandria in the 1890s, never reached Europe, with the exception of a small epidemic around Oporto (Portugal) in 1899; see Jo N. Hays, *Epidemics and Pandemics: Their Impacts on Human History* (Santa Barbara etc.: ABC-Clio, 2005), Chapter 36.

34 The name of smallpox derives from the distinction, made in the 15th century, with another disease that caused somewhat similar skin eruptions and that was labelled "the Great pox": syphilis. For a history of smallpox epidemics, see, e.g. Hirsch, *Handbook* vol. I, pp. 123–53.

high case fatality. In the 18th century, in the European countries or large cities that already kept cause-of-death statistics, smallpox accounted for around 10% of all deaths, and a much higher proportion of deaths among children.[35]

Yet, smallpox has gone: the last cases world-wide occurred in the 1970s, and smallpox largely disappeared from Europe in the 19th and first half of the 20th century, mainly as a result of vaccination.[36]

The core of this success story is well-known and can therefore be summarized in a few sentences. In Asia it had already been known for a long time that 'inoculation' of healthy persons with infected material from smallpox patients protected them from smallpox. In the early 18th century this procedure was imported into Europe from the Ottoman Empire, and although inoculation carried a substantial risk, it was used on a wide scale in England and several other European countries. In the early decades of the 19th century it was rapidly replaced by the safer procedure of 'vaccination', which was discovered at the end of the 18th century and used infected material from cows suffering from cowpox.[37]

Vaccination immediately became very popular, and was promoted by the medical profession, Royal Commissions, national parliaments and voluntary organizations all over Europe. While it is likely that inoculation already reduced mortality from smallpox in the 18th century, vaccination certainly and substantially reduced mortality from smallpox in the 19th century. Studies comparing the mortality rates from smallpox before and after the introduction of vaccination show a reduction of between 50 and 90%.[38]

Continuous series of cause-specific mortality spanning this period are rare, and limited to the Nordic countries and a few of Europe's largest cities. In Finland and Sweden, mortality from smallpox started to decline precipitously

---

35 See, e.g., Kari J. Pitkänen, James H. Mielke, and Lynn B. Jorde, "Smallpox and Its Eradication in Finland: Implications for Disease Control," *Population Studies* 43, no. 1 (1989): 95–111, on mortality from smallpox in 18th century Finland, and Mercer, *Disease* on mortality from smallpox in 18th century London.

36 It has been argued that vaccination coverage in European countries in the 19th centuries was not high enough to completely explain the decline of smallpox, and that spontaneous declines in virulence must also have played a role; see A.B. Christie, "Smallpox," in *World Geography of Human Diseases*, ed. G. Melvyn Howe (London etc.: Academic Press, 1977).

37 On the use of inoculation during the 18th century, see Peter Razzell, *The Conquest of Smallpox* (Firle: Caliban Books, 1977). The discovery of vaccination is associated with the name of the English physician Edward Jenner (1749–1823), who systematically tested the effectiveness of 'vaccination' and disseminated the results in a scientific publication (Edward Jenner, *An Inquiry into Causes and Effects of the Variolae Vaccinae* (London: Sampson Low, 1798)).

38 The studies cited relate to parts of Germany and the Austro-Hungarian Empire. See Mercer, *Disease*, table 3.2.

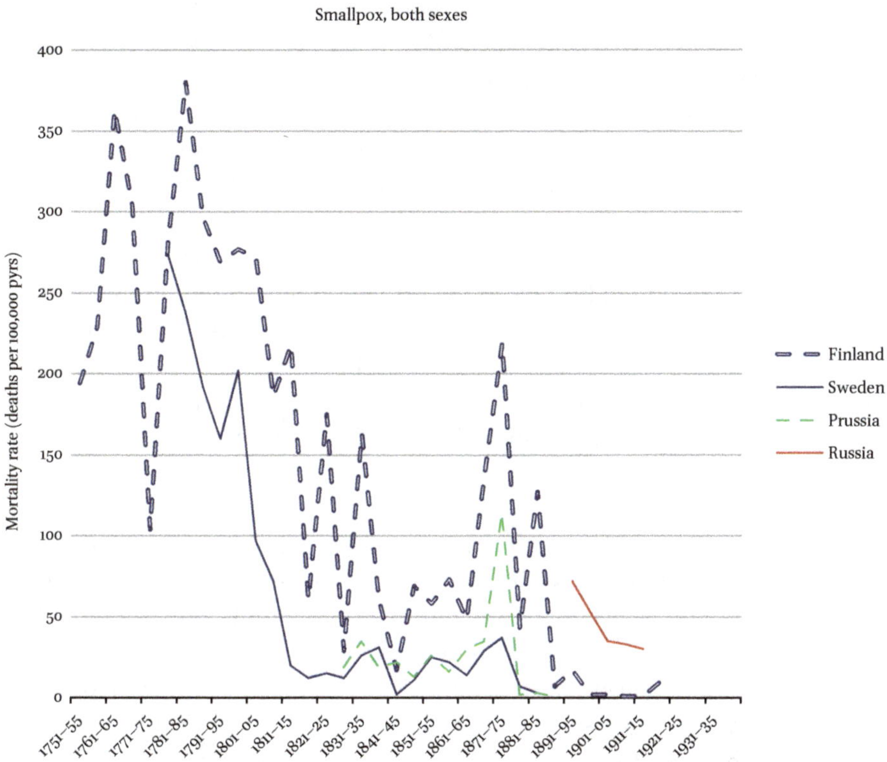

FIGURE 11 Trends in smallpox mortality in selected European countries, 1751–1935
Notes: Quinquennial data
SOURCE OF DATA: KARI J. PITKÄNEN, JAMES H. MIELKE, AND LYNN B. JORDE. "SMALLPOX AND ITS ERADICATION IN FINLAND: IMPLICATIONS FOR DISEASE CONTROL." *POPULATION STUDIES*. 43, NO. 1 (1989): TABLE 4

around the turn of the 19th century, but rose again during the severe 1870 pandemic. This struck many European countries, including the Netherlands and Prussia for which data are available from the 1860s onwards (Figure 11). The fact that smallpox mortality during this pandemic rose less in Sweden and Denmark than in Finland, the Netherlands and Prussia has been ascribed to the fact that in the former two countries vaccination was compulsory. In the latter three it was voluntary only, so that vaccination rates had gradually declined in the preceding decades when smallpox epidemics became less frequent.[39]

39 See Pitkänen et al., "Smallpox and Its Eradication in Finland" for an analysis of trends in Finland and other European countries. The comparison between countries with compulsory and voluntary vaccination has been made in Willibrord Rutten, *'De Vreselijkste Aller Harpijen'* (Wageningen: Afdeling Agrarische Geschiedenis, Landbouwuniversiteit Wageningen, 1997), table 11.6. The spread of smallpox during this epidemic was promoted by the demobilization of German and French troops after the 1871 Franco-Prussian War.

A similar decline of smallpox mortality can be seen in some of Europe's larger cities. While the London 'Bills of Mortality' show a modest reduction of mortality from smallpox during the 18th century, a precipitous decline started around the turn of the 19th century. The success of smallpox vaccination has contributed importantly to the suppression of mortality crises, and may have played an important role more generally in the decline of mortality in Europe during the 19th century.[40]

It took until the middle of the 20th century, however, before smallpox completely disappeared from Europe. In the first decades of the 20th century, there was still appreciable mortality from smallpox in Spain, Portugal, and Greece, as well as in Finland, and occasional deaths still occurred in many other countries. After World War II, Portugal was the last of the European countries in which smallpox mortality became a disease of the past.[41]

Typhus

More than the history of any other infectious disease, "[t]he history of typhus is written in those dark pages of the world's story which tell the grievous visitations of mankind by war, famine, and misery of every kind." The disease is characterized by high fever, headache and red spots on the skin (from which its other name, 'spotted fever', derives), and is caused by infection with *Rickettsia prowazeki*, a micro-organism transmitted between humans by the body louse.[42]

Because the symptoms of typhus are not very distinctive, it is difficult to trace its history, and before the middle of the 19th century it was often confused with what we now call 'typhoid', an intestinal infection. Bacteriologist Hans Zinsser, who wrote a classic history of typhus just before World War II (*Rats, Lice and History*), thinks that the disease arrived in Europe from Asia in the late 15th century, as a result of the movement of troops from Cyprus, where they had fought against the Turks, to Spain. From Spain, the disease eventually spread towards the North, but it may well have been introduced into Europe on several occasions, e.g., during confrontations with the Turks on the Austro-Hungarian front-line.

Over time, typhus spread to all parts of Europe, particularly during the many wars that were fought in the 17th century. It became endemic in Ireland, Italy and Russia where epidemics were frequent even in peace-time. Elsewhere, typhus epidemics mainly flared up whenever war erupted or famines occurred.

40 Some authors, such as Mercer, *Disease*, have claimed that smallpox vaccination was even the most important cause of mortality decline in this period.

41 As seen in Michael Alderson, *International Mortality Statistics* (New York: Facts on File, 1981), table 32.

42 The quote is from Hirsch, *Handbook*, vol. 1, p. 545.

Numbers of deaths were often enormous, and in several European wars more men were lost through typhus than through action on the battlefield. The well-known decimation by typhus of Napoleon's troops during the invasion of Russia is just one of many examples, as is the role of typhus in causing massive mortality during the 'Great Irish Famine'.[43]

Although improvements in personal hygiene, and the industrial production of soap for washing bodies and clothes, gradually reduced exposure to typhus in the more advanced European countries during the 19th century, targeted prevention became feasible only with the discovery in 1909 of its mode of transmission through the bites of the body louse. 'De-lousing' then proved an effective counter-strategy, and was at first carried out by a cumbersome process of bathing of bodies and heating of clothes. This was later replaced by the more practical 'fumigation' with DDT powder, which could be sprayed through sleeves and neck openings and did not require people to take off their clothes.[44]

A major typhus epidemic raged during the Balkan Wars (1912–13) and then again during World War I in Serbia, where 150,000 deaths occurred in a population of just 3 million, as well as 35,000 deaths among 70,000 Austrian prisoners-of-war. During and immediately after World War I, in the chaotic years following the October Revolution, an even more massive typhus epidemic accompanied Civil War and famine in Russia, and caused no less than 3 million deaths (Plate 9 and Suppl. Figure 8). This inspired Lenin to his famous appeal: "Comrades, we must concentrate everything on this problem. Either the lice will defeat socialism, or socialism will defeat the lice!". Large typhus epidemics also occurred in Poland, during the Russo-Polish war (1919–1922), and in Greece, due to the forced population movements during the expulsion of Greeks from Turkey (1922).[45]

Because these epidemics threatened to spread through Europe from East to West, an internationally coordinated action was mounted. Alarming reports by the Red Cross and the Rockefeller Foundation accelerated the formation of the

---

43 The fascinating history of typhus, including its role in deciding the outcome of wars, has been written several times, but most engagingly in Hans Zinsser, *Rats, Lice and History* (London etc.: Routledge [re-edition by Penguin Books in 2000], 1935). DNA testing of the remains of French soldiers of Napoleon's retreating army, buried in a mass grave in Vilnius, have confirmed the presence of *Rickettsia prowazekii* in their dental pulp; see Didier Raoult et al., "Evidence for Louse-Transmitted Diseases in Soldiers of Napoleon's Grand Army in Vilnius," *Journal of Infectious Diseases* 193, no. 1 (2006): 112–20.

44 For the history of soap, see John A. Hunt, "A Short History of Soap," *Pharmaceutical Journal* 263, no. 7076 (1999): 985–89. The development of de-lousing strategies and their benefits during World War I and II are described in John C. Snyder, "Typhus Fever in the Second World War," *California Medicine* 66, no. 1 (1947): 3–10. During World War II, a vaccine was developed, but this proved to be unsafe.

45 The quote from Vladimir Lenin can be found in his Collected Works, Vol. 30, p. 228.

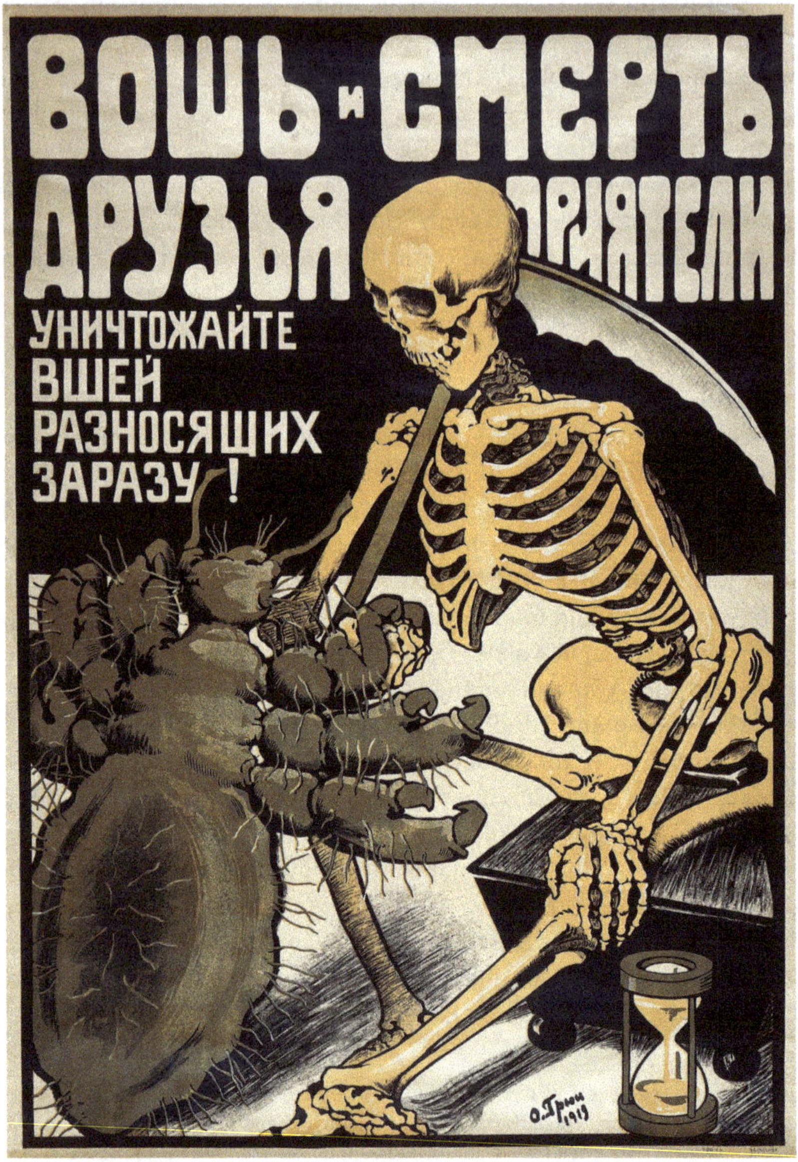
ВОШЬ и СМЕРТЬ
ДРУЗЬЯ ПРИЯТЕЛИ
УНИЧТОЖАЙТЕ
ВШЕЙ
РАЗНОСЯЩИХ
ЗАРАЗУ !
О. Грин 1919

PLATE 9 "The louse and death are friends." Russian poster warning against typhus, 1919
This poster dates from the Russian Civil War, in which the Bolsheviks fought the White Army defending the pre-Revolution status quo. This terrible war was accompanied by famine and epidemics, including a huge typhus epidemic. Translation of the Russian text: "The louse and death are friends and comrades. Kill all lice carrying infection!"
COLOUR LITHOGRAPH BY O. GRIN. WELLCOME COLLECTION

League of Nations Health Organization (LNHO) and its Epidemic Commission, which saw the control of typhus in Europe as one of its first priorities. With some international support, the government of newly independent Poland established a network of quarantine and de-lousing stations, in order to prevent further spread of typhus with the massive movements of people through its territory.[46]

After these episodes typhus kept returning to Europe, e.g., during the 1930s famine in Ukraine and Russia, during the Spanish Civil War (1936–39), and during World War II on the Eastern front, in German concentration camps, and in the Warsaw ghetto. Over-all, however, due to more effective countermeasures typhus made less casualties in and after World War II than in and after World War I.

Typhus is one of those diseases that easily lend themselves for metaphorical use, sometimes in a highly malicious way. The association with misery and lack of hygiene implied that typhus also occurred more frequently among the impoverished Jewish populations in Central and Eastern Europe. This was well-known in Germany, and in the 1930s and 1940s the Nazis used this association to reinforce antisemitism, and portrayed the Jews not only as bringers of typhus, but as a metaphorical typhus that needed to be eliminated. Gassing the Jews in concentration camps like Auschwitz thus – horrendously – became a form of 'de-lousing' the Aryan race.[47]

Malaria

Malaria is a very wide-spread disease. It can be caused by infection with four different species of *Plasmodium* parasites, which in their turn are transmitted by many different species of *Anopheles* mosquitoes. The disease probably originated in Africa, but after the Neolithic agricultural revolution established itself in the river basins of the civilizations of India, China, Mesopotamia and Egypt, from where it also reached the Mediterranean. From these original foci it spread to most of the tropical and to large parts of the temperate world.

In Europe, malaria has been prevalent nearly everywhere, even above the Arctic circle, but with a predilection for marshy regions. It occurred both in an endemic and an epidemic form. Malaria was endemic in many European regions, causing a general weakness and increased mortality from various

46 For the history of typhus control in Poland, see Francesca Piana, "Humanitaire et Politique, in Medias Res," *Relations Internationales* 2, no. 138 (2009): 23–38. Polish bacteriologist and public health pioneer Ludwik Rajchman (1881–1965) was the first chairman of the League of Nations Health Organization, and led some of the epidemic reconnaissance trips into Russia and Poland. For his biography, see Marta A. Balińska, *For the Good of Humanity* (Budapest: Central European University Press, 1998).

47 Weindling, *Epidemics*.

other causes in all years, particularly among children. It also occurred in epidemics which caused peaks of mortality even outside endemic regions. A first documented epidemic overran most of Europe in the 1550s, and again repeatedly thereafter, with at least four large epidemics in the 18th and five in the 19th century.[48]

Like epidemics of typhus, epidemics of malaria were often associated with warfare. Some of the last epidemics in Europe occurred after World War I in Southern, South-eastern and Eastern Europe. They were due to catastrophic social and medical conditions, large numbers of refugees carrying parasites, and infection of previously non-exposed populations. Some smaller epidemics occurred as recently as in World War II, even in the Netherlands.

In North-western Europe, malaria started to regress in the 18th century, with countries in the South and East following later, and some European countries were only declared malaria-free in the 1950s. Although the start of the decline long antedated the discovery of the malaria parasite in 1880, this regression was not spontaneous.

Much of the early decline was related to what we have called "changes in living conditions, pursued for reasons indirectly related to health" (Chapter 1). Expansion of agriculture required drainage of lands formerly infested with mosquitoes. Improvements in agricultural methods led to higher yields and better nutrition which increased human resistance, and where cattle breeding increased this reduced mosquito bites to humans. Over time, however, the role of disease control measures in the decline of malaria increased. This is clear from the fact that several of the malaria control measures that we now know to be effective, were already applied in the 19th century, on the basis of incomplete or even incorrect knowledge of the causes of this disease.

Five groups of effective measures are currently distinguished: (1) Prevention of mosquito bites, e.g., by screening of windows. (2) Reduction of mosquito-breeding by eliminating collections of water, e.g., by draining marshes. (3) Reduction of mosquito larvae, e.g., by applying chemicals to breeding waters. (4) Reduction of adult mosquitoes, e.g., by applying insecticides to housing areas. (5) Elimination of malaria parasites in the human host, e.g., by anti-malarial drugs. Scientific discussions on the best way to control malaria have continued

48 The information on trends and distribution of malaria in this section is based on Hirsch, *Handbook*, vol. I, pp. 197–315, and on Andrew T.A. Learmonth, "Malaria," in *World Geography of Human Diseases*, ed. G. Melvyn Howe (London etc.: Academic Press, 1977); Leonard J. Bruce-Chwatt and Julian De Zulueta, *The Rise and Fall of Malaria in Europe* (Oxford etc.: Oxford University Press, 1980); Randall M. Packard, *The Making of a Tropical Disease* (Baltimore: Johns Hopkins University Press, 2007).

throughout the 20th century, but it has been shown that in different settings different combinations of measures have worked well.[49]

As indicated above, in the 18th and 19th centuries draining marshes (strategy 2) was undertaken on a large scale, and while this was at first done mainly for economic reasons, later it was also done because of the known association between malaria and stagnant water. The effectiveness of quinine in reducing case fatality in malaria (strategy 5) was already discovered in the 17th century, and in the 19th century quinine was used extensively in the treatment of malaria.[50]

In the 20th century, malaria eradication has been in the focus of public health authorities in many European countries, and also of international organizations like the League of Nations and the Rockefeller Foundation, particularly in the period between the two World Wars. In the 1940s, the development of DDT, an insecticide which after a single spraying provided longer-term protection against mosquitoes, briefly suggested that malaria could be eradicated. Unfortunately, this turned out to be a false hope when mosquitoes became resistant.

Italy, under a fascist government, had an ambitious program to tackle malaria, which focused on drainage and land reclamation. Spain, another country where malaria was still endemic in large areas in the beginning of the 20th century, also had a national anti-malaria program which, despite resistance of large land-owners, gradually succeeded in pushing back the disease. For newly formed Yugoslavia, anti-malaria programs had a dual purpose: tackling malaria and showing the benefits of nationhood to the newly united Southern Slavs. Starting in the 1920s, the Soviet Union also had a massive program – admired by foreign observers – to push back malaria, carried out by a network of thousands of anti-malaria stations and temporary paramedical detachments.

These efforts gradually eradicated endemic malaria from Europe, as shown in Figure 12. Spain (marked in the graph), Portugal, Italy and Greece still had many cases each year during the 1930s, although a decline can already be seen in the late 1930s in Italy. Spain saw a resurgence starting during its Civil War, but this reversed into a rapid decline in the late 1940s. Russia and later the Soviet Union had millions of cases each year before and after World War I, culminating in almost 10 million cases in 1934, but rapidly got rid of malaria in the late 1940s and 1950s.

---

49 Patrick Zylberman, "A Transatlantic Dispute," in *Shifting Boundaries of Public Health*, ed. Susan Gross Solomon, Lion Murard, and Patrick Zylberman (Rochester: University of Rochester Press, 2008).

50 Medical scientists in the 19th century believed that many diseases that are now considered to be infectious, found their origins in a 'miasma': noxious air emanating from rotting organic material in the soil. The term 'malaria' (literally: "bad air") still refers to this theory which is now obsolete, but did inspire effective public health interventions.

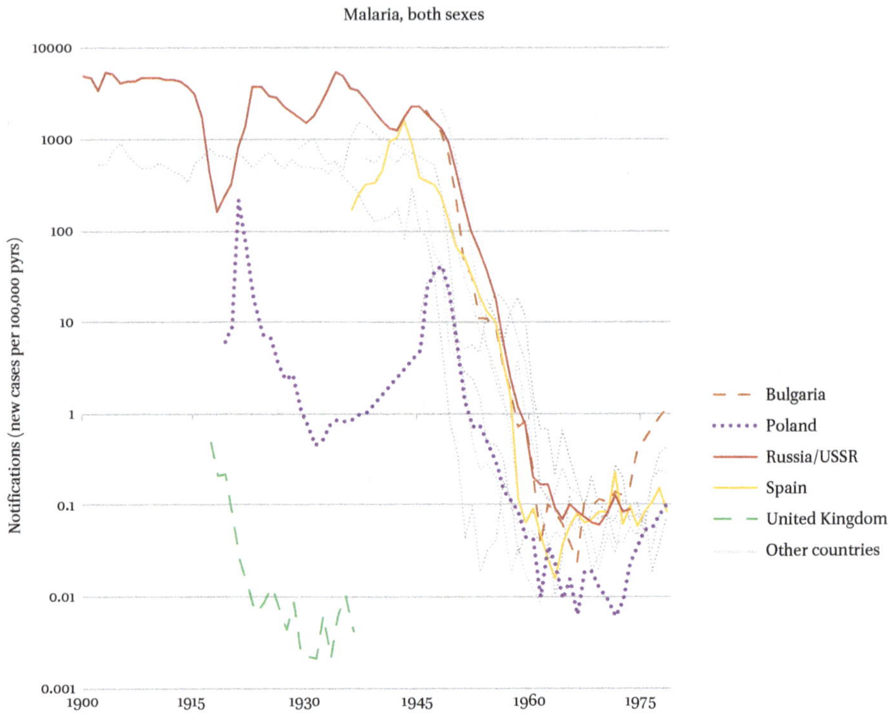

FIGURE 12 Trends in malaria incidence in Europe, 1900–1978
Notes: Logarithmic scale
SOURCE OF DATA: LEONARD J. BRUCE-CHWATT AND JULIAN DE ZULUETA. *THE RISE AND FALL OF MALARIA IN EUROPE* OXFORD ETC.: OXFORD UNIVERSITY PRESS, 1980. VARIOUS TABLES

The decline of malaria in Europe, which probably started in the 18th century, was accompanied – and not entirely coincidentally – by a rise of malaria at the other side of the world, i.e., in the larger Caribbean. The creation of sugar plantations in which black slaves from Africa were put to work, helped develop Europe's economy, but also introduced endemic malaria in the South-eastern United States, on Caribbean islands, and in North-eastern Brazil.[51]

More recently, the rise of global traveling increased the numbers of imported cases, and climate change threatens to bring endemic malaria back, particularly in Southern Europe.

51 John R. McNeill, *Mosquito Empires* (Cambridge etc.: Cambridge University Press, 2010).

CHAPTER 5

Health Problems of Industrializing Societies

In terms of population health, developments in Europe during the 18th and 19th centuries were not only positive. As a side effect of industrialization and urbanization, there was a rise in many diseases, which were only gradually brought under control. This chapter reviews the secular trends in a number of health conditions which first rose and then started to decline again in this period. These include a number of communicable diseases, as well as maternal and infant mortality, and some other, less easily classifiable diseases.

Communicable Diseases

Cholera, Dysentery, Typhoid

Cholera is one of the most extensively studied epidemic diseases of the 19th century. This is not only because it was such a deadly and frightening disease, but also because the experience of cholera played an important role in the genesis of public health as we know it today. It was particularly important for the acceptance of public health's most well-known method of prevention: 'sanitation'.[1]

Cholera was such a frightening disease because it gave symptoms of massive vomiting and diarrhoea and could be rapidly fatal, sometimes within 12 hours after symptom onset (Plate 10). Patients lost enormous amounts of body fluid, and because dehydration caused a change of the colour of the skin it became known as the 'blue disease'. It is caused by infection with the bacterium *Vibrio cholerae*, discovered as the cause of cholera in 1883 by German physician Robert Koch (1843–1910). It spreads by the faecal-oral route, and can nowadays be prevented by a vaccine and treated with oral rehydration therapy and antibiotics, but all this knowledge lay in the distant future when cholera first struck Europe in the 1830s.

The origins of cholera lie in the Indian subcontinent where it has been endemic for millennia. However, in the 19th century, probably as a result of an

1 A general history of cholera can be found in Christopher Hamlin, *Cholera: The Biography* (Oxford etc.: Oxford University Press, 2009). Before cholera pandemics reached Europe, the term 'cholera' referred to all kinds of diarrheal diseases. After the first pandemic reached Europe this 'new' cholera was referred to as 'Asiatic cholera'.

 | DOI:10.1163/9789004429130_006

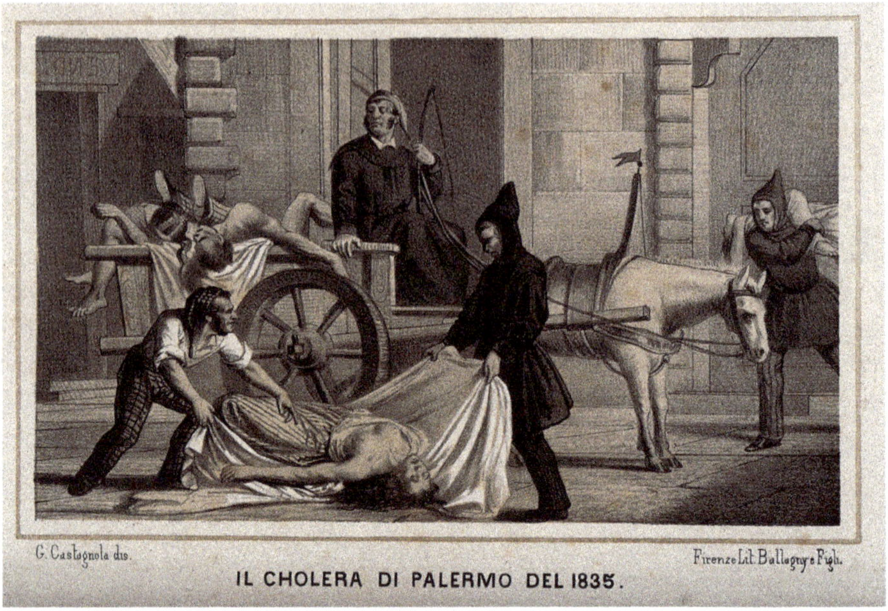

PLATE 10 Cholera victims being carried away in Palermo, 1835
Like many other cities in Europe, Palermo (on Sicily) was hit by the second cholera pandemic. Cholera sometimes struck so quickly that people died on the streets. This plate shows men in uniform picking up a corpse in the street and putting it on a wagon.
PRINT BASED ON DRAWING BY GABRIELE CASTAGNOLA. WELLCOME COLLECTION (CC BY 4.0)

increase in long-distance travel, the disease spread to other parts of the world in six large waves. The first of these pandemics (1817–24) did not reach Europe, with the exception of the region of Astrakhan at the South-eastern border of the Russian Empire. The other ones did reach Europe and caused large numbers of deaths, reminding people of the plague and shaking Europeans' confidence in progress. Epidemics spread along waterways, and later also and more rapidly along railways.[2]

The second pandemic (1829–37) reached Europe from India overland through Russia, from where it spread westwards, partly through troop movements in the on-going Russo-Polish War. It reached Western Europe in 1831 and 1832, and caused hundreds of thousands of deaths altogether (see Suppl. Table 7). The third pandemic (1846–60) followed a similar route and reached Europe

2 The spread of cholera during the pandemics has been documented in, e.g., Hirsch, *Handbook*, vol. 1, pp. 394–493, and in Reinhard Speck, "Cholera," in *Cambridge World History of Human Disease*, ed. Kenneth F. Kiple (Cambridge etc.: Cambridge University Press, 1993).

through Russia again. This was the most fatal of all European cholera epidemics, and caused more than one million deaths in Russia alone, perhaps because it coincided with a turbulent period in European political history and occurred immediately after the famines of the 1840s.[3]

The fourth pandemic (1863–75) followed a different route and arrived in Europe from Egypt. Its spread was again partly propagated by troop movements, in this case during the Austro-Prussian war of 1866. This was the last of the pandemics to cause large numbers of deaths in North-western Europe, because it stimulated many cities and countries to implement sanitation measures, in the form of piped drinking water and sewage systems. During the fifth pandemic (1881–96) the only larger North-western European city afflicted by cholera was Hamburg, where more than 8000 people died because the city had neglected to effectively filtrate its piped drinking water. However, this pandemic still caused large numbers of deaths in Southern and Eastern Europe.[4]

The gradual retreat of cholera continued during the sixth pandemic (1899–23), which mainly caused large-scale mortality in Russia and South-eastern Europe, but also – less well-known, because the Italian authorities tried to hide it – struck Naples and parts of Southern Italy in 1910–11. Whereas the rest of Europe was now reasonably well protected against the disease, the sixth pandemic still caused large numbers of deaths in South-eastern Europe during the Balkan Wars, and more than half a million deaths in Russia during the Civil war.[5]

What caused the decline (or non-return) of cholera? As the geographical variations illustrate, the implementation of effective sanitation measures certainly played an important role, together with improvements in personal hygiene. These changes were based on a better understanding of the causes of

3 K. David Patterson, "Cholera Diffusion in Russia, 1823–1923," *Social Science & Medicine* 38, no. 9 (1994): 1171–91. In Western Europe, the numbers were not as large as the ensuing panic suggests: deaths from cholera accounted for no more than 1% of total mortality in the 1848–72 period in England and Wales; see John Charlton and Mike Murphy, *The Health of Adult Britain 1841–1994. Decennial Supplement No. 12* (London: The Stationery Office, 1997), vol. 1, p. 32.

4 Weaving many interesting threads together, the fascinating story of the last cholera epidemic in Hamburg has been told in Richard J. Evans, *Death in Hamburg* (Oxford: Clarendon Press, 1987).

5 A combination of civic pride and fear of economic damage led the authorities to deny that a cholera epidemic occurred, and to fabricate health statistics to hide the 2600 cholera deaths in Naples and 14,000 deaths in Italy as a whole; see Frank M. Snowden, *Naples in the Time of Cholera, 1884–1911* (Cambridge etc.: Cambridge University Press, 1995). During the 20th century a seventh pandemic (1961–75), caused by the milder *Vibrio El Tor*, never reached Europe.

the disease and on gradual acceptance of intervention by the state, even if this interfered with personal freedom or commercial interests.[6]

Success was not immediate, however, as shown by the fact that cholera had to return at least three times before effective countermeasures were taken. When cholera first spread in Europe to the 1830s, it led to the imposition of quarantines and *cordons sanitaires*, which had been effective to contain plague epidemics. Yet, when epidemiological observations on the effects of these measures in Russia proved to be inconclusive, faith in contagion and the effectiveness of *cordons sanitaires* was lost.

Until the 1880s, when Robert Koch's discovery finally convinced (almost) everyone that cholera was contagious, cholera was a scientific battleground between those who believed that it somehow spread between humans ('contagionists'), and those who believed that cholera was not contagious but somehow emanated from the soil ('anti-contagionists'). The latter view could long be held not only because it was difficult to unambiguously prove that cholera was contagious, but also because anti-contagionism provided an argument for economically liberal governments to oppose restrictions on free trade.[7]

However, it did gradually become clear that cholera spread through contaminated drinking water. John Snow's (1813–1858) studies of cholera in London, leading to the famous removal of the handle of the Broad Street pump, were conducted during the third pandemic and published in 1855. Although his views were not immediately and widely accepted, studies by William Farr (1807–1883) of differences in cholera risks between different companies supplying London's drinking water during the fourth pandemic provided further evidence that contaminated drinking water was the culprit.[8]

---

6 See Patrice Bourdelais, *Épidémies Terrassées,* Chapter 3, for a nuanced synthesis of the various factors (medical, cultural, political, ...) contributing to the decline of cholera in Europe.

7 The classic history of anti-contagionism was written by Ackerknecht, "Anticontagionism." There is a clear analogy between anti-contagionism in the 19th century and 20th century forms of 'denialism' such as the denial of the harmful effects of smoking, both supported by commercial interests; see Mark Harrison, *Contagion* (New Haven and London: Yale University Press, 2012).

8 The history of the scientific disputes and eventual consensus on the causes of cholera is more complex than can be explained here; see Jan P. Vandenbroucke, H.M. Eelkman Rooda, and Harm Beukers, "Who Made John Snow a Hero?," *American Journal of Epidemiology* 133, no. 10 (1991): 967–73; George Davey Smith, "Commentary: Behind the Broad Street Pump," *International Journal of Epidemiology* 31, no. 5 (2002): 920–32; Alfredo Morabia, "Epidemiologic Interactions, Complexity, and the Lonesome Death of Max Von Pettenkofer," *American Journal of Epidemiology* 166, no. 11 (2007): 1233–38.

Convincing scientific evidence was certainly not the only condition which needed to be fulfilled for the implementation of large-scale sanitation measures that required enormous public investments. Another condition was that a degree of political consensus arose that this was necessary, or at least inevitable. As this was a period in which political conservatism and economic liberalism reigned supreme, this was far from self-evident and required an argumentation that fitted within the dominant way of thinking.

This can again be illustrated with the well-researched history of cholera prevention in Britain, where Edwin Chadwick (1800–1890) had published his *Report on The Sanitary Condition of the Labouring Population of Great Britain* in 1842, just before the third pandemic struck. This report showed that ill-health often caused poverty among the labouring classes, and was an important contributor to the high costs of public poverty relief. Chadwick therefore recommended to provide each house with a constant water supply and with water-closets that would discharge into sewers. These would carry faecal waste to rural areas where it could be spread on the land as manure, preventing rivers from becoming polluted. This 'sanitary idea' was soon adopted, and became popular throughout Europe.[9]

Strikingly, the second, third and fourth pandemics all occurred in periods of political upheaval in Europe, and in association with revolution and wars. This is probably not a coincidence: unrest produced cholera, and cholera produced unrest. As mentioned above, the spread of cholera was often promoted by mass movements of people, during war or in response to famines, although most spread was due to trade. Cholera could also produce unrest, as in the case of 'cholera riots' against the elites in Russia or civil protests against restrictions on movement and trade.[10]

In addition to cholera, many other intestinal infections played a role in the high death rates of industrializing societies. These other diseases were less eye-catching, but their accumulated death toll has been much larger than that of cholera. They must have become common as soon as humans adopted a sedentary lifestyle, and had assumed epidemic proportions in the 17th and 18th

---

9 Hamlin has argued that the health problems highlighted in Chadwick's *Report on The Sanitary Condition of the Labouring Population of Great Britain* could have been solved in other ways, e.g., by improving the economic situation of the lower classes. The choice for sanitation reflected a desire to stay away from politically less acceptable recommendations; see Christopher Hamlin, *Public Health and Social Justice in the Age of Chadwick: Britain, 1800–1854* (Cambridge etc.: Cambridge University Press, 1998).

10 Richard J. Evans, "Epidemics and Revolutions: Cholera in Nineteenth-Century Europe," *Past & Present*, no. 120 (1988): 123–46.

centuries. Within the larger family of diarrheal diseases, a few stand out as having been particularly important.

Dysentery, a disease mainly caused by *Shigella* bacteria, is characterized by a typical bloody diarrhoea and was therefore already recognized in antiquity. It caused major epidemics during military campaigns and famines, but as an endemic disease also caused many deaths among infants and children in 'normal' years.[11]

Typhoid fever, a disease caused by *Salmonella typhi* bacteria, had less distinctive symptoms, and was long confused with typhus (see Chapter 4). It was only in the 1830s that the difference between the two diseases was recognized, and it is therefore difficult to trace the history of this disease through the ages. Together with what we now call paratyphoid fever, due to infection by other members of the *Salmonella* family, it used to cause huge numbers of cases of disease and deaths. Dysentery, typhoid and the other intestinal infections are all spread by contaminated food and water, which was gradually discovered in the second half of the 19th century, often before the responsible micro-organisms were identified.[12]

In North-western Europe, mortality from intestinal infections started to decline around the middle of the 19th century, as a result of gradual improvements in sanitation (see Suppl. Figure 9). Very steep declines continued in the first half of the 20th century. As in the case of other diseases, declines in mortality in other European regions followed later. In the beginning of the 20th century, mortality rates from typhoid and paratyphoid fever were still very high in Spain, Italy and other Southern European countries, and undoubtedly also in South-eastern and Eastern Europe, although for these countries the data series start considerably later. In many countries, mortality from typhoid and paratyphoid rose during both World Wars, as it did in Spain during the Civil War.[13]

11 For a history of bacillary dysentery, see Hirsch, *Handbook*, Vol. III, pp. 284–370, and K. David Patterson, "Bacillary Dysentery," in *Cambridge World History of Human Disease*, ed. Kenneth F. Kiple (Cambridge etc.: Cambridge University Press, 1993).

12 For a history of typhoid fever, see Hirsch, *Handbook*, vol. I, pp. 617–87, and Dale Smith, "Typhoid Fever," in *Cambridge World History of Human Disease*, ed. Kenneth F. Kiple (Cambridge etc.: Cambridge University Press, 1993).

13 Long-term trends in mortality from intestinal infections have been analysed for England & Wales in Woods, *Demography*; Galbraith and McCormack, "Infection in England and Wales"; for the Netherlands in Judith H. Wolleswinkel-van den Bosch et al., "Cause-Specific Mortality Trends in the Netherlands, 1875–1992," *International Journal of Epidemiology* 26, no. 4 (1997): 772–81; and for Spain in Vicente Pérez Moreda, David S. Reher, and Alberto Sanz Gimeno, *La Conquista de la Salud* (Madrid: Marcial Pons, Ediciones de Historia, 2015).

Tuberculosis

The history of tuberculosis has been studied extensively – and for good reasons, because it was probably the most important cause of death in Northern and Western Europe during much of the 18th and 19th centuries. In cities like London, Paris, The Hague and Stockholm, respiratory tuberculosis, the most important form of this disease, accounted for between 10 and 25% of all deaths. Somewhat lower but still astonishingly high figures applied to countries as a whole when, in the course of the 19th century, national cause-of-death statistics became available. Because mortality was highest among young adults, the demographic, economic and social consequences were huge.[14]

Since then, tuberculosis mortality has declined enormously. The study of the causes of this decline has become something like a scientific battlefield, between those who have argued that the decline of tuberculosis mortality is mainly due to improvements in living standards, and those who have emphasized the contribution of public health and other interventions. Since the 1970s, when McKeown published his iconoclastic studies of the decline of mortality in England & Wales, the first point of view for some time had the upper hand, but the accumulated weight of the critiques of McKeown's analyses has gradually shifted the balance of opinion towards the second point of view.[15]

Tuberculosis is a disease that is caused by infection with *Mycobacterium tuberculosis*, which was discovered in 1882 by Robert Koch, who also discovered the causative agent of cholera. It usually enters the body through the lungs, where it may cause acute infection, but the bacterium may also lie dormant for a long time and still cause disease after many years, when the immune system fails as a result of stress, undernourishment, or – as has occurred more recently – HIV infection. While tuberculosis of the lungs and other respiratory organs is the most common form of the disease, many other organs may become affected, and without adequate treatment active tuberculosis has a high case fatality.

In the 19th century, another type of tuberculosis, caused by infection with *Mycobacterium bovis*, was also common, accounting for 20–30% of all nonpulmonary tuberculosis. This milder form of tuberculosis was transmitted in

14 Data for London are in Mercer, *Disease*. Data for Paris are in Victor K. Kuagbenou and Jean-Noel Biraben, *Introduction à l'Etude de la Mortalite par Cause de Décès à Paris dans la Première Moitié du XIXème Siècle* (Paris: Institut National d'Études Démographiques, 1998). Data for The Hague are in Pieter R.D. Stokvis, *De Wording van Modern Den Haag* (Zwolle: Waanders, 1987). Data for Stockholm are in Britt-Inger Puranen, *Tuberkulos: En Sjukdoms Förekomst och Dess Orsaker: Sverige 1750–1980*, vol. 7, Umeå Studies in Economic History, (Umeå: Umeå Universitet, 1984).

15 See Chapter 3 for a summary of this discussion.

cow's milk and mainly occurred among infants and young children. In the 20th century, it was eradicated by a combination of livestock sanitation (i.e., testing cattle for tuberculosis and destroying infected animals) and milk pasteurization.[16]

The term 'tuberculosis' refers to 'tubercles', i.e., the characteristic lumps of tissue which are found in the body of tuberculosis patients, and which contain tuberculosis bacteria. Before this term came in use, the disease was known under names like 'consumption', 'phthisis', and similar terms in national languages. These refer to a symptom characteristic of later stages of the disease, i.e., a state of exhaustion interrupted by temporary flare-ups, in which the patient appears to be 'consumed' by his or her illness.[17]

Before the discovery of the causative agent, it was widely believed, at least in Northern and Western Europe, that the main causes of tuberculosis were 'constitutional', i.e., that the disease found its origin in genetic and other characteristics of the diseased individual. It is not difficult to understand how this idea arose. Due to the slow progression of the disease it was not immediately obvious from where or whom individual cases arose, and tuberculosis was so common that often whole families fell ill. Yet, in Southern Europe tuberculosis was less common, and people generally believed that it was contagious even before the bacteriological revolution.[18]

Tuberculosis is an age-old human disease: traces of tuberculosis infection have been recovered from Egyptian and Peruvian mummies more than 1000 years old. The emergence of tuberculosis as an important infectious disease of humans is associated with the shift from hunting-gathering to the sedentary life of agriculturists, which greatly increased opportunities for transmission.[19]

However, as a result of industrialization and urbanization tuberculosis became much more prevalent, and much more important as a cause of death, in the 18th and 19th centuries. Overcrowded housing, exposure to dust in mining and other occupations, and a rise of excessive alcohol consumption – to name

16 Amy L. Fairchild and Gerald M. Oppenheimer, "Public Health Nihilism Vs Pragmatism," *American Journal of Public Health* 88, no. 7 (1998): 1105–17.

17 In the 19th century, these symptoms gave rise to a certain 'romanticization' of tuberculosis. The usual pallor of tuberculosis patients inspired a new beauty ideal, and because artists who died of tuberculosis sometimes produced great works of art during their flare-ups, it was thought that tuberculosis sparked genius; see René J. Dubos and Jean Dubos, *The White Plague* (Boston: Little, Brown & Company, 1952), Chapter 5.

18 As a result, tuberculosis patients from the North who came to the Mediterranean to heal, were sometimes refused access to hotels, as happened to Frédéric Chopin (1810–1849) on Mallorca; see Dubos and Dubos, *The White Plague*, 31–32.

19 Sharon Levy, "The Evolution of Tuberculosis," *BioScience* 62, no. 7 (2012): 625–29.

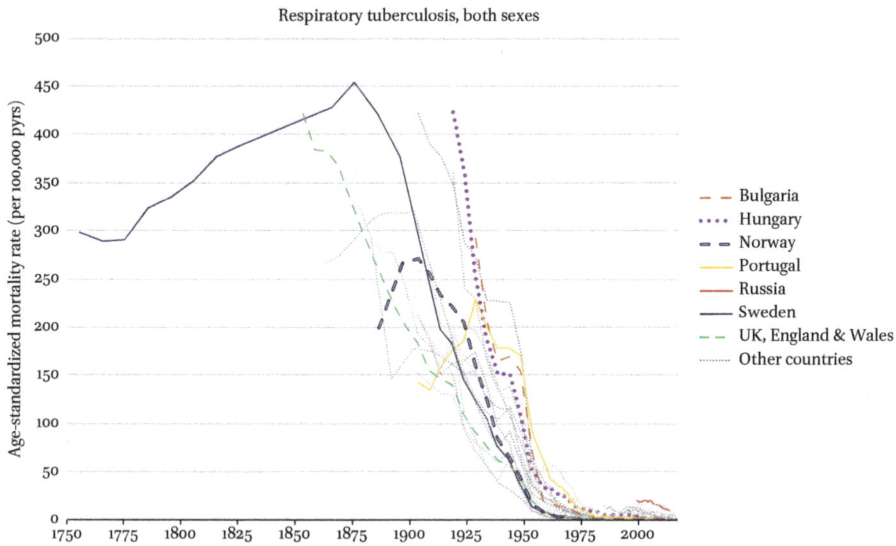

FIGURE 13 Trends in tuberculosis mortality in Europe, 1750–2015
Notes: Both sexes combined Before 1900: decadal or quinquennial data from various sources, calibrated using overlaps with data from Alderson for the first years of the 20th century. Between 1900 and 1960: quinquennial data
SOURCE OF DATA: BEFORE 1900: VARIOUS NATIONAL PUBLICATIONS; AFTER 1900: SEE SUPPL. TABLE 1

just a few side-effects of the Industrial Revolution – increased the likelihood of tuberculosis transmission as well as the likelihood of a fatal outcome of the disease. The resulting rise of mortality can clearly be seen in Swedish mortality data, which show an increase in mortality from respiratory tuberculosis between ca. 1750 and ca. 1850. In many other countries, this rise probably occurred before the start of national cause-of-death registration, but a rise can be witnessed in a few other European countries as well, such as Norway and Portugal where mortality rose until ca. 1900 and ca. 1930, respectively (Figure 13).[20]

In most countries, all we can see in the available data is a decline of tuberculosis mortality, and it is impossible to give a precise date to its start. McKeown

20 Long-term trends in mortality from tuberculosis in Sweden have been analysed in Puranen, *Tuberkulos*, 7; Britt-Inger Puranen, "Tuberculosis and the Decline of Mortality in Sweden," in *The Decline of Mortality in Europe*, ed. Roger S. Schofield, David S. Reher, and Alain Bideau (Oxford etc.: Clarendon Press, 1991). These publications show that tuberculosis mortality in Finland rose to a peak in the late 1800s, and then declined, but slower than in Sweden, in the 20th century.

thought that the decline in mortality from respiratory tuberculosis in England & Wales started around 1850, i.e., before sanitation and other public health interventions could be expected to have had an impact. Yet, as he himself noted, the timing is uncertain because of problems in cause-of-death classification and irregular fluctuations in the mortality rate. Others have argued that mortality decline did not start before the late 1860s, i.e., in a time when public health interventions may have started to have an effect.[21]

In addition to England & Wales, Sweden and the Netherlands also had a relatively early decline, i.e., a decline starting before or around 1875, but, as mentioned above, in some other European countries the decline started around the turn of the century or even later. As is clear from Figure 13, declines of mortality were generally precipitous, and although the rate of decline naturally slowed down in absolute terms as the mortality rate started to approach the null, in relative (or percentage) terms the rate of decline actually accelerated in the 1940s and 1950s in all European countries.[22]

Two other observations that can be made on Figure 13 – and which tuberculosis shares with several other causes of death – are that during most of the 20th century, countries in Southern and Central-eastern Europe lagged behind countries in Northern and Western Europe in their tuberculosis mortality decline. Countries in Central-eastern and Eastern Europe – for the latter, only post-World War II data are available – also experienced a renewed (but small) rise of tuberculosis mortality in the 1990s and 2000s.

As mentioned above, there are several competing explanations for this long-term decline of tuberculosis mortality. A first possibility to consider is a spontaneous, favourable change in the biological relationship between the 'agent' (*Mycobacterium tuberculosis*) and its 'host' (European citizens). This is an explanation that always needs to be considered when one deals with the time-course of infectious diseases, because these often become less severe over time. This can occur through selection of less virulent bacteria which, because they do not kill or incapacitate their hosts, have a greater likelihood to spread to other people. On a longer time-scale, it can also occur through selective survival of genetically more resistant hosts. However, although this may have played a role in the early declines of tuberculosis mortality, it is a less likely explanation for the continued decline in later stages, because changes in

21 For McKeown's analysis of the start of the decline in mortality from respiratory tuberculosis in England and Wales, see McKeown and Record, "Reasons for the Decline of Mortality in England and Wales." For a detailed critique, see Szreter, "Social Intervention."

22 As noted by McKeown, and later shown in interrupted time-series analyses in Finland (Hemminki and Paakkulainen, "Antibiotics") and The Netherlands (Mackenbach and Looman, "Secular Trends").

virulence of *Mycobacterium tuberculosis* have never been demonstrated in laboratory studies, and because effects of the disease on reproduction of tuberculosis patients were limited.[23]

Another autonomously operating, biological factor may have been more important. As soon as the incidence of tuberculosis mortality starts to decline, for example as a result of isolation of patients or less overcrowding, the number of patients who can spread the disease to others also becomes less. This will set in motion a self-propelling mechanism which, as has been shown in mathematical modelling studies, may well have been partly responsible for the continued rapid decline of the disease during the 20th century.[24]

A second factor to consider is a general improvement in living standards, which decreased the risks of transmission (e.g., through more spacious housing with less overcrowding) or the risk of becoming ill when infected (e.g., through better nutrition). Despite all the scientific criticisms of McKeown's work, in which this explanation was championed, there can be little doubt that, during the whole trajectory of mortality decline, nutrition and other factors linked to general living standards must indeed have played a role. For example, tuberculosis mortality in many European countries rose during World Wars I and II, even in those countries that stayed neutral, and studies have shown that the most likely explanation was food scarcity.[25]

Furthermore, while McKeown did not have data on changes in food consumption in England & Wales during the 19th century, and thus had to speculate about the role of this factor, later studies have shown that food availability in this country did rise between 1750 and 1800, then stagnated between 1800 and 1850, and rose again between 1850 and 1900. These changes roughly coincide with periods of rising, stagnating and again rising life expectancy at birth, and provide some support for the idea that improvements in nutrition may have helped to bring down tuberculosis mortality.[26]

---

23 See Puranen, "Tuberculosis" for an argumentation. On changes in virulence as an explanation for the decline of tuberculosis, see Woods, *Demography*, 332–40.

24 E. Vynnycky and P.E. Fine, "Interpreting the Decline in Tuberculosis: The Role of Secular Trends in Effective Contact," *International Journal of Epidemiology* 28, no. 2 (1999): 327–34.

25 War-related food shortages caused increases in tuberculosis mortality in, e.g., France during the Franco-Prussian War (1870–71), and in the Netherlands and Denmark during World War I (1914–1918); see Dubos and Dubos, *The White Plague*; Godias J. Drolet, "World War I and Tuberculosis. A Statistical Summary and Review," *American Journal of Public Health and the Nations Health* 35, no. 7 (1945): 689–97.

26 Bernard Harris, "Public Health, Nutrition, and the Decline of Mortality," *Social History of Medicine* 17, no. 3 (2004): 379–407. Periods of increasing and stagnating life expectancy also coincided with periods of increasing and stagnating height of British military

The third factor to consider – largely rejected by McKeown but increasingly accepted as an important contributory factor in the decline of tuberculosis mortality – is public health and medical interventions. Improvements in housing were not only a side-effect of increased living standards, but were also the result of stricter housing regulations and government investments in public housing projects, particularly after the turn of the 20th century. A similar point can be made for working conditions, which partly improved as a side-effect of changes in production and mining methods, but were also the result of labour union demands and labour protection laws.

Medical knowledge also helped to limit the spread of the disease, e.g., by educating patients not to spit, and by treating infective patients in hospitals or sanatoria instead of at home. Vaccination, first used in 1921, and outreaching facilities for prevention and treatment of tuberculosis, implemented in many European countries in the 1920s, were important as well.[27]

Even before the 1940s, treatment probably also contributed to mortality decline. Although the first highly effective medical treatment, antibiotics, only became available in the 1940s, previous generations of doctors had gradually worked out how to treat tuberculosis patients. In the course of the 19th century, the newly invented stethoscope helped to diagnose the condition more accurately. Some treatments, such as a combination of rest and a nutritious diet, or collapsing the affected lung by surgically creating an artificial pneumothorax, may already have helped to slow down the progression of the disease.

The first effective drugs against tuberculosis, such as streptomycin, arrived late in the course of tuberculosis mortality decline in England & Wales, and therefore made a relatively small contribution in this country, as well as in other North-western European countries where tuberculosis mortality was already well underway. However, as Figure 13 shows, in those countries where

---

recruits, lending further support to the idea that improved nutrition played a role in these secular trends (Floud et al., *Changing Body*, Chapter 4). Yet, the importance of nutrition should not be overrated, because as shown in Puranen, "Tuberculosis" in 18th century Sweden members of the royal family, who were well-fed, did not have lower tuberculosis mortality than their servants.

27 See Szreter, "Social Intervention" for a general overview. The decline of tuberculosis mortality in England & Wales in the second half of the 19th century was already studied by early 20th century scholars, who showed that segregation of poor people with tuberculosis in 'poorhouses' probably made an important contribution to mortality decline; see Arthur Newsholme, "An Inquiry into the Principal Causes of the Reduction in the Death-Rate from Phthisis During the Last Forty Years," *Journal of Hygiene (Camb.)* 6 (1906): 304–84; Leonard G. Wilson, "The Historical Decline of Tuberculosis in Europe and America," *Journal of the History of Medicine and Allied Sciences* 45, no. 3 (1990): 366–96.

tuberculosis mortality was still high, the precipitous declines in the 1940s and 1950s accounted for a much larger part of mortality decline.[28]

Although it has not been possible to disentangle the separate contribution of each of these three factors, a reasonable conclusion is that the decline of tuberculosis mortality reflects the combined and mutually reinforcing effect of all three. The relative importance of each factor has likely shifted over time, and has probably also been different between European countries, because they differed in their timing of tuberculosis mortality decline. Seen from a European perspective, it strikes one as a little odd that so much energy has been spent on finding the main factor driving tuberculosis mortality decline in England & Wales – a country unlikely to be representative for the wider European experience.

As can be seen in Figure 13, recent trends in tuberculosis have not been altogether favourable. During the 1990s, mortality from respiratory tuberculosis increased again in the former Soviet Union, and also in some South-eastern European countries (Bulgaria and Romania) and in Portugal. Because of the decoupling of mortality and incidence, trends in mortality no longer give an accurate picture of trends in incidence, and incidence has risen almost everywhere, also in Northern and Western Europe.[29]

This renewed rise of tuberculosis has a complex explanation. One immediate cause is the rise of drug-resistant, and then multi-drug resistant, and then extremely multi-drug resistant, strains of Mycobacteria. Another part of the story is that, after the successful push-back on tuberculosis in the 1940s and 1950s, tuberculosis control programs were neglected in many European countries.

However, wider societal factors also played a role. Immigration from countries outside Europe where tuberculosis was still endemic raised its incidence,

28 The effect of the introduction of antibiotic treatment is not only apparent from an acceleration of mortality decline (Hemminki and Paakkulainen, "Antibiotics"; Mackenbach and Looman, "Secular Trends") but also from a widening of the gap between incidence and mortality. Before the 1940s, trends for tuberculosis mortality and incidence ran in parallel, but after the 1940s mortality declined much faster than incidence; see Philippe Glaziou, Katherine Floyd, and Mario Raviglione, "Trends in Tuberculosis in the UK," *Thorax* 73 (2018): 702–03.

29 Rising trends in tuberculosis incidence in the 1990s were signalled in Mario C. Raviglione et al., "Secular Trends of Tuberculosis in Western Europe," *Bulletin of the World Health Organization* 71, no. 3–4 (1993): 297–306; Mario C. Raviglione et al., "Tuberculosis Trends in Eastern Europe and the Former USSR," *Tubercle and Lung disease* 75, no. 6 (1994): 400–16. For recent European trends, see European Centers for Disease Control, *Tuberculosis Surveillance and Monitoring in Europe 2019* (Copenhagen: WHO Regional Office for Europe, 2019).

as did the epidemics of injecting drug use and – partly related – AIDS. In the background, an increasing prevalence of homelessness, and increasing socio-economic inequality generally, made parts of the population more vulnerable. Increasing rates of incarceration, and inadequate control of tuberculosis in prisons, also contributed.[30]

In response to this (world-wide) surge of tuberculosis, strong international action has been mounted, and more recently tuberculosis incidence and mortality in Europe have declined again.[31]

Syphilis

The mortality trends for syphilis are somewhat similar to those for respiratory tuberculosis in the same period, with steep declines during most of the 20th century (see Suppl. Figure 10). In contrast to tuberculosis there has been no epidemic rise of mortality from syphilis in the 1990s, but in this case mortality trends are somewhat misleading. Syphilis mortality has become almost completely decoupled from syphilis incidence, even more so than tuberculosis mortality has become decoupled from tuberculosis incidence, and hiding below the flat trends in syphilis mortality in the second half of the 20th century are rises of syphilis incidence of epidemic proportions.

The available evidence on long-term trends in syphilis incidence in Europe suggests that trends since the beginning of the 20th century, when syphilis incidence and prevalence were still very high, can be characterized as an over-all decline interrupted by four periods of steep temporary increases. Incidence and prevalence of syphilis in the general population rose during World War I, then declined, rose again during and shortly after World War II, declined to its lowest level ever in the 1950s, then rose again during and after the 'sexual revolution' of the 1960s, declined in response to the AIDS epidemic of the 1980s, but rose again in the 1990s after the AIDS scare had disappeared.[32]

30 On the rise of extremely drug-resistant strains of Mycobacteria, see Mario C. Raviglione, "XDR-TB: Entering the Post-Antibiotic Era?," *International Journal of Tuberculosis and Lung Disease* 10, no. 11 (2006): 1185–87. On the failure of tuberculosis control in the former Soviet Union, see Olga S. Toungoussova, Gunnar Bjune, and Dominique A. Caugant, "Epidemic of Tuberculosis in the Former Soviet Union," *Tuberculosis* 86, no. 1 (2006): 1–10. On the role of immigration in the rise of tuberculosis incidence, see H.L. Rieder et al., "Tuberculosis Control in Europe and International Migration," *European Respiratory Journal* 7, no. 8 (1994): 1545–53. On the role of social factors in the recent rise of tuberculosis, see Paul Farmer, "Social Inequalities and Emerging Infectious Diseases," *Emerging Infectious Diseases* 2, no. 4 (1996): 259–69.

31 See European Centers for Disease Control, *Tuberculosis Surveillance and Monitoring in Europe*.

32 For trends in the 19th century we are skating on very thin ice, with some military statistics indicating a decline and other data indicating little systematic change in the population

Syphilis is a treacherous disease. After infection, it may lead to 'early infectious syphilis' with local ulceration a few weeks after infection, followed, after a few symptomless weeks, by a variety of a-specific signs of illness (skin rash, headaches, sore throat etc.). These symptoms usually disappear spontaneously, leading to a latent period of up to many years, but the disease may then return in the form of 'late syphilis' with serious cardiovascular and neurological complications, eventually leading to paralysis, dementia and even death. Syphilis is caused by infection with *Treponema pallidum* which was discovered in 1905. In contrast to many other infectious diseases, however, the contagious nature of syphilis was obvious to medical professionals and lay people long before the bacteriological revolution.[33]

The origins of syphilis have long been debated, but it is most likely that it was brought from the Americas to Europe by Columbus and other seafarers in the last decade of the 15th century. It spread rapidly, partly as a result of Europe-wide military campaigns, and originally had a violent and malignant

at large. Statistics on syphilis among young men enlisting for the army in the United Kingdom indicate a decline between 1870 and 1910 (O. Idsoe and Thorstein Guthe, "The Rise and Fall of the Treponematoses. 1. Ecological Aspects and International Trends. In Venereal Syphilis," *British Journal of Venereal Diseases* 43, no. 4 (1967): 227–43). However, it is unclear whether this can be extrapolated to the general British population, because reconstructions of trends in syphilis in Britain between the 1770s and 1911–12 found little change (Simon Szreter, "Treatment Rates for the Pox in Early Modern England," *Continuity and Change* 32, no. 2 (2017): 183–223). My summary of trends in the 20th century is mainly based on compulsory notification data on syphilis in the general population as found in Idsoe and Guthe, "The Rise and Fall of the Treponematoses. 1"; Inga Lind and Steen Hoffmann, "Recorded Gonorrhoea Rates in Denmark, 1900–2010," *BMJ Open* 5, no. 11 (2015): e008013; Thorstein Guthe, *Worldwide Epidemiological Trends in Syphilis and Gonorrhea* (Washington: World Health Organization, 1970); Annet Mooij, *Geslachtsziekten en Besmettingsangst* (Amsterdam: Boom, 1993). As recently as 1913–1916, around 8% (ranging between 4% in rural districts and 11% in London) of all men in their mid-thirties in England & Wales tested positive for syphilis; see Simon Szreter, "The Prevalence of Syphilis in England and Wales on the Eve of the Great War," *Social History of Medicine* 27, no. 3 (2014): 508–29.

33 Syphilis also spreads from mother to child during pregnancy, leading to congenital syphilis, which used to be a frequent cause of congenital anomalies and infant mortality in Europe in the early 20th century; see Lori Newman et al., "Global Estimates of Syphilis in Pregnancy and Associated Adverse Outcomes," *PLoS Medicine* 10, no. 2 (2013): e1001396. There is also an 'endemic' form of syphilis, spread by non-venereal routes and usually attracted in childhood. This was prevalent in poor, illiterate areas, as illustrated by Bosnia-Herzegovina where a campaign to eliminate the disease by serology surveys and penicillin treatment was necessary as recently as 1948–1955; see E.I. Grin and T. Guthe, "Evaluation of a Previous Mass Campaign against Endemic Syphilis in Bosnia and Herzegovina," *British Journal of Venereal Diseases* 49, no. 1 (1973): 1–19; Thorstein Guthe and O. Idsoe, "The Rise and Fall of the Treponematoses. II. Endemic Treponematoses of Childhood," *British Journal of Venereal Diseases* 44, no. 1 (1968): 35–48.

character. However, after a few decades it developed into the milder disease as we still know it today (illustrating a biological mechanism mentioned above in our discussion of the decline of tuberculosis mortality).[34]

Because syphilis is spread by sexual intercourse, attitudes to syphilis and syphilis control have always been strongly influenced by norms on sexual behaviour. Moralizing approaches have always competed with more pragmatic approaches to the control of syphilis and other sexually transmitted diseases (STDs).[35]

Historically, four phases in the approach to syphilis can be distinguished. In a first period (ca. 1490–ca. 1520), the sudden eruption of a very serious disease of unknown origins was commonly regarded as God's punishment for men's sins. In a second period (ca. 1520–ca. 1750), when it had become clear that syphilis spread through sexual intercourse, 'double standards' applied. Syphilis in lower class people was regarded as a punishment for their sins, whereas syphilis in higher class patients was seen as the acceptable risk of a frivolous life-style. In a third period (ca. 1750–ca. 1900), rejection and shame dominated the attitudes towards syphilis under the influence of the morality of the upcoming bourgeoisie, which regarded syphilis as a threat to family-life. Finally, in a fourth period (ca. 1900 to the present), a more pragmatic attitude came to prevail, with increasing involvement of the state, due to a recognition that syphilis was a threat to society as a whole, reducing the strength of the military, limiting successful procreation, etc.[36]

Syphilis control became an issue in the 19th century, mainly in the form of regulation of prostitution, but also of education of the public at large (including the military) about the dreadful disease that promiscuity could lead to.

---

34 That syphilis was part of the 'Columbian exchange', and did not exist in Europe before the discovery of America, is supported by paleoanthropological findings and contemporary reports (Alfred W. Crosby, "The Early History of Syphilis: A Reappraisal," *American Anthropologist* 71, no. 2 (1969): 218–27; Thomas A. Cockburn, "The Origin of the Treponematoses," *Bulletin of the World Health Organization* 24, no. 2 (1961): 221–28), and by molecular-genetic studies (Kristin N. Harper et al., "On the Origin of the Treponematoses: A Phylogenetic Approach," *PLoS Neglected Tropical Diseases* 2, no. 1 (2008): e148). On the change in character of the disease around the year 1500, see Eugenia Tognotti, "The Rise and Fall of Syphilis in Renaissance Europe," *Journal of Medical Humanities* 30, no. 2 (2009): 99–113.

35 See, for example, Allan M. Brandt, *No Magic Bullet* (Oxford etc.: Oxford University Press, 1987); Mooij, *Geslachtsziekten*. The reverse is true as well: STDs have often been used for the promotion of conservative or liberal ideas about sexuality, the family, and gender roles.

36 These stages in the response to syphilis have been proposed by Owsei Temkin, "Zur Geschichte von 'Moral und Syphilis,'" *Archiv für Geschichte der Medizin* 19, no. 4 (1927): 331–48.

These efforts may have contributed to some decline of syphilis in the second half of the 19th century. Prostitution was very wide-spread, perhaps due to the disruption of family life caused by industrialization and urbanization which had brought many single men into Europe's larger cities. It was more or less accepted that these men's 'sexual urges' had to find an outlet in prostitution, so that bourgeois girls and women could remain chaste, but in order to limit prostitution's medical and social risks it had to be strictly regulated.

This regulation implied that prostitutes were only allowed to work in brothels, which were placed under municipal and medical supervision. They had to be tested regularly for signs of venereal disease, and when they were found to be infected, they were prohibited from working until they were free of symptoms again. Treatment options were limited in the 19th century, and mainly consisted of various applications of mercury, which have never been shown to be effective but did have very unpleasant side-effects. The regulatory approach to prostitution started in the early 1800s in Paris, under the influence of the socio-medical studies of Alexandre Parent-Duchâtelet, and was later adopted in many other European countries.[37]

A change in approach occurred around 1900, involving a turn away from prostitution as the main or only source of syphilis infection, and towards more pragmatic strategies of syphilis control, in what mattered most was effectiveness and not morality. This turn coincided with the discovery of salvarsan (1909), which proved to be much more effective against syphilis than mercury, and created opportunities for a more medically oriented approach. In many European countries, venereal disease clinics and dispensaries were set up, which offered treatment free of charge and also offered testing and treatment of contacts of syphilis patients.

Other social-hygienic measures included targeted prevention and treatment facilities for military and naval personnel (Plate 11), deployment of specially trained nurses and social workers for active contact tracing, and screening and treatment of pregnant women to protect their babies from congenital syphilis. Although it remains unclear whether salvarsan as such reduced mortality, the combination of advances in treatment with outreaching service

37 For the history of prostitution in the 19th century, see Alain Corbin, *Les Filles de Noce* (Paris: Flammarion, 1982). Parent-Duchâtelet's work gives s shocking picture of the working conditions of Parisian prostitutes: Alexandre Parent-Duchâtelet, *De la Prostitution dans la Ville de Paris, Considérée sous le Rapport de l'Hygiène Publique, de la Morale et de l'Administration* (Paris: J.-B. Baillière et fils, 1836).

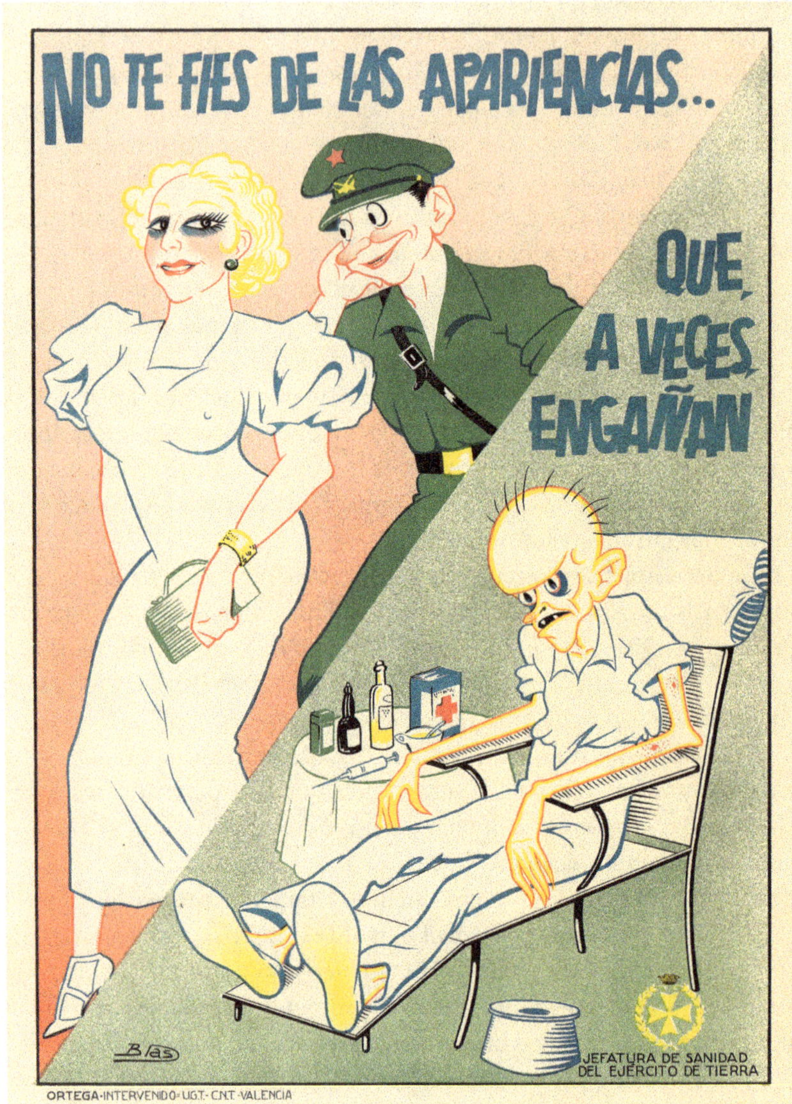
NO TE FIES DE LAS APARIENCIAS...
QUE, A VECES, ENGAÑAN
BLAS
JEFATURA DE SANIDAD DEL EJERCITO DE TIERRA
ORTEGA-INTERVENIDO-U.G.T.-C.N.T.-VALENCIA

PLATE 11 "Do not trust appearances." Spanish poster warning against syphilis, 1938
Soldiers have always been at risk for sexually transmitted diseases, which were not only a threat to their personal health but also to army strength. Translation of the Spanish text: "Do not trust appearances ... Sometimes they cheat." Poster published by the Health headquarters of the Republican army during the Spanish Civil War.
LITHOGRAPH BY BLAS. WELLCOME COLLECTION (CC BY 4.0)

facilities almost certainly contributed to the general decline of syphilis incidence and mortality in the first decades of the 20th century.[38]

In the 1940s, partly as a result of stepped-up research efforts because of the war, penicillin became available and proved to be much more effective than salvarsan. Several studies have shown that the introduction of penicillin coincided with an acceleration of syphilis mortality decline. The wide spread in syphilis mortality curves in the post-war period suggests, however, that delays were common.[39]

Starting in the late 1940s, the incidence of 'early infectious syphilis' declined to a historical low in many European countries, briefly plateaued in the late 1950s, and then turned upwards again. Fortunately, and probably thanks to penicillin, this was not followed by a rise in 'late syphilis' and/or syphilis mortality, but it was worrying enough. Contemporary analyses pointed to a complex of causes that have since been summarized under the heading of the 'sexual revolution'. The rise of syphilis and other STDs resulted from an increase in pre-marital sex, an increase in homosexual intercourse, and an increase in promiscuity generally. This 'sexual enthusiasm' was promoted by cultural change and the advent of safe oral contraceptives in the early 1960s. The increasing share of men-having-sex-with-men (MSM) among syphilis patients was particularly striking in this period.[40]

In Northern and Western European countries, the rise of syphilis abruptly reversed in the second half of the 1980s, probably as a result of the AIDS scare and campaigns to promote 'safe sex'. However, when AIDS became a treatable disease in the 1990s, 'safe sex' practices declined and syphilis rose again.[41]

---

38 Treatment options continued to expand in the 1920s and 1930s, with neo-salvarsan, bismuth, and fever therapies. For the history of syphilis control measures in the 20th century in a few European countries, see Tana Green, M.D. Talbot, and R.S. Morton, "The Control of Syphilis, a Contemporary Problem: A Historical Perspective," *Sexually Transmitted Infections* 77, no. 3 (2001): 214–17; Mooij, *Geslachtsziekten*; Roger Davidson, *Dangerous Liaisons* (Amsterdam & Atlanta: Rodopi, 2000).

39 See Suppl. Figure 10. The acceleration of decline in the late 1940s can easily be seen when the mortality rates are plotted on a logarithmic scale; see Mackenbach and Looman, "Secular Trends."

40 Guthe, *Worldwide Epidemiological Trends*; Idsoe and Guthe, "Rise and Fall of the Treponematoses. I." That syphilis and other STDs could now be treated with antibiotics may also have played a role. On the rise of 'sexual enthusiasm', see Paul Robinson, *The Modernization of Sex* (Oxford etc.: Harper & Row, 1976).

41 Irena Jakopanec et al., "Syphilis Epidemiology in Norway, 1992–2008," *BMC Infectious Diseases* 10, no. 1 (2010): 105. The rise of syphilis and other STDs since the late 1950s, the loosening of sexual norms during the 1960s, and the 'informalization of manners' more generally, has by some been interpreted as a reversal of the 'civilising process'; see Cas Wouters, "Formalization and Informalization: Changing Tension Balances in Civilizing Processes,"

Scarlet Fever, Measles, Whooping Cough, Diphtheria

The four diseases that have been clustered in this section were important causes of childhood mortality in the 19th century. Scarlet fever, measles, whooping cough and diphtheria were diseases of crowding: they spread by airborne droplets and intimate contact. Their incidence therefore was higher when population density in an area was higher, and when families lived together in more cramped housing conditions.[42]

The frequency with which these diseases occurred, increased when European countries started to industrialize and urbanize. Mortality from these diseases peaked in the 19th century before starting to decline again. For example, in the Netherlands mortality from measles, whooping cough and diphtheria was still very high in the last decades of the 19th century, but started to decline in the 1890s (see Suppl. Figure 11). Currently, the likelihood that a child will die from one of these diseases is almost nil, but behind us lies a time in which 5–10% of all children died from one of these diseases before reaching their 15th birthday.[43]

Mortality from these diseases fluctuated from year to year in regular cycles. These oscillations were due to the fact that after an epidemic had occurred, and all surviving children had been naturally immunized, it took a few years before a new group of susceptible children had been born and had become large enough to allow a new epidemic to occur.[44]

Mortality from these four conditions reached negligible levels in most European countries in the 1960s. These declines were due to a combination of factors: a 'spontaneous' decline in virulence of the infectious agent; 'side-effects'

Theory, Culture & Society 3, no. 2 (1986): 1–18. A similar hypothesis has been proposed for the rise of homicide (see Chapter 4).

42 See Woods, *Demography*, Chapter 7, for an analysis of mortality from these diseases in Victorian Britain. Woods' analysis shows that the causes of childhood mortality were different from the causes of infant mortality, and that – in Britain – the start of the decline of childhood mortality preceded that of infant mortality.

43 The distinction between these diseases was only gradually made. For example, the term 'croup', used in early cause-of-death statistics, referred to a laryngitis that could be due to diphtheria, whooping cough, scarlet fever, measles, and other infectious diseases; see Hirsch, *Handbook*, vol. III, pp. 50–51.

44 For an analysis of the periodicity of childhood epidemic diseases, see Roy M. Anderson, Bryan T. Grenfell, and R.M. May, "Oscillatory Fluctuations in the Incidence of Infectious Disease and the Impact of Vaccination," *Epidemiology & Infection* 93, no. 3 (1984): 587–608. The length of the inter-epidemic period depends on both biological and social factors; see C.J. Duncan, S.R. Duncan, and Susan Scott, "The Dynamics of Measles Epidemics," *Theoretical Population Biology* 52, no. 2 (1997): 155–63.

of modernization which reduced exposure, or increased resistance, to infection; and the introduction of effective methods of prevention and treatment.

One important 'side-effect' of modernization which played a role in the decline of mortality from childhood infections was fertility control. When families became smaller, the likelihood of transmission of infection within the family became smaller, which reduced the incidence of infectious diseases. It probably also reduced case fatality, because a lower force of infection led to a higher age of infection, at which children were less vulnerable.[45]

Other important factors which – as part of the socioeconomic modernization of European societies – reduced mortality from childhood infections were better nutrition (undernutrition increased case fatality), better education (educated mothers provided better care for their children), and better housing (more space and better ventilation reduced risks of infection). Some of these changes were definitely intentional, with better well-being or even better health in mind; others would simply not have occurred if the effects on well-being or health had been negative.[46]

Finally, medical advances contributed to mortality decline. At the end of the 19th century, medical science gained momentum. The discovery of the microbiological origin of these diseases not only allowed more targeted advice on how to prevent infection, but was also a spring-board for the development of prophylactics such as vaccinations, and therapies such as immune sera and antibiotics.

The relative importance of each of these three groups of factors differs between the four diseases, and is also likely to differ between countries, because in a country where decline started later the scope for a contribution from medical advances was larger. We will now briefly discuss the history of the four childhood infectious diseases one-by-one, to illustrate when, where and why their decline occurred.

45 For an analysis of the effect of lower fertility on average age at infection and case fatality, see Randall Reves, "Declining Fertility in England and Wales as a Major Cause of the Twentieth Century Decline in Mortality," *American Journal of Epidemiology* 122, no. 1 (1985): 112–26. Lower infection pressure may also have directly reduced case fatality; see Peter Aaby et al., "Severe Measles in Sunderland, 1885," *International Journal of Epidemiology* 15, no. 1 (1986): 101–07.

46 For a comprehensive analysis of the factors contributing to childhood mortality decline in Britain. see Woods, *Demography*, Chapters 7 and 8, and Hardy, *Epidemic Streets*, Chapters 1 to 4. Although children of better educated mothers had lower risks of dying from infectious diseases, schooling itself may have helped the spread of infectious diseases. The need to control infection in schools was one of the reasons why some countries tried to institute compulsory notification by teachers; see Mooney, *Intrusive Interventions*, Chapter 4.

Scarlet fever is a disease with symptoms of a sore throat, fever, headache and a typical skin rash. It may cause fatal complications such as anaemia, meningitis, and sepsis, particularly in young children. It is due to infection by haemolytic ("blood-cell destroying") streptococci which spread by intimate contact, and which may also have spread by contaminated milk.

This is one of the few diseases for which there is reliable evidence that its severity has spontaneously changed over time. In Western Europe, there was a rise of a virulent form of scarlet fever from the 1820s onwards, making scarlet fever the leading cause of death among the childhood infectious diseases in mid-century. Thereafter, it declined in severity, first in England and other Western European countries, and much later in Central-eastern and Eastern Europe.[47]

While a 'spontaneous' decline in virulence was probably the most important factor in the decline of scarlet fever mortality in the 19th century, other factors have made additional contributions in the 20th century. These include smaller families, more spacious housing and – from the 1930s and 1940s onwards – the introduction of sulphonamides and antibiotics. The latter resulted in an acceleration of the decline in scarlet fever mortality, as well as in the mortality from other streptococcal infections, such as erysipelas and puerperal fever, and the mortality from the sequelae of streptococcal infections (acute rheumatic fever and acute nephritis).[48]

Measles is a disease with symptoms of fever, cough, and (again) a typical skin rash. It may cause potentially fatal complications such as pneumonia,

47 There are many different strains of haemolytic streptococcus, which differ in virulence, and whose prevalence has varied over time. For an introduction to the history of scarlet fever, see Anne Hardy, "Scarlet Fever," in *Cambridge World History of Human Disease*, ed. Kenneth F. Kiple (Cambridge etc.: Cambridge University Press, 1993) and Francis B. Smith, *The People's Health, 1830–1910* (Canberra: Australian National University Press, 1979), pp. 136–42. The rise and fall of scarlet fever in England during the 19th century has been shown in Galbraith and McCormack, "Infection in England and Wales"; Alex Mercer, "Relative Trends in Mortality from Related Respiratory and Airborne Infectious Diseases," *Population Studies* 40, no. 1 (1986): 129–45. Mercer has argued, on the basis of a correlation between declines of scarlet fever and of dysentery and typhoid in Britain, that the apparent decline in streptococcal virulence was due to improvements in water supply and sewerage and the greater resistance against respiratory infections that this produced (Mercer, *Infections*, Chapter 8).

48 For the effect of sulphonamides and antibiotics, see Galbraith and McCormack, "Infection in England and Wales"; Mackenbach and Looman, "Secular Trends." The decline of acute rheumatic fever has been particularly spectacular; see Edward F. Bland, "Declining Severity of Rheumatic Fever: A Comparative Study of the Past Four Decades," *New England Journal of Medicine* 262, no. 12 (1960): 597–99; Leon Gordis, "The Virtual Disappearance of Rheumatic Fever in the United States," *Circulation* 72, no. 6 (1985): 1155–62.

encephalitis (infection of the brain), and severe diarrhoea, and case fatality may be as high as 5–10% among malnourished children. It is one of the most highly communicable diseases, and caused by infection with the *Morbilli* virus which is transmitted through the air and by direct contact. Measles needs a population of a substantial size to secure a continuous chain of susceptibles. It is thought to have arisen around 2500 BCE, when a similar virus in domesticated animals, perhaps rinderpest, jumped the species barrier after humans had started to live in cities.[49]

Measles occurred in large epidemics in the 18th and 19th centuries, and struck very dramatically. It caused huge numbers of deaths when it arrived on virgin soil, for example (and famously) on the Faeroe islands in 1846 which had been free of measles for 65 years. Mortality from measles remained high throughout the 19th century, partly as a negative side-effect of increased schooling which provided new reservoirs of infection.[50]

Mortality from measles started to decline in the first decades of the 20th century, not because incidence declined but because case fatality declined. Because case fatality was influenced by crowding, undernutrition, and previous respiratory infections, it is likely that the general improvement in living conditions helped to reduce case fatality. From the 1930s and 1940s onwards, sulphonamides and antibiotics helped to reduce deaths among measles patients as a result of secondary bacterial infections. The incidence of measles only started to decline when mass vaccination was gradually introduced in European countries from the 1960s onwards.[51]

Whooping cough, also known as pertussis, is a disease characterized by terrifying paroxysms of coughing. These culminate in a prolonged inspiration with a typical sound that gave the disease its name. Its potentially fatal complications include collapsed lungs, lack of oxygen and secondary bacterial infections, and it used to have a case fatality of around 10%. It is caused by infection with *Bordetella pertussis*, which has an airborne transmission.

49 For a general history of measles, see Robert J. Kim-Farley, "Measles," in *Cambridge World History of Human Disease*, ed. Kenneth F. Kiple (Cambridge etc.: Cambridge University Press, 1993) and Smith, *The People's Health*, pp. 142–48.

50 The epidemic on the Faeroe islands was famously analysed by Danish physiologist Peter Panum (1820–1885); see Peter L. Panum, *Lagttagelser, Anstillede under Maesllinge-Epidemien Paa Faeroerne I Aaret 1846* [*Observations Made During the Epidemic of Measles on the Faroe Islands in the Year 1846*] (Copenhagen: Bibiliothek for Laeger, 1847). For the likely connection with schooling, see Smith, *The People's Health*, pp. 142–48.

51 An in-depth analysis of the reasons for the decline of measles mortality in England and Wales can be found in Woods, *Demography*, pp. 319–23. For the effect of measles vaccine on measles incidence see, e.g., Heikki Peltola et al., "Measles, Mumps, and Rubella in Finland," *Lancet Infectious Diseases* 8, no. 12 (2008): 796–803.

Like the other childhood infections discussed in this section, its frequency as a cause of death rose in the 18th and 19th centuries. It reached a peak in the last decades of the 19th century, and then declined, at first because case fatality declined (from 10% in the 1880s to 1% during World War II, and then to only 0.1% in recent years), and more recently because incidence declined as well.[52]

As mentioned above, the decline in case fatality in the first half of the 20th century may be partly due to smaller families. This shifted the age group experiencing the highest incidence of pertussis from very young to older children, among whom case fatality was lower. It may also have been partly due to better housing and diet and better nursing care. An effective vaccine was introduced in the 1930s and was in wide-spread use from the late 1940s onwards, leading to a decline in incidence and an acceleration of mortality decline.[53]

Unfortunately, this success story was followed by several temporary, but severe, setbacks. In Britain, a vaccine scare led to a decline in vaccine uptake in the mid-1970s, leading to a rise in whooping cough incidence around 1980. In many European countries, there was a resurgence of whooping cough in the late 1990s due to decreasing vaccine efficacy, possibly because of an evolutionary change in the micro-organism and/or the shift to an acellular vaccine which had fewer side-effects but proved less effective.[54]

Diphtheria is a disease with symptoms of sore throat, coughing, fever, and a swollen neck. It derives its name from a characteristic membrane that forms on the tonsils and in the throat, and that obstructs the airways. It is caused by infection with *Corynebacterium diphtheriae* which spreads through airborne droplets, intimate contact and contaminated milk. When the bacterium itself is infected by a phage virus, it excretes a powerful toxin that may damage the heart and the nervous system. Case fatality can then be in the order of 30–50%.

52 For a general history of whooping cough, see Hardy, "Whooping Cough," and Smith, *The People's Health*, pp. 104–11. In addition to the factors mentioned in the main text, a decline of rickets, which reduced the child's stamina in coping with whooping cough, may also have played a role; see Hardy, *Epidemic Streets*, Chapter 1. For long-term trends in whooping cough in England and Wales, see Galbraith and McCormack, "Infection in England and Wales."

53 On the causes of the decline in case fatality in the first half of the 20th century, see Edward A. Mortimer Jr and Paul K. Jones, "An Evaluation of Pertussis Vaccine," *Reviews of Infectious Diseases* 1, no. 6 (1979): 927–34. See Galbraith and McCormack, "Infection in England and Wales" for the effect of vaccination.

54 On this 'vaccine scare' and its effects in Britain, see Ingrid Wolfe, "Child Health," in *Successes and Failures of Health Policy in Europe*, ed. Johan P. Mackenbach and Martin McKee (Maidenhead: Open University Press, 2013). On the decrease in vaccine efficacy and its possible causes, see, e.g., Douglas W. Jackson and Pejman Rohani, "Perplexities of Pertussis," *Epidemiology & Infection* 142, no. 4 (2014): 672–84.

Diphtheria already occurred in antiquity, but became more common in Europe in the 17th and 18th centuries, before mortality peaked in the second half of the 19th century.[55]

This is the only of the four diseases for which an effective treatment was already developed in the 19th century. 'Antitoxin' – that is, passive immunization on the basis of serum from horses which had been infected with human diphtheria – became available in the 1890s. Together with tracheostomy – that is, creating an opening in the neck in order to place a tube into the child's windpipe – antitoxin reduced case fatality and mortality from diphtheria in the first half of the 20th century. Other factors mentioned above (smaller families, more spacious housing, etc.) likely also played a role.[56]

In the 1920s active immunization with a vaccine was developed and shown to be effective, after which it spread rapidly in the US and Canada in the 1930s. Vaccination in Western Europe started to spread in the 1940s, even during World War II. Mass vaccination covering the entire population of children generally started in the 1950s, with the exception of Portugal where it started in 1966. Vaccination reduced diphtheria incidence, and accelerated the decline of diphtheria mortality.[57]

---

55 For a general history of diphtheria, see Ann Carmichael, "Diphtheria," in *Cambridge World History of Human Disease*, ed. K.F. Kiple (Cambridge etc.: Cambridge University Press, 1993) and Smith, *The People's Health*, pp. 148–152. The emergence of diphtheria has been reconstructed in Hirsch, *Handbook*, vol. III, p. 73 ff.

56 For the development of antitoxin and its effects, see F.M. Lévy, "The Fiftieth Anniversary of Diphtheria and Tetanus Immunization," *Preventive Medicine* 4, no. 2 (1975): 226–37; Mercer, *Disease*; Carmichael, "Diphtheria." Others have noted, however, that the introduction of antitoxin in the 1890s coincided with a shift in virulence which also contributed to the decline in diphtheria mortality; see Hardy, *Epidemic Streets*; Thorvald Madsen, "Diphtheria in Denmark from 23,695 to 1 Case: Post or Propter? I. Serum Therapy," *Danish Medical Bulletin* 3, no. 4 (1956): 112–15.

57 On the efficacy of diphtheria vaccination, see Lévy, "The Fiftieth Anniversary of Diphtheria and Tetanus Immunization." For the early spread of vaccination, see W.T. Russell, "Epidemiology of Diphtheria During the Last Forty Years," (London: His Majesty's Stationery Office, 1943); Jane Lewis, "The Prevention of Diphtheria in Canada and Britain 1914–1945," *Journal of Social History* 20, no. 1 (1986): 163–76, on the United Kingdom, and Dick Hoogendoorn, *Over de Diphtherie in Nederland* (Zwolle: Tijl, 1948) on the Netherlands. For the effect of mass vaccination, see Galbraith and McCormack, "Infection in England and Wales" on England and Wales, and Maarten van Wijhe et al., "Quantifying the Impact of Mass Vaccination Programmes on Notified Cases in the Netherlands," *Epidemiology & Infection* 146, no. 6 (2018): 716–22 on the Netherlands. On the introduction of mass vaccination in Portugal, see M.C. Gomes, J.J. Gomes, and A.C. Paulo, "Diphtheria, Pertussis, and Measles in Portugal before and after Mass Vaccination," *European Journal of Epidemiology* 15, no. 9 (1999): 791–98.

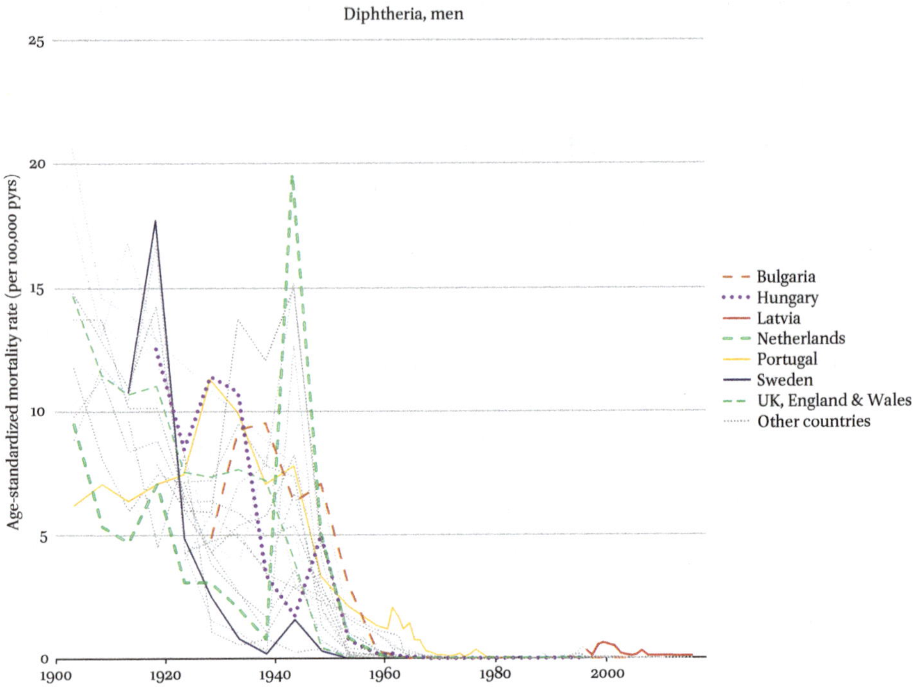

FIGURE 14 Trends in diphtheria mortality in Europe, 1900–2015
Notes: Between 1900 and 1960: quinquennial data
SOURCE OF DATA: SEE SUPPL. TABLE 1

While Figure 14 clearly shows the over-all decline of diphtheria mortality in European countries (and the delayed decline in Portugal), it also shows a massive epidemic during World War II, and a setback in Eastern Europe in the 1990s. The diphtheria epidemic during the war struck many European countries, both warring and neutral, and both German-occupied and non-occupied. In the Netherlands this was the most serious epidemic of diphtheria ever. It may have been due to a particularly virulent strain of diphtheria that was already circulating in Western and Central-eastern Europe in the late 1930s, and/or to a decrease in natural immunity as a consequence of war-time conditions.[58]

58 Gaylord W. Anderson, "Foreign and Domestic Trends in Diphtheria," *American Journal of Public Health and the Nations Health* 37, no. 1 (1947): 1–6; Bo Vahlquist, "Studies on Diphtheria. 1. The Decrease of Natural Antitoxic Immunity against Diphtheria," *Acta Paediatrica* 35, no. 1–2 (1948): 117–29.

In the Soviet Union, mass vaccination against diphtheria (and other childhood infections) was implemented in the 1950s, and this effectively controlled the disease. However, the incidence of diphtheria slowly rose again in the 1980s. A serious epidemic broke out around 1990, coinciding with the collapse of communism and the transition to a new political and economic order. The weakening of state structures led to declines in vaccine coverage and an epidemic of diphtheria with thousands of deaths, many of whom were adults.[59]

Russia did not report diphtheria deaths to the World Health Organization in this period, but Figure 14 does show the rise of diphtheria mortality in Latvia, where a serious epidemic occurred as well. With international support, aggressive countermeasures were taken in 1995, which within a few years brought diphtheria mortality down again in the countries of the former Soviet Union.[60]

Pneumonia, Influenza

Like the diseases treated in the previous section, pneumonia and influenza form part of a larger group of acute respiratory infections which were important causes of mortality in Europe before the middle of the 20th century. Trends in mortality from pneumonia and influenza are illustrated in Figure 15, together with trends in a few other respiratory diseases. The data come from the Netherlands, but similar trends have been found elsewhere. Please note that, in order to fit these diseases with very different mortality rates in the same graph, the vertical axis has a logarithmic scale.[61]

Mortality from all the acute respiratory conditions (pneumonia, influenza, otitis, laryngitis) has declined, in contrast to mortality from chronic respiratory conditions (chronic bronchitis, emphysema and asthma, taken together under its modern heading 'Chronic Obstructive Pulmonary Disease'). In the

59 Wolfe, "Child Health"; Charles R. Vitek and Melinda Wharton, "Diphtheria in the Former Soviet Union: Reemergence of a Pandemic Disease," *Emerging Infectious Diseases* 4, no. 4 (1998): 539–50.

60 On Latvia, see Aija Griskevica et al., "Diphtheria in Latvia, 1986–1996," *Journal of Infectious Diseases* 181, no. Supplement 1 (2000): S60–S64. On countermeasures and their effect, see Sieghart Dittmann et al., "Successful Control of Epidemic Diphtheria in the States of the Former USSR," *Journal of Infectious Diseases* 181, no. Supplement 1 (2000): S10–S22.

61 For trends in mortality from these conditions in other countries, see, e.g., Galbraith and McCormack, "Infection in England and Wales"; Clare Griffiths and Anita Brock, "Twentieth Century Mortality Trends in England and Wales," *Health Statistics Quarterly* 18, no. 2 (2003): 5–17. Trends in the Netherlands have been analysed in Wolleswinkel-van den Bosch et al., "Cause-Specific Mortality."

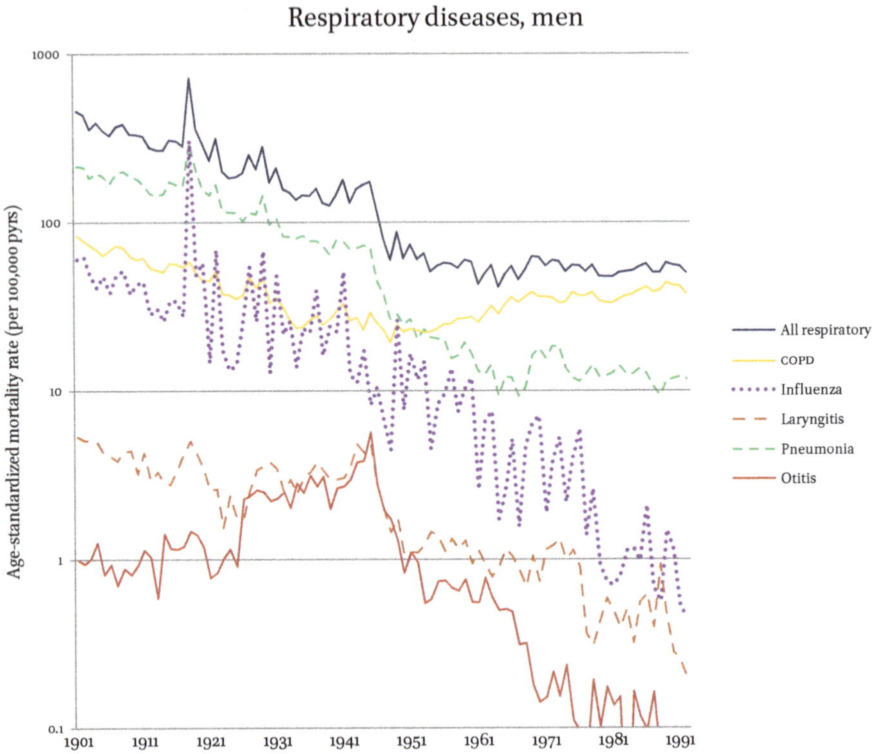

FIGURE 15 Trends in respiratory disease mortality in the Netherlands, 1901–1992
Notes: Logarithmic Y-axis. COPD = *Chronic Obstructive Pulmonary Diseases*
SOURCE OF DATA: JUDITH H. WOLLESWINKEL-VAN DEN BOSCH. *THE EPIDEMIOLOGICAL TRANSITION IN THE NETHERLANDS*. ERASMUS UNIVERSITY, 1998

Netherlands, as well as in many other European countries, mortality from COPD started to rise in the early 1950s, due to the smoking epidemic.[62]

The over-all decline of mortality from acute respiratory conditions has been far from smooth. This applies particularly to mortality from influenza, which has oscillated in cycles of between two and six years, reflecting periodic

62 Trends in COPD mortality in European countries have been complex, largely reflecting the diffusion of smoking and smoking cessation. There is also an association with poverty in childhood, perhaps via higher exposure to acute respiratory infections. For international overviews, see Peter G.J. Burney et al., "Global and Regional Trends in Copd Mortality, 1990–2010," *European Respiratory Journal* 45, no. 5 (2015): 1239–47; Alan D. Lopez et al., "Chronic Obstructive Pulmonary Disease: Current Burden and Future Projections," *European Respiratory Journal* 27, no. 2 (2006): 397–412.

changes in virulence and immunity. Mortality from influenza had an exceptionally high peak in 1918 during the well-known pandemic of 'Spanish flu'. But trends for the other diseases have also been quite volatile. For example, mortality from pneumonia and several other respiratory infections peaked in 1944, due to war-time conditions in the Netherlands, and mortality from laryngitis and otitis temporarily rose in the 1930s, due to a rise in streptococcal virulence.[63]

We will now discuss the trends for pneumonia and influenza in more detail, focussing on the explanation of mortality decline and temporary setbacks, and incorporating the experience of a wider range of European countries.

Pneumonia, particularly in its classic form of 'lobar pneumonia' in which a complete lobe of the lung was affected, was a very serious disease, with a case fatality of up to 30%. It was most commonly caused by infection with *Streptococcus pneumoniae* (also called the 'pneumococcus'), discovered in 1880 by French biologist Louis Pasteur (1822–1895). However, it may also be caused by a range of other bacteria and by viruses.[64]

Antisera were introduced in the 1920s but had limited effectiveness, and so the sulphonamides, discovered in the 1930s, and penicillin, discovered in the early 1940s, were the first life-saving treatments for pneumonia. Figure 15 shows that mortality from pneumonia in the Netherlands declined abruptly in the late 1940s, and then continued to decline at a faster speed than in the 1920s and 1930s, until the early 1960s. A similarly abrupt decline, and/or acceleration of pre-existing decline, has been noted in many countries.[65]

However, the quantitative impact, and the contribution of these new medical treatments to over-all decline of pneumonia mortality, differed importantly between European countries. This depended on whether or not pneumonia mortality had already reached a low level before they were introduced. Around 1930, pneumonia mortality was already quite low in Northern and Western

63 The rise in mortality from laryngitis and otitis coincided with a rise in mortality from scarlet fever, puerperal fever, and several other streptococcal infections, and has been attributed to a rise in virulence of the streptococcus (see section on scarlet fever above).

64 Pneumonia is one of the oldest diagnosed diseases, whose symptoms and physical signs were well known to doctors long before the discovery of its bacteriological origins (see Hirsch, *Handbook*, vol. III, Chapter VI). For an introduction to the history of pneumonia, see Jacalyn Duffin, "Pneumonia," in *Cambridge World History of Human Disease*, ed. Kenneth F. Kiple (Cambridge etc.: Cambridge University Press, 1993).

65 See Mackenbach and Looman, "Secular Trends" for an interrupted time-series analysis of mortality from pneumonia and other acute respiratory infections in the Netherlands. See Griffiths and Brock, "Twentieth Century Mortality Trends in England and Wales"; Galbraith and McCormack, "Infection in England and Wales" for pneumonia mortality trends in England.

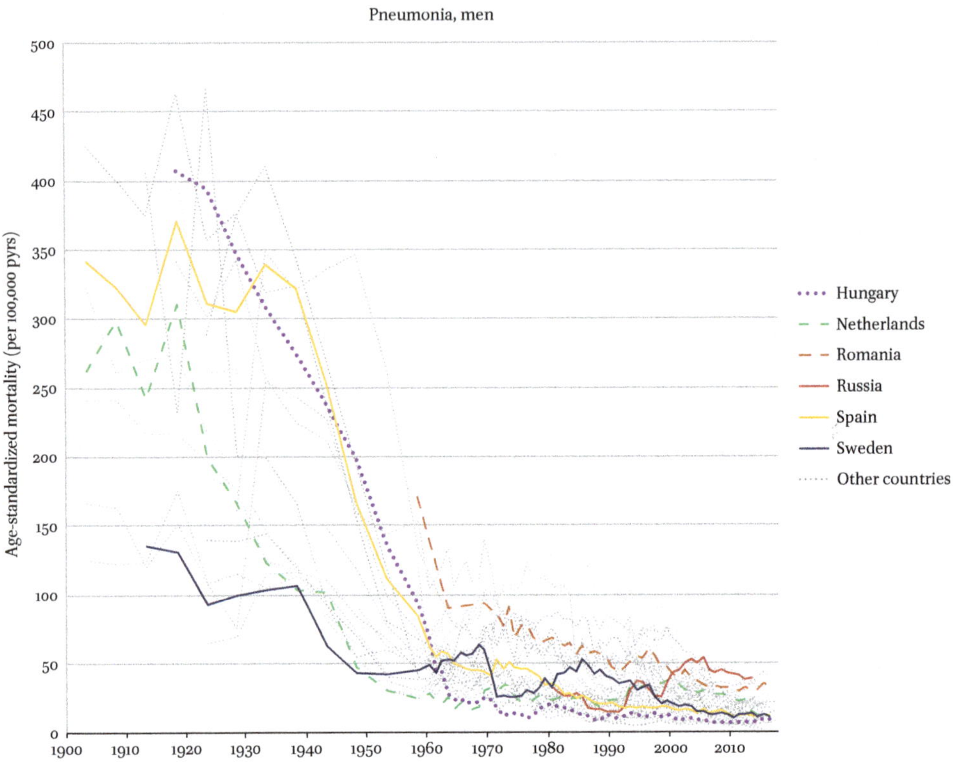

FIGURE 16 Trends in pneumonia mortality in Europe, 1900–2015
Notes: Quinquennial data before 1960
SOURCE OF DATA: SEE SUPPL. TABLE 1

Europe, whereas it was still high in the rest of Europe, so that the introduction of effective medical treatment could make a much larger contribution elsewhere (Figure 16).

For example, in countries like Sweden, Norway, England, the Netherlands, and Switzerland pneumonia mortality declined from 100–150 per 100,000 in 1930 to 25–50 per 100,000 in 1960 – certainly a most impressive decline. However, in countries like Italy, Spain, Greece, Czechoslovakia, and Hungary, pneumonia mortality declined from 250–350 per 100,000 in 1930 to 50–100 per 100,000 in 1960. Their decline was larger in both relative and absolute terms, and formed a much larger part of the over-all decline in pneumonia mortality during the 20th century.[66]

66 For example, in the Netherlands age-standardized pneumonia mortality was 262 in 1900, 123 in 1930 and 28 in 1960, implying a relative decline between 1930 and 1960 of 77% and

Although mortality from pneumonia has declined, it is still a common cause of death, particularly among the elderly. A deceleration of pneumonia mortality decline occurred in the 1960s in the Netherlands (Figure 15), and around the same time in many other countries (Figure 16). This may partly be a manifestation of the decreased efficacy of antibiotics after the emergence of penicillin resistance. It probably also reflects increasing survival of people with chronic conditions, among whom pneumonia is one of the few remaining gateways to death. This also implies that the validity of pneumonia as an underlying cause of death has become somewhat doubtful.[67]

Recently, several European countries have introduced vaccination against pneumococcal pneumonia, but whether this is effective against pneumonia mortality is uncertain.[68]

Influenza is a disease of humans, but also of pigs, horses, swine and birds, and is extremely contagious. During pandemics, it may infect more than half of the world's population. This has given the disease its Italian name: the Italians blamed its massive occurrence on the 'influence' of the stars. Case fatality is usually low (below 1%) and death mainly occurs among the very young, the very old, and the immune-compromised. Yet, because of the enormous numbers of infected persons, influenza mortality can be very high.

Influenza is caused by a virus which was discovered in 1933 and which changes all the time, making permanent immunity impossible. These changes may occur through mutation of the virus in humans, through mutation of a virus in animals that crosses the species barrier, or through recombination between a human and an animal virus. Often these changes are small, but

---

an absolute decline of 95 per 100,000, which is 41% of the total decline between 1900 and 1960. In Italy, age-standardized pneumonia mortality was 425 in 1900, 376 in 1930 and 62 in 1960, implying a relative decline between 1930 and 1960 of 84% and an absolute decline of 314 per 100,000, which is 87% of the total decline between 1900 and 1960. Data from Alderson, *International Mortality Statistics*, table 103.

67 For the deceleration of pneumonia decline, see Griffiths and Brock, "Twentieth Century Mortality Trends in England and Wales"; Galbraith and McCormack, "Infection in England and Wales." For the role of pneumonia as a cause of death in other conditions, see, e.g., Eric M. Mortensen et al., "Causes of Death for Patients with Community-Acquired Pneumonia," *Archives of Internal Medicine* 162, no. 9 (2002): 1059–64. For the recent increase in community-acquired pneumonia, see, e.g., Mette Søgaard et al., "Nationwide Trends in Pneumonia Hospitalization Rates and Mortality, Denmark 1997–2011," *Respiratory Medicine* 108, no. 8 (2014): 1214–22; A.B. van Gageldonk-Lafeber et al., "Time Trends in Primary-Care Morbidity, Hospitalization and Mortality Due to Pneumonia," *Epidemiology & Infection* 137, no. 10 (2009): 1472–78.

68 Systematic reviews have concluded that effectiveness of the vaccine has not been proven; see, e.g., Anke Huss et al., "Efficacy of Pneumococcal Vaccination in Adults: A Meta-Analysis," *Canadian Medical Association Journal* 180, no. 1 (2009): 48–58.

sometimes they are more radical causing a pandemic, i.e., an epidemic affecting a large part of the world.[69]

Europe had several large-scale epidemics of influenza in the 16th and 17th centuries, and there were at least three documented pandemics in the 18th century (1729–30, 1732–33, 1781–82). The last of these three arrived in Europe from Russia, and spread by sea routes. Three-quarters of the European population fell ill, and despite the fact that case fatality was low, it caused hundreds of thousands of deaths. There were also at least three pandemics in the 19th century (1830–31, 1833, 1889–90). The last was called the 'Russian flu', because it arrived again from the East. It spread by steamship over sea, and by train over land, and caused between 250,000 and 300,000 deaths in Europe.[70]

However, the greatest influenza pandemic of all – and the one that eclipses all others in popular memory – was the 'Spanish flu' which killed around 1% of the European population between Spring 1918 and Spring 1919. There were around 2.5 million deaths in Europe, and at least 50 million deaths world-wide. In contrast to most other influenza epidemics it killed many young adults, perhaps because these had not experienced the 1889–90 influenza and therefore had no natural immunity.

There has been much speculation about a relationship between this pandemic and World War I. Was it a coincidence that it started in the last year of the 'Great War'? Even the remotest countries on earth were struck by this pandemic, so it may have occurred anyway. But the war also increased transmission of the virus (due to massive troop movements, often in crowded ships), reduced human resistance (due to other diseases and other war-related suffering), and reduced collective capacity for countermeasures (due to countries'

69 For a general history of influenza, dating the first influenza epidemics in Europe to the 16th century, see Alfred W. Crosby, "Influenza," in *Cambridge World History of Human Disease*, ed. Kenneth F. Kiple (Cambridge etc.: Cambridge University Press, 1993). For contemporary theories on how changes in the influenza virus occur, see Christopher W. Potter, "A History of Influenza," *Journal of Applied Microbiology* 91, no. 4 (2001): 572–79; Martha I. Nelson and Michael Worobey, "Origins of the 1918 Pandemic: Revisiting the Swine 'Mixing Vessel' Hypothesis," *American Journal of Epidemiology* 187, no. 12 (2018): 2498–502. There are three types of human influenza virus: A, B, C. Influenza A, which naturally occurs in wild aquatic birds, has been involved in pandemics. Important serotypes include H1N1 ('Spanish flu' in 1918, 'Swine flu' in 2009), H2N2 ('Asian flu' in 1957), H3N3 ('Hong Kong flu' in 1968), and H5N1 ('Bird flu' in 2004).

70 For a history of influenza pandemics in the 18th and 19th centuries, see K. David Patterson, *Pandemic Influenza, 1700–1900* (Totowa: Rowman & Littlefield 1986).

focus on the war, and the collapse of some governments at the end of the war).[71]

Mortality from influenza was considerably higher in Europe than in the US. This has been attributed to the fact that the public health response in the US was more vigorous, by closing schools and other measures that lowered the mortality peak. The death toll also differed importantly between European countries (see Suppl. Figure 12). Northern and Western Europe experienced far lower influenza mortality than Southern and South-eastern Europe. One possible explanation is that, as we have seen in previous sections, the latter countries still had a higher disease burden from other respiratory conditions (such as respiratory tuberculosis, pneumonia, …), and that the higher prevalence of co-morbidity increased influenza's case fatality.[72]

After the 1918 pandemic, several other pandemics occurred, but although influenza mortality kept oscillating, none of the later pandemics really stands out with an exceptional death toll. This is probably not only due to lesser virulence of the virus, but also to better medical treatment, including antibiotics for secondary bacterial pneumonia, and better supportive care. Nevertheless, influenza has remained an important cause of death, particularly in cold winters and among the elderly.[73]

---

71 It was called the 'Spanish flu' because contemporaries mistakenly thought it originated in Spain. On the history of 'Spanish flu', see John M. Barry, *The Great Influenza* (Harmondsworth: Penguin, 2005); Cécile Viboud and Justin Lessler, "The 1918 Influenza Pandemic: Looking Back, Looking Forward," *American Journal of Epidemiology* 187, no. 12 (2018): 2493–97. For the death toll, see Niall P.A.S. Johnson and Juergen Mueller, "Updating the Accounts: Global Mortality of the 1918–1920 'Spanish' Influenza Pandemic," *Bulletin of the History of Medicine* 76, no. 1 (2002): 105–15.

72 On lower excess mortality from influenza in the US, see Stephen S. Morse, "Pandemic Influenza: Studying the Lessons of History," *Proceedings of the National Academy of Sciences* 104, no. 18 (2007): 7313–14. On a more fatalistic attitude in Britain, see Sandra M. Tomkins, "The Failure of Expertise: Public Health Policy in Britain During the 1918–19 Influenza Epidemic," *Social History of Medicine* 5, no. 3 (1992): 435–54. For an analysis of between-country differences in excess deaths, see S. Ansart et al., "Mortality Burden of the 1918–1919 Influenza Pandemic in Europe," *Influenza Other Respiratory Viruses* 3, no. 3 (2009): 99–106. Aspects of the high death toll in Portugal were analysed in B. Nunes et al., "The 1918–1919 Influenza Pandemic in Portugal," *American Journal of Epidemiology* 187, no. 12 (2018): 2541–49.

73 For analyses of recent influenza trends, see G.C. Donaldson and W.R. Keatinge, "Excess Winter Mortality: Influenza or Cold Stress?," *British Medical Journal* 324, no. 7329 (2002): 89–90; Martin W. Brinkhof et al., "Influenza-Attributable Mortality among the Elderly in Switzerland," *Swiss Medical Weekly* 136, no. 19–20 (2006): 302–09. Officially registered deaths from influenza underestimate the total death toll.

Whether the introduction of mass vaccination of the elderly and other high-risk groups has contributed to a decline in the incidence and/or mortality from influenza is uncertain. This was successfully introduced in several European countries in the 1990s, and may have contributed to further mortality decline in recent years. Yet, studies comparing trends of influenza mortality with trends in vaccine uptake have not found a clear relationship.[74]

Despite progress in the prevention and treatment of influenza, some experts believe that there is still a serious risk that a new pandemic, with a much more virulent influenza virus, will arise and cause large numbers of deaths. So far, however, nothing of the sort has happened, despite world-wide scares of 'bird flu' in 2004 (which only caused a few hundred deaths world-wide) and 'swine flu' in 2009 (which perhaps caused 30,000 deaths in Europe, including excess deaths from other causes).[75]

Maternal, Infant and Perinatal Mortality

Maternal Mortality

Maternal mortality – defined as "the death of a woman while pregnant or within 42 days of termination of pregnancy, from any cause related to or aggravated by the pregnancy or its management" – nowadays is very rare. In 2015, the maternal mortality rate was far below 1 per 10,000 births in almost all European countries, down from more than 100 per 10,000 births three centuries ago.[76]

---

74 For the history of influenza vaccine development, see I. Barberis et al., "History and Evolution of Influenza Control through Vaccination," *Journal Prevention Medical Hygiene* 57, no. 3 (2016): e115-e20. Evidence on the effectiveness of influenza vaccination among the elderly is not entirely convincing; see Alexander Domnich et al., "Effectiveness of Mf59-Adjuvanted Seasonal Influenza Vaccine in the Elderly," *Vaccine* 35, no. 4 (2017): 513–20. Introduction of influenza vaccination coincided with declines in influenza mortality in the Netherlands (Angelique G. Jansen et al., "Decline in Influenza-Associated Mortality among Dutch Elderly," *Vaccine* 26, no. 44 (2008): 5567–74), but not in Italy (Caterina Rizzo et al., "Influenza-Related Mortality in the Italian Elderly," *Vaccine* 24, no. 42–43 (2006): 6468–75).

75 'Swine flu' was originally called 'Mexican flu'. For a model-based estimate of the number of excess deaths, see Fatimah S. Dawood et al., "Estimated Global Mortality Associated with the First 12 Months of 2009 Pandemic Influenza a H1N1 Virus Circulation," *Lancet Infectious Diseases* 12, no. 9 (2012): 687–95.

76 Even then, because death from other causes was so frequent, maternal mortality did not account for more than 10% of total mortality among women of child-bearing age. Yet, because women had many children the life-time risk could be in the order of 10%; see Irvine Loudon, *Death in Childbirth* (Oxford etc.: Oxford University Press, 1992).

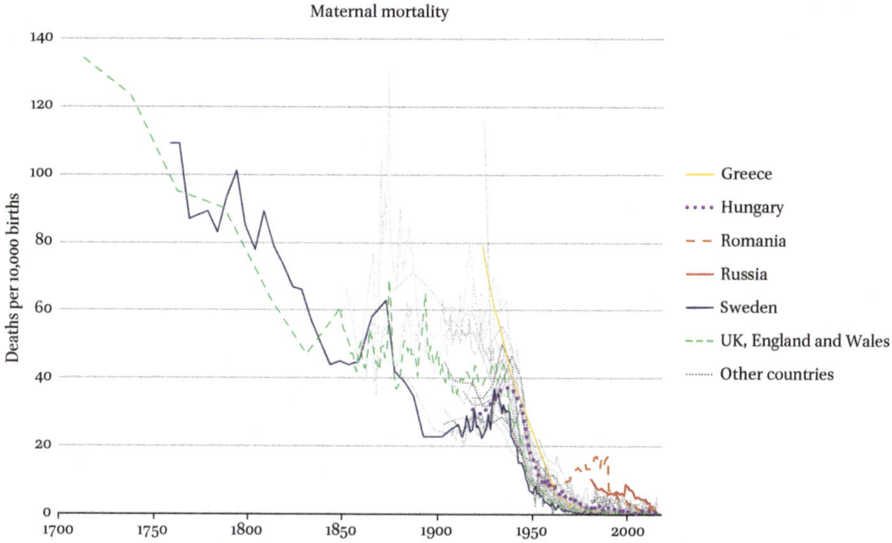

FIGURE 17 Trends in maternal mortality in Europe, 1700–2015
Notes: Sparse data in many countries before 1900
SOURCE OF DATA: SEE SUPPL. TABLE 1

As Figure 17 illustrates, this is one of the most breath-taking trends ever seen in population health, with the steepest decline occurring in the 1940s and shared by all European countries. Only few countries have data on maternal mortality going back to the 18th century or before. However, national data from Sweden and nationally representative data from English family reconstitution studies show that the maternal mortality rate in these two countries was above 100 per 10,000 births in the first half of the 18th century. The English study actually found an even higher rate, of more than 150 per 10,000 births, in the late 17th century. Regional data from France confirm this with estimates of between 100 and 200 maternal deaths per 10,000 births in the 17th and 18th centuries.[77]

At this time medical assistance of child-birth was still rare: most parturient women were assisted by female neighbours, family members and/or lay birth assistants. When complications arose, such as breech presentation, too narrow birth canal, post-partum haemorrhage or puerperal fever, little could be done.

77 Historical data for Sweden are in Loudon, *Death in Childbirth*, appendix 6. Data for England are in E. Anthony Wrigley et al., *English Population History from Family Reconstitution 1580–1837* (Cambridge etc.: Cambridge University Press, 1997), table 6.21. Data for regions in France are in Hector Gutierrez and Jacques Houdaille, "La Mortalité Maternelle en France au XVIIIe Siècle," *Population* (*French Edition*) 36, no. 6 (1983): 975–94, tables 1 and 2.

It is likely, therefore, that a maternal mortality rate of 100 deaths per 10,000 births or more represents the risk of maternal death in the absence of any professional assistance.[78]

In Sweden and England, maternal mortality already declined importantly between 1700 and 1850, to around half its original level. After 1850 we have data from many more European countries, which show highly variable levels and trends. In contrast to the pre-1850 period, for many countries we now have annual (instead of quinquennial or decadal) mortality data, which show very 'spikey' patterns up to the 1930s.

More generally, the maternal mortality trends in Europe are not altogether favourable between 1850 and the 1930s. The main exception is a group of countries consisting of Sweden, Norway, Denmark and the Netherlands. In these countries, maternal mortality declined strongly in the second half of the 19th century, reached comparatively low levels of just above 20 deaths per 10,000 births around the year 1900, but then rose somewhat again in the first decades of the 20th century, before starting a precipitous decline around 1935.

In all other European countries, including England and other parts of the United Kingdom, maternal mortality declined less or not at all in the second half of the 19th century, and several European countries had 'spikes' of maternal mortality exceeding a rate of 60 deaths per 10,000 births even in the first decades of the 20th century.

However, in the late 1930s and 1940s maternal mortality declined strongly all around Europe, to reach levels of ca. 10 per 10,000 deaths in 1950, with slower but continuous declines until the present day. The main exception is Romania, which experienced an epidemic of maternal mortality in the 1960s to 1980s, ending with a steep decline in 1989, coinciding with the fall of the communist regime.

As we will see in the next section, long-term trends of maternal mortality are remarkably different from those of infant mortality, particularly in the late 19th and early 20th century when infant mortality showed a more consistent decline (Figure 18). Trends are more similar between maternal mortality and late foetal mortality (Figure 19), suggesting common determinants between maternal and late foetal mortality, but not between maternal and infant mortality.

78 See Ulf Högberg, Stig Wall, and Göran Broström, "The Impact of Early Medical Technology on Maternal Mortality in Late 19th Century Sweden," *International Journal of Gynecology & Obstetrics* 24, no. 4 (1986): 251–61. This paper cites a maternal mortality rate of 87 per 10,000 births in 1975–1982 among women from a religious group in the U.S. who avoided antenatal and obstetric care.

Those who have studied possible explanations for the trends of maternal mortality have come to the conclusion that most of the decline can be attributed to improvements in obstetric practice. As always in these historical analyses, definite proof is impossible to obtain, but the available evidence is rather compelling. While improvements in living standards, general improvements in women's health, and declines in fertility have also played a role, the main factor has probably been more effective medical assistance. Yet, this has not been a smooth trajectory.[79]

It is during the 18th century that the old style of childbirth started to change, both with regard to who attended the birth and to what was known and done. Medical doctors and surgeons became interested in pregnancy and childbirth, wrote treatises on how to deal with complications, and started to assist women from the higher social classes as their 'man-midwife' or '*accoucheur*'. In several European countries, such as Sweden and France, governments started to promote a formal education of lay birth assistants, based on an increased understanding of the anatomy of the uterus and the mechanics of delivery, as a result of which the number of trained 'midwives' gradually increased.

While it is likely that improvements in obstetric care contributed to the decline of maternal mortality during the 18th and first half of the 19th century, the decline stalled around 1850, with the exception of the Nordic countries and the Netherlands. This was due to a combination of factors. The increased involvement of medical doctors in child-birth, particularly within so-called lying-in hospitals, actually increased the risk of puerperal fever; and not all countries regulated community midwifery in such a way that all births outside hospital were attended by well-trained midwives.

The main difference between the Nordic countries and the Netherlands on the one hand, and most other European countries on the other hand was in the second factor. In the second half of the 19th century, most deliveries in these

79 The most extensive analysis, relying on time-trend analyses and in-depth comparisons between countries, is Loudon, *Death in Childbirth*. It has been summarized in, e.g., Irvine Loudon, "Maternal Mortality: 1880–1950. Some Regional and International Comparisons," *Social History of Medicine* 1, no. 2 (1988): 183–228; Irvine Loudon, "The Transformation of Maternal Mortality," *British Medical Journal* 305, no. 6868 (Dec 19–26 1992): 1557–60. The Swedish experience has been analysed in several papers: Ulf Högberg, "The Decline in Maternal Mortality in Sweden: The Role of Community Midwifery," *American Journal of Public Health* 94, no. 8 (2004): 1312–20; Högberg et al., "The Impact of Early Medical Technology on Maternal Mortality." A good general overview can also be found in Vincent De Brouwere, "The Comparative Study of Maternal Mortality over Time," *Social History of Medicine* 20, no. 3 (2007): 541–62.

countries still occurred at home, and were attended by qualified midwives who were able to apply new insights in their obstetric practice, such as the importance of antisepsis for the prevention of puerperal fever.[80]

In the 19th century, puerperal fever was the most important single cause of maternal mortality, accounting for up to half of all maternal deaths. We now know that it is mostly caused by infection with *Streptococcus pyogenes*, a bacterium with high variable behaviour, generally present in people's noses and throats, and involved in a range of diseases, including pharyngitis, otitis, erysipelas, scarlet fever, and acute rheumatic fever. During child-birth it can enter the woman's body through her wounds, and when it caused puerperal sepsis this was often fatal before the advent of sulphonamides and antibiotics in the 1930s and 1940s.

Puerperal fever has probably occurred throughout human history, but became epidemic with the increased involvement of medical practitioners in child-birth. This was because they could unwittingly introduce the bacterium during their interventions, for example after having done a vaginal examination on another woman in a lying-in hospital, after having conducted an autopsy on a woman who had died from puerperal fever, or simply because they carried the bacterium in their own nose and throat. It was a well-known fact that some doctors were tragically followed by epidemics of puerperal fever among the women they attended. The spikes in maternal mortality seen in Figure 17 were probably due to epidemics of puerperal fever.

The discovery of the aetiology of puerperal fever is traditionally associated with the name of Ignaz Semmelweis (1818–1865). Semmelweis was a medical doctor of Hungarian descent who worked in the lying-in part of the *Allgemeines Krankenhaus* in Vienna. By comparing two parts of this clinic, he discovered the connection between puerperal fever and previously conducted autopsies by the same doctors who assisted in deliveries. He published his findings in 1860, but his views on the aetiology of puerperal fever remained controversial until the end of the 19th century. So were similar views propagated by others, some of whom had discovered the contagious nature of puerperal fever long before Semmelweis.

The idea that puerperal fever had a simple aetiology only became widely accepted, after Louis Pasteur (1822–1895) had demonstrated that infection was caused by living organisms, and after Joseph Lister (1827–1912) had demon-

80 Högberg, "The Decline in Maternal Mortality in Sweden"; Mart J. van Lieburg and Hilary Marland, "Midwife Regulation, Education, and Practice in the Netherlands During the Nineteenth Century," *Medical History* 33, no. 3 (1989): 296–317; Loudon, "The Transformation of Maternal Mortality."

strated that 'antisepsis' with carbolic acid and other chemicals could prevent wound infection. Application of these new ideas led to a rapid reduction of the frequency of puerperal fever in the last decades of the 19th century, but unfortunately adoption was not universal, even in countries where these new ideas were widely diffused.

Instead of accelerating, the decline of maternal mortality stagnated in England and other parts of the United Kingdom in the second half of the 19th century and first decades of the 20th century (Figure 17). This has been attributed to the fact that, in contrast to midwives in the Nordic countries and the Netherlands, British midwives were not well-trained and did not adequately apply the lessons of the 'bacteriological' and 'antiseptic' revolutions. This coincided with a probable rise in the virulence of *Streptococcus pyogenes* in the first decades of the 20th century, which led to a rise in puerperal fever mortality in many European countries. It was the arrival of sulphonamides and penicillin that finally brought the mortality rate drastically down.[81]

The rapid, and almost simultaneous decline in maternal mortality in the late 1930s and 1940s can, however, not be explained by the reduction of puerperal fever mortality alone. Other causes of maternal mortality also started to decline rapidly. In the 19th century and first decades of the 20th century, the most important other causes of maternal mortality were haemorrhage (e.g., due to problems with the placenta praevia), pregnancy-induced hypertension (which may in severe forms lead to 'toxaemia' or 'eclampsia'), and the complications of induced abortion. In a detailed analysis for England it was shown that all three declined in the late 1930s and 1940s, but with subtle differences in timing related to the timing of the interventions involved.

For example, while puerperal fever started to decline in the late 1930s, coinciding with the introduction of the sulphonamides, maternal mortality from haemorrhage started to decline in the early 1940s. This coincided with the introduction of ergometrine (a drug that helps the uterine blood vessels to contract), blood transfusion, and the transformation of the health service to better accommodate emergency cases during World War II. Caesarean sections, which were too dangerous before the advent of blood transfusion and antibiotics, now also could be applied on a larger scale.[82]

---

81 For the history of puerperal fever from classical times to the late 19th century, see Hirsch, *Handbook*, vol. II, pp. 416–75. The history of the discovery of the aetiology of childbed fever and the causes of its final retreat have been described in Irvine Loudon, *The Tragedy of Childbed Fever* (Oxford etc.: Oxford University Press, 2000). For the causes of the stagnation of the decline from puerperal fever in England, see Loudon, *Death in Childbirth*.

82 See Loudon, *Death in Childbirth*, Chapter 15.

The simultaneous decline of maternal mortality during the late 1930s and the 1940s in so many European countries can only be understood if we assume that the diffusion of these new insights and methods took place very rapidly. The only country that forms an exception to the favourable trends in the post-War period is Romania, where the brutally pro-natalist policies of the Ceausescu regime caused an epidemic of maternal mortality. Starting in 1966, the Romanian government tried to raise the birth rate by forbidding both contraceptives and induced abortion, as a result of which many women resorted to illegal abortion, often with fatal consequences.[83]

Despite the fact that, seen from a historical perspective, levels of maternal mortality are generally very low in Europe, there are still relevant variations, which point to differences in the quality of antenatal and perinatal care.[84]

Infant Mortality

Declines in infant mortality – deaths occurring in the first year of life – have been extremely important for the increase in life expectancy in Europe. The contribution of declines in infant mortality to the total increase in life expectancy since the 19th century exceeds that of any other age-group. This is not only because saving the life of an infant adds more years to life than saving the life of an older child or adult, but also because declines of mortality in the first year of life have been larger than those in other age-groups.[85]

It is difficult to grasp the enormity of these changes – and the enormity of the social and psychological impact infant mortality must have had in the past. Around 1870, before infant mortality started to decline, the infant mortality rate in most European countries ranged between 150 and 300 per 1000 live-born children. In 2015, the likelihood that a child would die before its first birth-day had declined to below 10 per 1000 everywhere – only Turkey had an infant mortality rate that was still slightly above 10 per 1000.

These high death rates were mainly due to the fact that many babies died from diarrheal and respiratory diseases. These were caused by a combination

83 Another consequence was a dramatic rise in the number of unwanted children, many of whom ended up in orphanages. See Charlotte Hord et al., "Reproductive Health in Romania: Reversing the Ceausescu Legacy," *Studies in Family Planning* 22, no. 4 (1991): 231–40; Patricia Stephenson et al., "Commentary: The Public Health Consequences of Restricted Induced Abortion – Lessons from Romania," *American Journal of Public Health* 82, no. 10 (1992): 1328–31.

84 Katherine Wildman and Marie-Helene Bouvier-Colle, "Maternal Mortality as an Indicator of Obstetric Care in Europe," *British Journal of Obstetrics and Gynaecology* 111, no. 2 (2004): 164–69.

85 See Suppl. Figure 2.

of unhygienic living conditions and inadequate infant care, e.g., overcrowded housing, lack of clean water, too early weaning, and bacterial contamination of food and milk. In many European countries, infants' high risk of infection was also due to the fact that mothers often did not breast-feed their infants, but gave them animal milk, gruels or other artificial foods, or relied on poor 'wet nurses' in the country-side. Many factors played a role, ranging from a taboo on sexual intercourse during lactation to a complete lack of understanding of infants' dietary needs. Also, breast-feeding was often impossible when women had to work outdoors, which became more common as a result of low wages in the industry and high cost of living in cities.[86]

Around 1870, about one-third of infant deaths occurred during the first month of life ('neonatal mortality'), whereas two-thirds occurred in the remaining eleven months ('post-neonatal mortality'). Since then, because the decline of post-neonatal mortality has been much stronger than that of neonatal mortality, the distribution has reversed: nowadays, neonatal mortality accounts for two-thirds, and post-neonatal mortality for one-third of infant mortality.

A similar shift has occurred *within* the first month of life: deaths in the first week ('early neonatal mortality') used to account for only one-third of all neonatal deaths, but now far outnumber those in the remaining three weeks ('late neonatal mortality'). This shift tells us something important: the causes of death in the first week of life are different from those in the rest of the first year of life, and have been much more difficult to tackle.

Death in the first week of life occurs among babies who are born in a suboptimal manner (e.g., because they are born prematurely, or because they are damaged during childbirth), and among babies who are already compromised during pregnancy (e.g., because they do not grow well, or have a congenital anomaly). These are health problems that need a different approach from what worked against the digestive and respiratory diseases which dominated infant mortality before 1870.[87]

---

86 In many European regions, only a small minority of infants were breast-fed, despite the fact that infant mortality was much higher among wet-nursed or artificially fed infants. For a history of infant feeding practices from 1500 to 1800, see Valerie Fildes, *Breasts, Bottles and Babies* (Edinburgh: Edinburgh University Press, 1986). For short histories of infant feeding in the 18th and 19th centuries, see Emily E. Stevens, Thelma E. Patrick, and Rita Pickler, "A History of Infant Feeding," *Journal of Perinatal Education* 18, no. 2 (2009): 32–39; Ian G. Wickes, "A History of Infant Feeding: Part Iii: Eighteenth and Nineteenth Century Writers," *Archives of Disease in Childhood* 28, no. 140 (1953): 332–40.

87 There is little information on the causes from which infants died in their first weeks of life in the 19th century. Prematurity, low birth weight and congenital malformations were

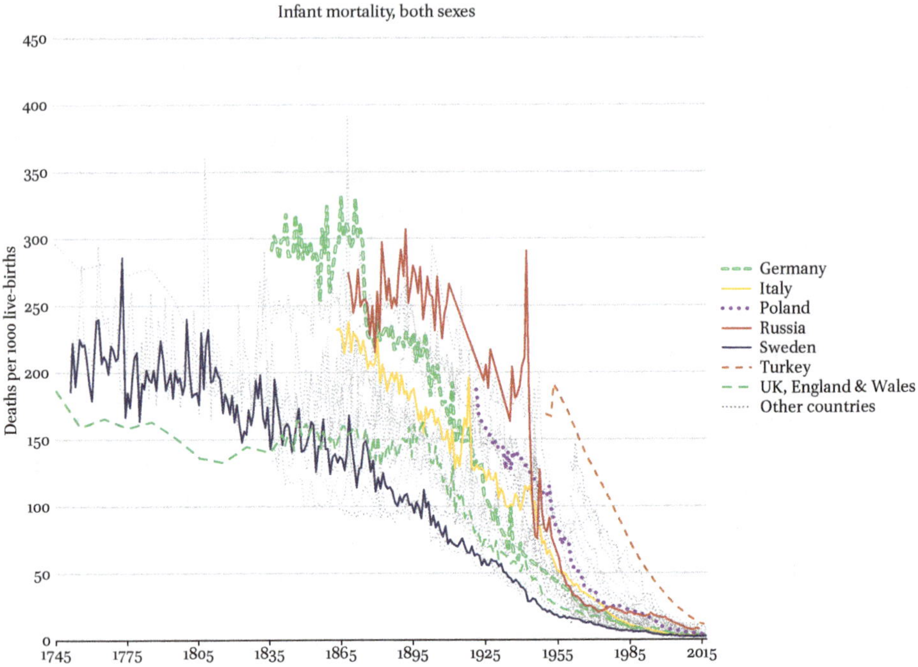

FIGURE 18 Trends in infant mortality in Europe, 1745–2015
Notes: Decadal data for England & Wales before 1840
SOURCE OF DATA: SEE SUPPL. TABLE 1

The historically slower decline of first-week mortality is mirrored by a similarly slow decline of the still-birth rate, or the 'late foetal mortality rate'. This is the death rate among unborn babies who are considered viable, i.e., who are developed well enough to be able to survive independently of their mother. As a result of its slow decline, the still-birth rate has become relatively more important as an object of concern, just like the early neonatal mortality rate. In the late 1940s this resulted in the promotion of the 'perinatal mortality rate' (which is the sum of late foetal and early neonatal mortality) as an additional indicator for monitoring the health of infants.[88]

probably already important; see Alice Reid and Eilidh Garrett, "Doctors and the Causes of Neonatal Death in Scotland in the Second Half of the Nineteenth Century," *Annales de Démographie Historique*, no. 1 (2012): 149–79.

88 If we combine still-births with all deaths in the first year of life, and calculate proportions of all deaths occurring between 28 weeks of gestation and the first birth-day, we find that around 1870 still-births accounted for one-quarter, neonatal deaths for one-quarter, and post-neonatal deaths for one-half. Nowadays, these proportions are one-half, one-third, and one-sixth, showing that the share of still-births has doubled over time (data from

We will review the history of both infant and perinatal mortality in Europe, using – as elsewhere in this book – a compilation of data from national statistics. More than in the case of other statistics, these need to be interpreted with caution, because criteria for the registration of infant and perinatal mortality have varied, both over time and between countries, and because under-registration has been and still is common.[89]

Figure 18 illustrates the long-term trends of infant mortality in Europe. Like the decline of the all-ages mortality rate that we saw in Figure 2, the decline of infant mortality has not followed a smooth path. Although there has been a dramatic net decline, this has been interrupted by huge spikes, such as in Finland in 1868 when more than 400 out of 1000 infants died during the last great famine, and in Russia in 1942, when almost 300 out of 1000 infants died during the worst years of World War II.

The Nordic countries already started national registration of infant mortality in the 18th century, reflecting an early interest in the fate of their new-borns among politicians and medical professionals. Sweden's infant mortality rate has been highlighted in Figure 18, and had already started to decline by the beginning of the 19th century. Since then, it has been declining almost continuously. The same applies to Norway and Denmark. These early declines have been attributed to the promotion of breast-feeding, partly through community midwives, high levels of literacy, early uptake of smallpox vaccination, and other measures reducing exposure to infection. Due to their early and persistently rapid decline, Sweden's and Norway's infant mortality rate have been among the lowest in Europe throughout the 19th and 20th centuries.[90]

Norway presented in Robert Woods, *Death before Birth* (Oxford etc.: Oxford University Press, 2009), fig. 4.2).

89 For sources of under-registration and registration differences between European countries, see G. Gourbin and Godelieve Masuy-Stroobant, "Registration of Vital Data: Are Live Births and Stillbirths Comparable All over Europe?," *Bulletin of the World Health Organization* 73, no. 4 (1995): 449–60; Wilco C. Graafmans et al., "Comparability of Published Perinatal Mortality Rates in Western Europe," *BJOG: An International Journal of Obstetrics & Gynaecology* 108, no. 12 (2001): 1237–45. Registration criteria have also changed over time, reflecting the increasing possibilities of keeping babies with a short gestational age alive. More comparable data on perinatal mortality in European countries were collected in EURO-Peristat Project, *European Perinatal Health Report* (n.p.: EURO-Peristat Project, 2018).

90 For an analysis of trends in infant mortality in the five Nordic countries, see Sören Edvinsson, Ólöf Garðarsdóttir, and Gunnar Thorvaldsen, "Infant Mortality in the Nordic Countries, 1780–1930," *Continuity and Change* 23, no. 3 (2008): 457–85. Finland also experienced an early decline, but infant mortality remained higher than in Sweden and Norway; see Oiva Turpeinen, "Les Causes des Fluctuations Annuelles du Taux de Mortalité Finlandais entre 1750 et 1806," *Annales de Démographie Historique* (1980): 287–96. Infant mortality in

Other countries in which infant mortality rates can be followed since the 18th century are France and England. France experienced a decline in the last decades of the 18th century but, in contrast to Sweden, this was followed by stagnation of infant mortality during most of the 19th century. The early decline has been attributed to *"la première médicalisation de la petite enfance à l'époque des lumières"* [the first medicalisation of infancy in the age of Enlightenment]. In this period, physicians started to promote breast-feeding, safer methods of delivery assistance, and regular bathing of infants, which may already have helped to bring infant mortality down from ca. 300 to ca. 200 deaths per 1000 live-born.[91]

Infant mortality trends in England (highlighted in Figure 18) can also be followed over a very long period, partly thanks to family reconstitution studies. England had relatively low infant mortality in the 18th and early 19th centuries, perhaps because artificial feeding had become less wide-spread than elsewhere. Yet, the secular decline of infant mortality started later than in other European countries. English trends were unfavourable in the second half of the 19th century, probably due to rapid urbanization which exposed increasing numbers of infants to the sanitary problems of England's larger cities. The decline that started in the late 1890s has been studied extensively, and has been attributed to a combination of declining fertility, improvements in women's education, sanitary reform, and improved milk supply and food hygiene.[92]

Similar factors must have played a role in the first phase of infant mortality decline elsewhere, but with national variations in timing which have, unfortu-

---

Iceland only started to decline around 1870, after breast-feeding had been promoted; see Loftur Guttormsson and Ólöf Garðarsdóttir, "The Development of Infant Mortality in Iceland, 1800–1920," *Hygiea Internationalis* 3, no. 1 (2002): 151–76. For an individual-level study showing the effect of public health measures and trained midwives on infant mortality decline, see Volha Lazuka, Luciana Quaranta, and Tommy Bengtsson, "Fighting Infectious Disease: Evidence from Sweden 1870–1940," *Population and Development Review* 42, no. 1 (2016): 27–52.

91 The causes of the late 18th century decline in France have been discussed in Marie-France Morel, "Les Soins Prodigués aux Enfants: Influence des Innovations Médicales et des Institutions Médicalisées (1750–1914)," *Annales de Démographie Historique* (1989): 157–81.

92 On advances in obstetrics and their (modest) impact on infant mortality in the 18th century in England, see Robert Woods and Chris Galley, *Mrs Stone & Dr Smellie: Eighteenth-Century Midwives and Their Patients* (Liverpool: Liverpool University Press, 2014). On the causes of stagnation and decline of infant mortality in England & Wales in the late 19th and early 20th centuries, see Robert Woods, Patricia A. Watterson, and John H. Woodward, "The Causes of Rapid Infant Mortality Decline in England and Wales, 1861–1921. Part I," *Population Studies* 42, no. 3 (1988): 343–66; Robert Woods, Patricia A. Watterson, and John H. Woodward, "The Causes of Rapid Infant Mortality Decline in England and Wales, 1861–1921. Part II," *Population studies* 43, no. 1 (1989): 113–32.

nately, never been satisfactorily explained. National studies have revealed many of the factors involved in national infant mortality decline, but explaining why some countries (other than the Nordic countries) had earlier infant mortality decline than others has remained guesswork. Despite considerable research efforts, the same applies to the explanation of national variations in the timing of another important component of the demographic transition, fertility decline.[93]

In the second half of the 19th century, infant mortality was high and rising in the Netherlands, and even higher in Germany and Austria, probably because of unhygienic conditions and wide-spread artificial infant feeding in all three countries. However, infant mortality started to decline precipitously in the 1870s, due to a combination of changes in infant care, partly driven by cultural change (breast-feeding, modern hygienic practices) and the start of large-scale public sanitation.[94]

In France and Switzerland, infant mortality also started to decline in the 1870s. Spain and Italy followed in the 1880s, England and Scotland towards the end of the 1890s, and Hungary, Bulgaria, Romania, Yugoslavia, Russia, and Portugal after the year 1900.[95]

---

93 The timing of the onset of fertility decline in European countries has been studied in the Princeton European Fertility Project. This concluded that the decline started simultaneously throughout Europe in the 1870s, suggesting that cultural diffusion of new ideas about fertility control was the main explanation; see Ansley J. Coale and Susan C. Watkins, eds., *The Decline of Fertility in Europe* (Princeton: Princeton University Press, 1986). Other theories have emphasized economic determinants, such as a "reversal of intra-familial wealth flows" due to the increasing importance of education which made children expensive instead of a source of income; see Karen Oppenheim Mason, "Explaining Fertility Transitions," *Demography* 34, no. 4 (1997): 443–54; John C. Caldwell, *Theory of Fertility Decline* (New York: Academic, 1982).

94 Infant mortality was high in the Netherlands due to a combination of low breast-feeding and contaminated surface water. The onset of infant mortality decline has been attributed to cultural factors, such as the spread of modern hygienic practices and breast-feeding; see Evert W. Hofstee, *De Demografische Ontwikkeling van Nederland in de Eerste Helft van de 19de Eeuw* (Deventer: Van Loghum Slaterus, 1978); Wolleswinkel-van den Bosch et al., "Determinants of Infant and Early Childhood Mortality Levels." For timing of decline of infant mortality in Germany, and the role of sanitary improvements in this decline, see Jorg Vogele, "Urbanization, Infant Mortality and Public Health in Imperial Germany," in *The Decline of Infant and Child Mortality*, ed. Carlo A. Corsini and Pier P. Viazzo (Dordrecht: Martinus Nijhoff, 1997). For decline of infant mortality in Austria, see Josef Kytir, Christian Köck, and Rainer Münz, "Historical Regional Patterns of Infant Mortality in Austria," *European Journal of Population/Revue européenne de Démographie* 11, no. 3 (1995): 243–59.

95 For an overview of the timing of infant mortality decline in different European countries, see Godelieve Masuy-Stroobant, "Infant Health and Infant Mortality in Europe," in *The*

Underlying the specific causes of infant mortality decline, such as the promotion of breast-feeding and sanitary reform, was often a broader national movement to reduce the appallingly high levels of infant mortality. This is clear in the case of the Nordic countries, where both early registration of mortality and training of midwives were inspired by a political desire to strengthen the population. It also applies in varying degrees and at different points in time to other countries. For example, in France during the last decades of the 19th century a concern with both social justice and the national interest led the government to enact a series of laws to protect infants (e.g., a law regulating nanny care), to organize the distribution of pasteurized milk, and – somewhat later – to set up a system of home visiting.[96]

This public concern with the health of infants continued and strengthened during the first decades of the 20th century, and led to an expanding system of child health and social services, with child health clinics, food supplements, child benefits, antenatal clinics, etc. in all European countries. Mean-while, improvements in obstetric care, a shift from home to hospital deliveries, the introduction of antibiotics, and later the creation of neonatal intensive care units and other advanced medical treatments made the medical component of these systems more and more effective, with all factors together helping to continue the decline of infant mortality.[97]

After World War II, infant mortality continued to decline, and ultimately all national rates converged around values of between 2 and 10 per 1000. This also applies to the communist and post-communist countries of Europe, although in the Balkans it took more time than elsewhere. In the 1980s, infant mortality rates above 30 per 1000 were still registered in North Macedonia, Serbia, Kosovo and Albania, but in these (now independent) countries infant mortality rates have since declined to lower levels. Registration issues may, however, apply, both before and after 1991. For example, under-registration of infant mortality has been documented for the Soviet Union before 1991, and for many

Decline of Infant and Child Mortality, ed. C.A. Corsini and P.P. Viazzo (Dordrecht: Martinus Nijhoff, 1997). For in-depth studies of infant mortality decline and its causes in France, Central-Spain and Italy, see other chapters in the same book.

96 Catherine Rollet-Echalier, "La Politique à l'Egard de la Petite Enfance sous la IIIe République," *Population (French Edition)* 46, no. 2 (1991): 349–58.

97 For a review of the contribution of technological innovations see Steven L. Gortmaker and Paul H. Wise, "The First Injustice: Socioeconomic Disparities, Health Services Technology, and Infant Mortality," *Annual Review of Sociology* 23, no. 1 (1997): 147–70.

countries of the former Soviet Union as well as several countries in Central-eastern Europe after 1991.[98]

Still-births

The long-term trend in the still-birth rate does not at all resemble the trend in the infant mortality rate. In some of the Nordic countries, the still-birth rate can be followed since the 18th or early 19th century – again illustrating the early public engagement with the health of new-borns – and seems to have fluctuated in large waves, without indications for a consistent decline until the 1940s (Figure 19).[99]

Whereas the decline of the infant mortality rate has taken more than a century, the decline of the still-birth rate is of more recent date and appears to be concentrated in a short period of time starting around 1940. The decline coincides with the sudden decline of the maternal mortality rate that occurred in the same period.

This also applies to the perinatal mortality rate which, in some countries, can be traced since the second or third decade of the 20th century. In Sweden, Denmark, England & Wales and the Netherlands, perinatal mortality started to decline in the late 1930s or early 1940s, and has further declined without major interruptions until the present day. Similar declines have been registered in the post-war period for other European countries. Before World War II, the perinatal mortality rate was around 50 per 1000: 50 still-born and first-week deaths per 1000 still- and live-born taken together. Currently, the perinatal mortality rate is below 10 per 1000 almost everywhere.[100]

98 For under-registration of infant mortality in the Soviet period, see Ellen Jones and Fred W. Grupp, "Infant Mortality Trends in the Soviet Union," *Population and Development Review* 9, no. 2 (1983): 213–46. Infant mortality rose in the 1970s and 1980s, due to environmental pollution, smoking and drinking in pregnancy, and changes in parity distribution; see Jones and Grupp, "Infant Mortality Trends." For under-registration in the post-Soviet period, see Nadezhda Aleshina and Gerry Redmond, "How High Is Infant Mortality in Central and Eastern Europe and the Commonwealth of Independent States?," *Population Studies* 59, no. 1 (2005): 39–54.

99 The history of still-birth registration in the Nordic countries has been described in Woods, *Death before Birth*, Chapter 4. Midwives had to report still-births to the parish priest. As is clear from Figure 19, Sweden had lower still-birth rates in the 19th century than the few other countries for which data are available. This was probably due to birth assistance by trained midwives; see Tobias Andersson, U. Hogberg, and S. Bergstrom, "Community-Based Prevention of Perinatal Deaths: Lessons from Nineteenth-Century Sweden," *International Journal of Epidemiology* 29, no. 3 (2000): 542–48.

100 On trends in perinatal mortality, see Signild Vallgårda, "Trends in Perinatal Death Rates in Denmark and Sweden, 1915–1990," *Paediatric and Perinatal Epidemiology* 9, no. 2 (1995): 201–18; Geoffrey Chamberlain, "Abc of Antenatal Care. Vital Statistics of Birth," *British*

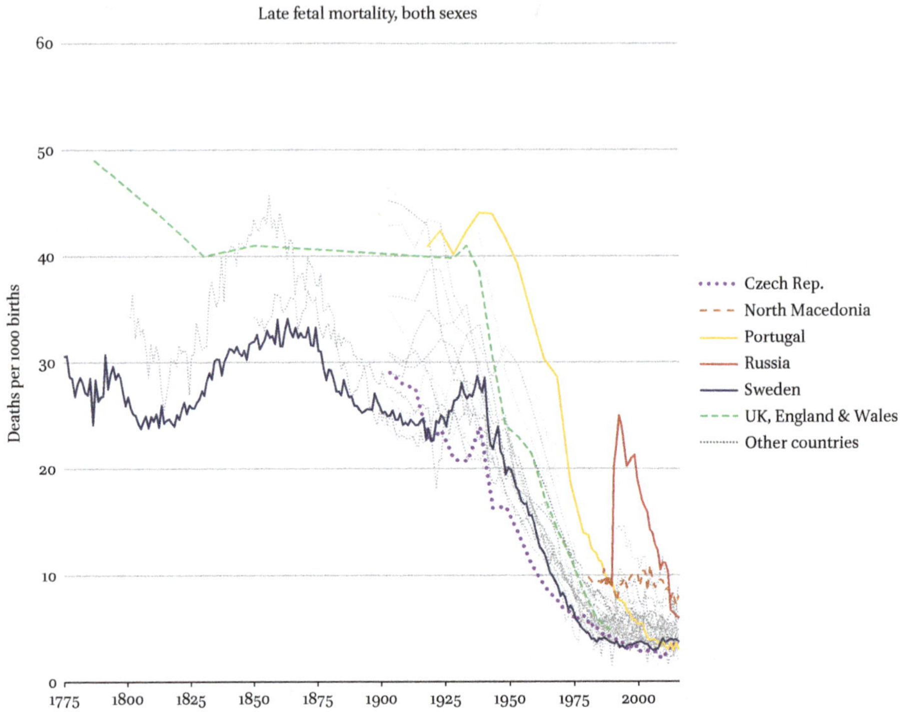

FIGURE 19 Trends in still-births in Europe, 1775–2015
Notes: Sparse data for England & Wales before 1928; quinquennial data for many countries before 1980
SOURCE OF DATA: SEE SUPPL. TABLE 1

The co-occurrence of the decline in the still-birth rate with the rapid decline in maternal mortality in the middle of the 20th century suggests that both had the same causes, i.e., improvements in obstetric care. That is indeed what different authors on this topic have concluded. Antibiotics not only saved mothers from puerperal infection, but together with the advent of blood transfusion also reduced the risk of infection of operative procedures. As caesarean sections became less risky for the mother, they could now also be performed to save the life of her baby. Improvements in how midwives and specialized obstetricians

Medical Journal 303, no. 6795 (1991): 178–81; J.H. de Haas-Posthuma and J.H. de Haas, *Infant Loss in the Netherlands* (Washington: National Center for Health Statistics, 1968). For recent trends, see Jennifer Zeitlin et al., "Declines in Stillbirth and Neonatal Mortality Rates in Europe between 2004 and 2010," *Journal of Epidemiology and Community Health* 70, no. 6 (2016): 609–15.

handled childbirth and its complications probably also helped, as did the introduction of systematic antenatal care, in which women at risk were identified, counselled and, increasingly, referred for in-hospital delivery.[101]

Improvements in antenatal and perinatal care continued during the second half of the 1960s, and the continued decline of perinatal mortality reflects the combined effect of a wide range of favourable trends. These include important behavioural changes, such as less unwanted pregnancies, less teenage and multiparous pregnancies, less smoking in pregnancy, and better nutrition (e.g., more fresh fruits and vegetables, leading to less neural tube defects). Important advances in care for mother and child occurred as well. Advances in the antenatal period include screening for congenital anomalies followed by induced abortion and more wide-spread and systematic use of antenatal care. Advances in care during and immediately after child-birth included initiating delivery in overdue pregnancies, increased use of caesarean sections for babies at risk, regionalization of care, and creation of neonatal intensive care units.[102]

Not all trends were favourable, however, and the decline of perinatal mortality occurred despite the continued high frequency of premature birth. The latter even increased in some European countries in the past decades. Several factors, some of which are the result of more medical intervention, have contributed to an upward pressure on the preterm birth rate. There is an elevated risk of preterm birth in multiple pregnancies, and these have increased as a result of the application of in vitro fertilization. There has also been an increase in artificially induced early childbirth, aiming to protect the baby against the risks of a longer stay in the womb, for example in the case of eclampsia (severe pregnancy hypertension). In addition, the prevalence of some risk factors for preterm birth has risen as well, such as higher age and obesity of pregnant women. Although survival of preterm babies has improved, long-term consequences are often severe, and include cerebral palsy and difficulties at school.[103]

---

101 An overview of risk factors for still-birth can be found in Joy E. Lawn et al., "Stillbirths: Rates, Risk Factors, and Acceleration Towards 2030," *Lancet* 387, no. 10018 (2016): 587–603. See Woods, *Death before Birth* for an overview of the causes of the decline in still-births. See Anne Løkke, "The Antibiotic Transformation of Danish Obstetrics," *Annales de Démographie Historique*, no. 1 (2012): 205–24, for an analysis of how antibiotics transformed obstetric care, with direct and indirect benefits for mother and child.

102 On the role of antenatal and perinatal care to declines in perinatal mortality, see Jennifer Zeitlin, Beatrice Blondel, and Babak Khoshnood, "Fertility, Pregnancy and Childbirth," in *Successes and Failures of Health Policy in Europe*, ed. Johan P. Mackenbach and Martin McKee (Maidenhead: Open University Press, 2013).

103 For an analysis of trends in prematurity in European countries and an overview of factors involved in rising rates, see Jennifer Zeitlin et al., "Preterm Birth Time Trends in Europe:

The remarkable rise of the still-birth rate in Russia (and also Ukraine, see Figure 19) during the 1990s illustrates the sensitivity of these rates to registration practices. In the Soviet Union, the official criteria for registering still-births, live-births, and deaths among the live-born differed in subtle but relevant ways from the criteria recommended by the World Health Organization, to the effect that infant and perinatal mortality rates were underestimated. This changed in the 1990s, when Russia and the newly independent states started to harmonize their criteria with those of the WHO. The steep but temporary rise of the still-birth rate probably reflects an abrupt change, and later correction, in registration practices, and cautions against taking the currently low perinatal mortality rates in Eastern Europe at face-value.[104]

Other Health Problems of Industrializing Societies

Pellagra, Rickets, Goitre

Nutrient deficiencies used to be common, and an important cause of disease throughout Europe. One important group of such diseases are 'avitaminoses', i.e., diseases due to a lack of vitamins. Vitamins are essential dietary elements that are necessary in small quantities for the proper functioning of the organism. Although vitamins and their role in health and disease were only discovered in the first decades of the 20th century, the diseases caused by a lack of vitamins have been recognized for a long time. These include beriberi (now known to be due to lack of vitamin B1), pellagra (vitamin B3), scurvy (vitamin C) and rickets (vitamin D). Other important nutrient deficiencies were iodine-deficiency (leading to goitre and cretinism) and iron-deficiency (leading to anaemia). In this section, we will briefly illustrate the European history of this group of diseases with the long-term trends of pellagra, rickets, and goitre.

Pellagra is a disease of people living on a diet mainly consisting of maize. It is characterized by dermatitis (*'pelle agra'* meaning rough skin), diarrhoea and dementia (Plate 12). Before its cause was discovered, it could be highly fatal.

A Study of 19 Countries," *BJOG: An International Journal of Obstetrics & Gynaecology* 120, no. 11 (2013): 1356–65.

104 It is not known what the precise change was. It may reflect an increase in the completeness of the registration of still-births, as a result of harmonization with WHO criteria, but even then the peaks in Russia and Ukraine look improbably high. Perhaps early neonatal deaths were registered as still-births to create a flattering picture of the infant mortality rate; see Aleshina and Redmond, "How High Is Infant Mortality."

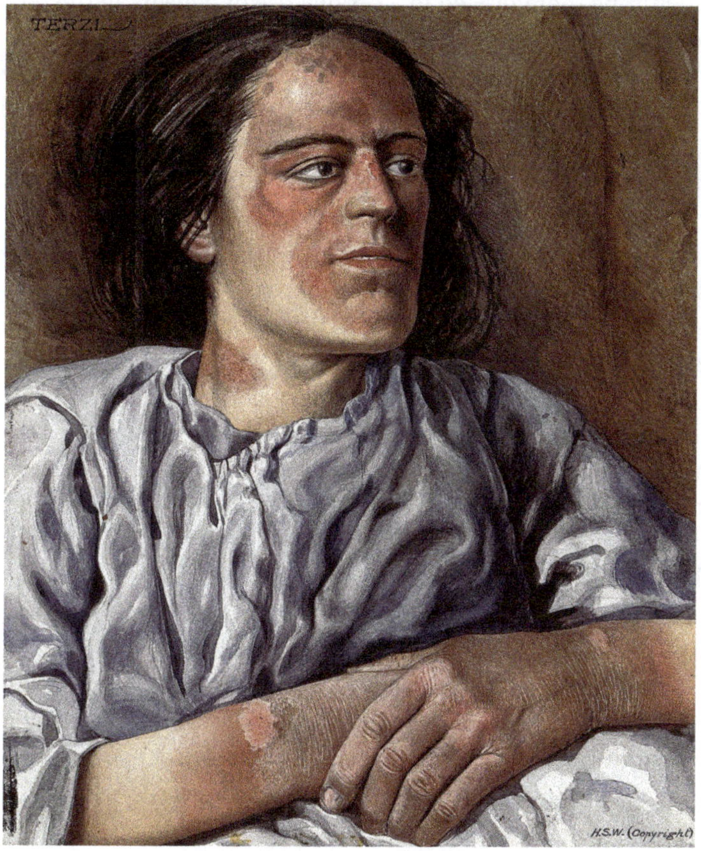

PLATE 12 A woman suffering from chronic pellagra. Watercolour, ca. 1925
This picture shows an Italian woman suffering from pellagra, showing the typical skin abnormalities. These are due to the fact that the effects of niacin deficiency are felt most in body parts with high rates of cell turnover, such as the skin. However, chronic pellagra also caused serious neurological symptoms, and Italian mental hospitals once housed many pellagra patients.
WATERCOLOUR BY A.J.E. TERZI. WELLCOME COLLECTION (CC BY 4.0)

Like potatoes, maize was brought to Europe from the New World in the 16th and 17th centuries. Maize grew easily in Southern Europe, and replaced wheat as a staple food for the poor in rural areas of Spain, Portugal, Southern France, Northern Italy, Yugoslavia, and Romania. Maize porridge (polenta) and other preparations of maize contain very little niacin (vitamin B3), particularly if maize is not treated in the traditional American-Indian way. The adoption of a monotonous maize diet among poor farmers and land labourers in Southern and South-eastern Europe therefore led to a serious rise of pellagra in the 18th and 19th centuries.[105]

Quantitative data on long-term trends in pellagra are scarce – most countries where pellagra occurred were underdeveloped at the time and did not keep registers or conduct surveys. The main exception is Italy, where the Ministries of Agriculture and Internal Affairs conducted several large-scale surveys of pellagra. In 1879, the total number of cases in Italy as a whole was still around 100,000 (3.4% of the population). In the last decades of the 19th century, prevalence declined strongly, to 42,000 cases (1.2% of the population) in 1909. In 1954, only 25 cases were left in the country as a whole. Strong declines have also occurred elsewhere, creating another striking picture of a disease's 'rise-and-fall'.[106]

In Italy as in other European countries, the decline of pellagra was partly caused by the improvements in nutrition that accompanied the general rise in living standards and diversification of diets. Yet, deliberate interventions to prevent and treat pellagra also played a crucial role. The link with a monotonous maize diet had already been recognized by some in the 19th century, leading to early attempts to change diets for the better, and to improve the miserable living conditions of poor agricultural workers. It had also already been found that yeast (later shown to be rich in niacin) could cure pellagra. More precisely targeted interventions, such as food fortification for the prevention of pellagra, and vitamin injections for its treatment, became possible in the late 1930s, after the scientific demonstration that the disease was due to a lack of niacin.[107]

---

105 For a general history of pellagra, see Elisabeth W. Etheridge, "Pellagra," in *Cambridge World History of Human Disease*, ed. Kenneth F. Kiple (Cambridge etc.: Cambridge University Press, 1993). For the social history of pellagra, see Daphne A. Roe, *A Plague of Corn* (London: Cornell University Press, 1973). For political aspects, see, e.g., Alfred J. Bollet, "Politics and Pellagra: The Epidemic of Pellagra in the US in the Early Twentieth Century," *Yale Journal of Biology and Medicine* 65, no. 3 (1992): 211–21.

106 Quantitative data for Italy can be found in Renato Mariani-Costantini and Aldo Mariani-Costantini, "An Outline of the History of Pellagra in Italy," *Journal of Anthropological Sciences* 85 (2007): 163–71; Monica Ginnaio and Amy Jacobs, "Pellagra in Late Nineteenth Century Italy: Effects of a Deficiency Disease," *Population (French edition)* 66, no. 3 (2011): 583–609.

107 France was ahead of other Southern European countries in the fight against pellagra, as a result of early studies demonstrating the combined role of diet and poverty, and subsequent advocacy for dietary change and social reform, by Théophile Roussel (1816–1903) (see Roe, *Plague of Corn*, Chapter 6). For analyses of the decline of pellagra, see Youngmee K. Park et al., "Effectiveness of Food Fortification in the United States: The Case of Pellagra," *American Journal of Public Health* 90, no. 5 (2000): 727–38; Mariani-Costantini and Mariani-Costantini, "An Outline of the History of Pellagra in Italy."

Rickets is another nutrient deficiency disease that rose strongly and then fell precipitously during the socioeconomic modernization of European societies. Its name has an unknown origin, and is synonymous with '*rachitis*'. Rickets is due to faulty ossification of bones, which leads to weak bones that fracture easily, bowed legs, stunted growth, and various other abnormalities, including mental retardation. It was a disease of growing infants and children, caused by a lack of dietary vitamin D combined with insufficient exposure to sunlight. It was first described in the 17th century, apparently because the disease then started to occur more frequently, first in England, then in other countries in North-western Europe. It has remained uncommon in Southern Europe.

Rickets already occurred in prehistory and in antiquity, but became very common in the 18th and 19th centuries as a result of industrialization and urbanization. The rise was due to the increasing numbers of children growing up in crowded and air-polluted urban centres, with inadequate diets and very little exposure to sunlight. Sunlight is needed to make active vitamin D from vitamin D precursors in the skin. In the absence of active vitamin D, dietary calcium cannot be properly absorbed in the intestines, leading to the skeletal and other abnormalities mentioned above. Because England was ahead of other countries in its industrialization and urbanization, it also led the world in rickets, which was therefore often called 'the English disease'.[108]

As in the case of pellagra, quantitative data on long-term trends in rickets are hard to find. It was not a directly fatal disease, but did appear in the London Bills of Mortality as a cause of 2 to 3% of all deaths by the mid-17th century, to disappear again in the first half of the 18th century. In the 19th century, rickets prevalence among children must have been very high, as shown by hospital statistics. Data on admissions to children's hospitals, or visits to policlinics of children's hospitals in Europe's large cities, show that in the 1860s to 1880s the prevalence of rickets ranged between 8 and 30% of all children below the age of 5 years in Copenhagen, Basel, Dresden, Berlin, Frankfurt-on-Main, London, Manchester and Prague. Mild forms of rickets were present in even higher percentages of children.[109]

---

108 For a general history of rickets, see, e.g., R. Ted Steinbock, "Rickets and Osteomalacia," in *Cambridge World History of Human Disease*, ed. Kenneth F. Kiple (Cambridge etc.: Cambridge University Press, 1993); A. White Franklin, "Rickets," in *The History and Conquest of Common Diseases*, ed. Walter R. Bett (Norman: University of Oklahoma Press, 1954). The first description is by Whistler in 1645, in a thesis entitled (translated from Latin) *On the disease of English children which is commonly called the rickets.*

109 Mortality from rickets in the London Bills of Mortality can be found in Mercer, *Disease*, App. 2a. Children's hospital statistics on rickets were compiled by Hirsch, *Handbook*, vol. III, p. 735.

Although vitamin D was only identified in 1922, the role of lack of sunlight had already been established in the late 19th century. The beneficial effects of cod-liver oil, which is naturally rich in vitamin D, was known even earlier, and treatment with cod-liver oil was already applied sporadically in the 19th century. An experimental study among children in Vienna in 1919–1922 definitely showed that addition of cod-liver oil to their diets prevented the occurrence of rickets, and that cod-liver oil also cured the disease among rachitic children. From then onwards, cod-liver oil has been used prophylactically in millions of children in North-western Europe. As a result of improvements in housing conditions and diet, and of these specific prevention efforts, rickets has disappeared almost completely. However, it has recently returned in Europe as a disease among migrants (due to culturally prescribed whole-skin covering or to dark skins, in which the weaker sun-rays of Northern latitudes cannot sufficiently penetrate) and among families following unusual diets (e.g., infants on a vegan diet).[110]

Goitre, an enlargement of the thyroid that is due to iodine-deficiency, is different from the previous two diseases in that it has not followed a clear pattern of 'rise-and-fall'. It also had a peculiar geographic distribution across Europe, with a high prevalence of the disease in, for example, the Alps, Pyrenees and Apennines, and a number of circumscribed areas in Scandinavia, Yugoslavia, Hungary and Romania. This is probably due to the fact that drinking water in these areas does not naturally contain iodine, a mineral necessary for the synthesis of thyroid hormones.[111]

The enlargement of the thyroid results from attempts of the organism to increase the production of thyroid hormone. More serious than the goitre itself are some of the other consequences of a lack of thyroid hormone, such as growth retardation, mental retardation, fatigue and depression. Iodine deficiency in pregnancy can lead to cretinism in offspring, a congenital form of the disease that is characterized by severely stunted physical growth (dwarfism). Epidemiological studies conducted in European regions where goitre was endemic, showed that in the 1920s to 1940s the prevalence of the disease was as

110 For the history of cod-liver oil, see White Franklin, "Rickets." The story of the Vienna study has been retold in Harriette Chick, "Study of Rickets in Vienna 1919–1922," *Medical History* 20, no. 1 (1976): 41–51. For the current understanding of rickets, see Thomas O. Carpenter et al., "Rickets," *Nature Reviews Disease Primers* 3 (2017): 17101.

111 Good introductions to the history of goitre and cretinism can be found in Henschen, *History*, pp. 183–95, and in Clark T. Sawin, "Goiter," in *Cambridge World History of Human Disease*, ed. Kenneth F. Kiple (Cambridge etc.: Cambridge University Press, 1993).

high as 20 to 50% of all children, and that the prevalence of cretinism was as high as 0.1 to 1%.[112]

Iodine was discovered in the early 19th century, as part of the rise of modern chemistry. A possible role of iodine deficiency in causing goitre was already suspected in the 19th century, but side effects of iodine prophylaxis and treatment did not encourage its wide-spread use. It was in the early 1920s that the effectiveness of small doses of iodine was proven experimentally, after which iodization of table salt was gradually introduced as a public health measure to prevent goitre. Switzerland was the first European country to apply this policy, and to eliminate goitre and cretinism. Many other countries followed, and goitre and cretinism have since receded greatly.[113]

Unfortunately, low-grade iodine deficiency has returned in the 1980s and 1990s, when almost half of all European children and adults were shown to have insufficient iodine intake. This reversal has occurred partly because iodization of table salt is no longer strictly enforced, partly because table salt is no longer the main source of salt in the diet. The rise of iodine deficiency was particularly strong in Eastern Europe, where the political disruption after the collapse of the Soviet Union also disrupted these countries' iodization policies. The main health risk now is that this may cause cognitive impairment in children, who are born from mothers with low-grade iodine deficiency during pregnancy. Although the World Health Organization has tried to improve the situation, progress is unsatisfactory in many countries.[114]

Peptic Ulcer, Appendicitis

Peptic ulcer (i.e., stomach and duodenal ulcer) and appendicitis have been combined in one section, because both have a very striking 'rise-and-fall'

112 Figures cited from Henschen, *History*, pp. 186–89.

113 Quantitative data on long-term trends are again hard to find. Although goitre was not a common cause of death, trends in mortality can be followed over time in several European countries since the 1920s or 1930s. These data show that in the 1940s to 1950s, rates were still relatively high in the Alpine countries Austria and Switzerland, as well as in Hungary. Rates declined rapidly everywhere during the 20th century (data from Alderson, *International Mortality Statistics*, table 68).

114 For the recent history of iodine deficiency in Europe, see Liselotte Schaefer Elinder and Caroline Bollars, "Food and Nutrition," in *Successes and Failures of Health Policy in Europe*, ed. Johan P. Mackenbach and Martin McKee (Maidenhead: Open University Press, 2013). Epidemiological data can be found in Michael B. Zimmermann and M. Andersson, "Prevalence of Iodine Deficiency in Europe in 2010" (paper presented at the Annales d'Endocrinologie, 2011). For a review of recent (lack of) progress in tackling the problem, see John H. Lazarus, "Iodine Status in Europe in 2014," *European Thyroid Journal* 3, no. 1 (2014): 3–6.

pattern within the same, relatively short time-frame. Mortality data show a steep rise of both conditions until the 1930s, and an equally steep decline thereafter. The rising legs of these mortality curves are due to a rising incidence of these diseases, whereas the declining legs reflect a combination of decreasing incidence and decreasing case fatality.

In the case of peptic ulcer, a strong 'birth cohort effect' underlies these trends. In many European countries, mortality from gastric and duodenal ulcer increased among consecutive generations born during the second half of the 19th century, and then decreased in generations born around the turn of the 20th century and later. Such a 'birth cohort effect' suggests an influence of changes in early-life exposure to environmental factors, which influence disease risks throughout subsequent life-course. However, after the 1960s declines in peptic ulcer mortality were no longer due to birth cohort effects, but occurred as 'period effects', i.e., simultaneously in all birth cohorts. This points more in the direction of treatment effects, or other immediately operating changes affecting all birth cohorts at the same time (see Suppl. Figure 13).[115]

The causes of ulcers of the stomach and duodenum, and of the increased acid secretion in the stomach that produces these ulcers, have long remained mysterious. Because of the rise of these diseases in the 19th century, their causes were first sought in changes in nutrition or exposure to psychosocial stress. It was only in the 1980s that it was discovered that infection with *Helicobacter pylori* played a crucial role. Since then, treatment with antibiotics has been added to the management of the disease, which previously mainly focused on lowering acid-production (and surgical removal of parts of the stomach and duodenum in very severe cases).

Infection with *Helicobacter pylori*, and more specifically a shift in the ages at which children become infected with this micro-organisms, also provides a plausible explanation for the birth cohort effects just mentioned. According to this hypothesis, generations born before the later 19th century became infected with *H. pylori* as toddlers, and developed 'atrophic gastritis' (inflammation

115 The birth-cohort effect in peptic ulcer mortality was discovered by American epidemiologists Mervyn Susser and Zena Stein, and used to argue that peptic ulcer was not simply a 'disease of civilization'; see Mervyn Susser and Zena Stein, "Civilisation and Peptic Ulcer," *Lancet* 279, no. 7221 (1962): 116–19. The existence of strong cohort effects was confirmed for six European countries (Amnon Sonnenberg, "Time Trends of Ulcer Mortality in Europe," *Gastroenterology* 132, no. 7 (2007): 2320–27), but in more recent mortality declines cohort effects no longer play a role (Carlo La Vecchia et al., "The Impact of Therapeutic Improvements in Reducing Peptic Ulcer Mortality in Europe," *International Journal of Epidemiology* 22, no. 1 (1993): 96–106).

of the stomach with reduced acid secretion) which protected them from peptic ulcer in their later lives. As a result of improved hygiene and lower risks of transmission within the household, however, later born generations were infected with *H. pylori* at an older age. This made them develop less severe gastritis with less reduction of acid secretion, or even an increase in acid secretion, causing an increase in peptic ulcer incidence in their later lives. Finally, generations who were born even later, benefited from further improved hygiene and a lesser risk of infection with *H. pylori,* which explains the later decline of the incidence of peptic ulcer.[116]

The evidence for this explanation is largely circumstantial, and although the explanation fits the cohort patterns, other factors may have played a role as well. The striking pattern of 'rise-and-fall' may also be partly due to increased recognition of the disease in the early decades of the 20th century (contributing to its apparent rise), and improvements in treatment during the decline of the disease (surgery, blood transfusions, ...). The introduction of effective acid-lowering drugs (cimetidine and other H2-receptor-antagonists) has caused further mortality declines from the 1970s onwards – explaining why recent mortality trends no longer exhibit a birth cohort pattern.[117]

Surprisingly, trends in mortality from appendicitis are roughly similar to those for peptic ulcer: mortality started to rise in the late 19th century, peaked around the 1930s, and declined steeply thereafter (Figure 20). However, in contrast to peptic ulcer, no clear birth-cohort patterns have been identified. There are two competing hypotheses about the explanation of the rise and fall of this disease.

The first is the 'dietary fibre' hypothesis. Traditional diets contain large amounts of fibre, which produce large and soft stools that traverse the intestine rapidly. This decreases the risk of obstruction and subsequent infection of the appendix. In this hypothesis, the rise of the incidence of appendicitis is due to a change from a traditional diet rich in vegetables and cereals to a diet rich in refined food, meat and sugar. Yet, because the decline in the incidence of appendicitis does not coincide with an increase in fibre intake, this hypothesis cannot explain the declining leg of the trend curve, for which other factors have to be invoked. These include the increased use of antibiotics (which may unintentionally have decreased the incidence of appendicitis) and

116 Amnon Sonnenberg, "Causes Underlying the Birth-Cohort Phenomenon of Peptic Ulcer," *International journal of epidemiology* 35, no. 4 (2006): 1090–97.

117 La Vecchia et al., "Impact."

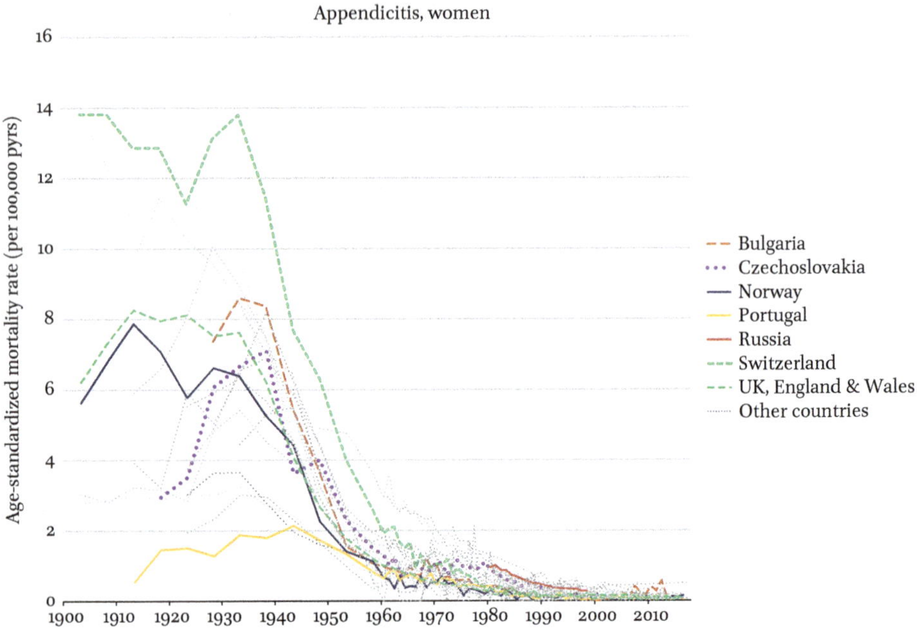

FIGURE 20 Trends in appendicitis mortality in Europe, 1900–2015
Notes: Quinquennial data before 1960
SOURCE OF DATA: SEE SUPPL. TABLE 1

improvements in medical care (safer and more effective surgery, which has certainly reduced the case fatality of the disease).[118]

The second hypothesis is – again – a shift in the age-distribution of infection with intestinal bacteria. Due to improved hygiene and decreased risks of transmission within the households, children born since the late 19th century have experienced intestinal infections at a later age, at which the lymphoid tissue surrounding the appendicular orifice is more developed, which may then upon infection more often lead to obstruction of the appendix. According to this hypothesis, the decline of appendicitis after the 1930s is due to further improved hygienic standards, which reduced risk of infections and/or shifted the age of infection even further upwards. Here again, the decline in mortality of the disease may reflect a combination of decreased incidence and decreased case fatality due to improvements in treatment.[119]

118 The 'dietary fibre' hypothesis was proposed in Trowell and Burkitt, *Western Diseases*.

119 The 'hygiene' hypothesis was proposed in David J. Barker, "Acute Appendicitis and Dietary Fibre: An Alternative Hypothesis," *British Medical Journal* 290, no. 6475 (1985): 1125–27. It

Lung Diseases Caused by Occupational and Environmental Exposures

That many diseases are man-made certainly applies to the diseases caused by the work people do. Working is indispensable to provide for the necessities of life, and so is perhaps some wear-and-tear as a result of the bodily and mental effort that work requires, but many forms of work cause specific health problems that go well beyond such wear-and-tear. Additionally, the actual production processes may lead to pollution of the environment affecting the health of residents of surrounding areas.

Rises-and-falls of health problems linked to occupational and environmental exposures have therefore accompanied European countries' economic development over the past three centuries. However, as explained in Chapter 1, secular changes in these health problems are difficult to capture in a disease-specific approach. This section, although focused on lung diseases caused by occupational and environmental exposures, is therefore somewhat different from other sections.

That working conditions sometimes cause health problems must have been the case throughout human history. Many pre-modern occupations had health risks that were so obvious that Bernardo Ramazzini (1633–1714) could describe more than 50 hazardous occupations in his famous *De Morbis Artificum Diatriba* (On the Diseases of Artisans) – the first book ever on occupational diseases, published in 1700.[120]

However, the following centuries brought a massive increase of occupational diseases and injuries, because industrial modes of production exposed workers to hazardous physical forces and chemical compounds on a scale never seen before. For example, mines for the extraction of coal, iron and other minerals became deeper and more dangerous, and use of steam and electrical power to mechanize work processes increased the risk of injuries, and released dusts and fumes that upon inhalation could cause lung disease.[121]

---

also covers several other diseases including poliomyelitis, see Barker, "Rise." Poliomyelitis originally was a mild disease without paralysis occurring in very young children, but when sanitation improved the average age of infection increased, and the disease became more serious. Poliomyelitis caused major epidemics in 1916 and in the late 1940s and early 1950s; see Hays, *Epidemics and Pandemics*, p. 377 ff. and 411 ff.

120 Giuliano Franco, "Ramazzini and Workers' Health," *Lancet* 354, no. 9181 (1999): 858–61.

121 For a history of occupational diseases from Roman times to the 1940s, with some comparative data for several European countries, see Ludwig Teleky, *History of Factory and Mine Hygiene* (New York: Columbia University Press, 1948).

Because of the enormous variety in physical and chemical exposures to which economic modernization led, the number of occupational diseases has become overwhelmingly large. *Hunter's Diseases of Occupations*, currently the standard textbook in this area, describes hundreds of diseases caused by exposure to specific metals, gases, noise, vibration, heat or cold, barometric pressure, radiation, repeated movements, infections and stress.[122]

Often, it took many years of labour union and public health activism to demonstrate these dangers, and then many years again to enforce countermeasures against often powerful commercial interests. Due to laws, regulations and technical fixes which ultimately made work in mining and manufacturing more safe, and due to the rise of the service sector which reduced the number of people working in mining and manufacturing, many occupational diseases and injuries are much less frequent today than they were in the 19th century. Here again, therefore, we encounter many examples of the 'rise-and-fall' of diseases.

Occupational exposures may cause diseases in any organ system, but play a particularly prominent and specific role in some diseases of the respiratory system, probably because inhalation leads to more intense contact with hazardous substances than other forms of bodily contact. Diseases of the airways and lungs that may be caused by occupational exposures include asthma, chronic obstructive pulmonary disease, pneumoconiosis, lung cancer, and mesothelioma, of which we will only discuss pneumoconiosis and mesothelioma in some detail. Unfortunately, availability of European-wide data on trends in the occurrence of these diseases is seriously limited, so we will have to mainly rely on reports in the scientific literature.[123]

Pneumoconiosis is a disease caused by accumulation of dust in the lungs, and dependent on the type of dust involved is given more specific names, such as silicosis (due to inhalation of silica dust), anthracosis (due to inhalation of coal dust), and asbestosis. Pneumoconiosis leads to an increasing and disabling shortness of breath, and may ultimately lead to death.

That miners, stonecutters and similar occupations exposed to dust have an increased risk of lung disease had been known for a long time. However, the increase in mining, particularly of coal, and the increasing use of power-driven

122 The tenth edition appeared in 2010; see Peter J. Baxter et al., *Hunter's Diseases of Occupations* [*Tenth Edition*] (London: Arnold 2010).

123 The World Health Organization, Eurostat and the International Labour Organization all collect information on aspects of occupational health, but between-country comparability of these data is usually low, and time-series are short.

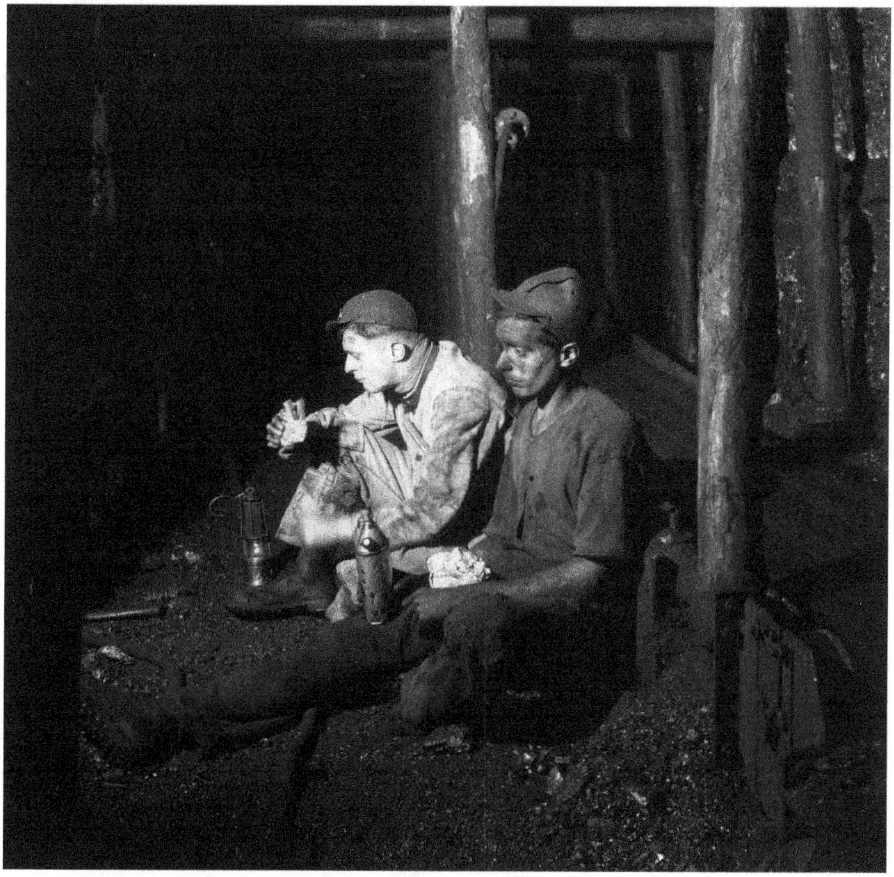

PLATE 13 Miners during their lunch-break in a coal mine in Limburg, 1945
Work in coal mines, often deep under the ground, was warm and dangerous, and inhalation of coal dust caused 'black lung disease,' which was later recognized as one of the pneumoconioses. On this photograph, two miners in the Staatsmijn Wilhelmina (province of Limburg, the Netherlands), covered in coal dust, eat their lunch.
COLLECTION REGIONAAL HISTORISCH CENTRUM LIMBURG (FOTOCOLLECTIE STAATSMIJNEN/DSM). REPRODUCED WITH PERMISSION

tools for grinding in the 19th century led to a big rise in occupational lung disease (Plate 13). This was first noted in England, where industrialization was farthest advanced, but other European countries such as Germany and France followed soon.[124]

124 Andrew Meiklejohn, "History of Lung Diseases of Coal Miners in Great Britain: Part I, 1800–1875," *Occupational and Environmental Medicine* 8, no. 3 (1951): 127–37.

Because other respiratory diseases, such as tuberculosis, were also common among workers in these occupations, it took a long time before pneumoconiosis was recognized as a separate disease. During most of the 19th century, the respiratory diseases of dust-exposed workers were regarded as a form of 'phthisis' or 'consumption' to which they were particularly sensitive.

The bacteriological revolution, which successfully uncovered the bacteriological origins of tuberculosis and many other respiratory diseases, made it seem plausible, that the high disease rates among dust-exposed workers were due to their poor personal hygiene and unsanitary living conditions. As a result, research into the effect of dust stopped for a while, and it was claimed that quartz lungs, coal lungs and the like "belong[ed] rather in a cabinet of curiosities than in industrial hygiene."[125]

It was only in the 1920s and 1930s that the specific aetiology of these diseases was finally recognized. This was mainly due to studies among miners – and to miners' social and political struggle to receive compensation for the health risks to which they were exposed. Mortality statistics in England & Wales showed increasingly high mortality among miners around the turn of 20th century, which led to government studies and official committees, to labour union activism, and to technical improvements in mining in the 1930s which finally reduced the risk of pneumoconiosis.[126]

Occupational exposures are also an important cause of cancer. Many agents to which workers in various industries may be exposed have been classified as carcinogenic, including asbestos, heavy metals, mineral dusts, polycyclic aromatic hydrocarbons and ionizing radiation. The contribution of occupational

125 The quote is from the Swiss hygienist Vogt, reproduced in Teleky, *History*, p. 199. For the recognition of pneumoconioses as separate disease entities, see David Rosner and Gerald Markowitz, "Consumption, Silicosis, and the Social Construction of Industrial Disease," *Yale Journal of Biology and Medicine* 64, no. 5 (1991): 481–98; Gerald Markowitz and David Rosner, "The Illusion of Medical Certainty: Silicosis and the Politics of Industrial Disability, 1930–1960," *Milbank Quarterly* 67, no. Suppl. 2 (1989): 228–53.

126 Andrew Meiklejohn, "History of Lung Diseases of Coal Miners in Great Britain. Part Iii, 1920–1952," *Occupational and Environmental Medicine* 9, no. 3 (1952): 208–20. In addition to lung disease, miners were at risk of many other potentially fatal problems, such as explosions of methane gas. These had to be prevented by ventilation of mine shafts and by the use of safety lamps, which reduced explosion-related deaths among miners In Great Britain and Germany in the first decades of the 20th century; see Teleky, *History*, pp. 238–252.

exposures to cancer occurrence in the population as a whole is in the order of 1–4%, but among workers in the relevant industries it may be up to 20%.[127]

Here we have space for just one illustration: *mesothelioma*, a cancer of (mostly) the lining of the lungs and chest wall that is caused by occupational exposure to asbestos. Asbestos has physical properties which make it attractive for the construction industry, e.g., to insulate buildings, ships, and electrical equipment. There is often a delay of 30 years or more between first exposure to asbestos and the incidence of mesothelioma, and the disease is almost uniformly fatal.

The association between asbestos exposure and mesothelioma was first noted in 1960, but regulatory efforts to reduce and ultimately eliminate asbestos exposure often took a long time to be enacted. Most countries in Northern and Western Europe adopted a ban on asbestos in the 1980s or 1990s, to be followed by many countries in Southern and Central-eastern Europe in the first decade of the 21st century. Many Eastern European countries still have no ban at all, and although asbestos use has declined there as well, it is still comparatively high.[128]

Asbestos use peaked around 1980, and had by then caused an epidemic of mesothelioma in Northern and Western Europe which started in the 1970s and 1980s, and which has been predicted to level off and then decline in the 2010s or 2020s. International data on mesothelioma mortality are only available since the early 1990s (Suppl. Figure 14).[129]

---

127 Doll and Peto estimated the contribution of occupational exposures to the occurrence of cancer in the US in the 1970s to be 4% – much lower than earlier reports had claimed; see Richard Doll and Richard Peto, "The Causes of Cancer: Quantitative Estimates of Avoidable Risks of Cancer in the United States Today," *JNCI: Journal of the National Cancer Institute* 66, no. 6 (1981): 1192–308. This estimate was later revised even further downwards, to 1% among non-smokers, to reflect reductions in exposure since the 1970s; see Julian Peto, "Cancer Epidemiology in the Last Century and the Next Decade," *Nature* 411, no. 6835 (2001): 390–95. Yet, these risks are concentrated in a small fraction of the population; see Paolo Boffetta, "Epidemiology of Environmental and Occupational Cancer," *Oncogene* 23, no. 38 (2004): 6392–403.

128 For asbestos use in Europe, see Takashi Kameda et al., "Asbestos: Use, Bans and Disease Burden in Europe," *Bulletin of the World Health Organization* 92 (2014): 790–97. A shift in marketing from high-income countries to the former Soviet Union was signalled in Laurie Kazan-Allen, "Asbestos and Mesothelioma: Worldwide Trends," *Lung Cancer* 49 (2005): S3–S8. In the 1980s, the Soviet Union had the highest asbestos use in Europe; see Fabio Montanaro et al., "Pleural Mesothelioma Incidence in Europe," *Cancer Causes & Control* 14, no. 8 (2003): 791–803.

129 Mesothelioma mortality started to rise in the 1970s in England and Wales; see Julian Peto et al., "Continuing Increase in Mesothelioma Mortality in Britain," *Lancet* 345, no. 8949

Rates of mesothelioma mortality have remained low in other parts of Europe (with the exception of Italy), which is somewhat surprising in view of the considerable levels of asbestos use in Southern, Central-eastern and Eastern Europe. This may partly be due to use of a less carcinogenic form of asbestos, but may also be a matter of under-registration (or of a rise-still-to-come).[130]

Most of the rise of mesothelioma in Northern and Western Europe could have been avoided if earlier action had been taken. This can be illustrated with the contrasting experiences of Sweden and the Netherlands. Whereas Sweden had its first asbestos regulation in 1964, followed by increasingly stricter rules on the use of asbestos in the 1970s and a ban in 1989, the Netherlands only started to act in the 1970s. This not only led to a decade's delay before the peak in asbestos use was reached, but also to a much higher peak in asbestos use in the Netherlands than in Sweden.[131]

At present, other health problems than the specific diseases listed in *Hunter's Diseases of Occupations* dominate the statistics of sickness absenteeism and work disability: common musculoskeletal diseases like arm and shoulder complaints and low back pain, and common mental health problems like depression. The first are partly due to the repetitive and sedentary work that is common in service economies, and the second are partly due to the equally common combination of high job demands and low job control.[132]

(1995): 535–39. For Sweden, see Bengt Järvholm and Alex Burdorf, "Emerging Evidence That the Ban on Asbestos Use Is Reducing the Occurrence of Pleural Mesothelioma in Sweden," *Scandinavian Journal of Public Health* 43, no. 8 (2015): 875–81. For the Netherlands, see O. Segura, Alex Burdorf, and Caspar Looman, "Update of Predictions of Mortality from Pleural Mesothelioma in the Netherlands," *Occupational and Environmental Medicine* 60, no. 1 (2003): 50–55.

130 Countries in Central-eastern and Eastern Europe Eastern mainly used chrysotile which is less carcinogenic than other types of asbestos; see Montanaro et al., "Pleural Mesothelioma."

131 For the effect of the early ban on mesothelioma in Sweden, see Järvholm and Burdorf, "Emerging Evidence." For comparison between Sweden and the Netherlands, see Alex Burdorf, Bengt Järvholm, and Anders Englund, "Explaining Differences in Incidence Rates of Pleural Mesothelioma between Sweden and the Netherlands," *International Journal of Cancer* 113, no. 2 (2005): 298–301.

132 On occupational musculoskeletal disorders, see, e.g., Bruno R. Da Costa and Edgar Ramos Vieira, "Risk Factors for Work-Related Musculoskeletal Disorders," *American Journal of Industrial Medicine* 53, no. 3 (2010): 285–323. For a review of the health effects of job demands and job control, see, e.g., Wilmar B. Schaufeli and Toon W. Taris, "A Critical Review of the Job Demands-Resources Model," in *Bridging Occupational, Organizational and Public Health*, ed. Georg F. Bauer and Oliver Hämmig (Dordrecht: Springer, 2014).

Although this shows that work may still pose a risk to health, being out of work currently poses an even greater risk to health. Due to the improvement of working conditions, the health promoting effects of having employment, e.g., as a result of the income, social contacts and/or self-fulfilment it provides, now generally outweigh its health risks.[133]

The Industrial Revolution not only increased workers' exposure to hazardous conditions, but also created health risks for the general population. It led to large-scale changes in the physical environment, many of which hold potential risks for human health. The clearest example is the burning of fossil fuels, which allowed humans to multiply their energy use, but also led to massive air pollution. Also, rivers were dammed, water tables depleted, and fresh water sources polluted. Forests were felled, seas and oceans over-fished, and natural environments replaced by sprawling megacities. Humans themselves became a significant geological agent, by mining the Earth, moving rocks, and eroding the soil.[134]

Like in the case of occupational exposures, this is too large a topic to be covered completely, and we will therefore focus on just one, but extremely important, aspect: long-term trends in *air pollution* and its health consequences. Currently, air pollution is the most important cause of health problems in Europe linked to the physical environment, accounting for around 2.5% of deaths and 1% of disability-adjusted life-years lost. It is much more important than other health risks in the physical environment, such as exposure to lead or other metals. It is also much more important than occupational exposures, but considerably less important, in terms of the associated disease burden, than behavioural risk factors such as smoking, excessive alcohol consumption and obesity.

The most obvious effects of air pollution are on the risks of respiratory diseases such as Chronic Obstructive Pulmonary Disease and respiratory infections, but it has increasingly become clear that inhalation of various air pollutants also increases the risk of cardiovascular diseases (ischaemic heart disease, cerebrovascular disease) and lung cancer.[135]

---

133 See, e.g., Maaike van der Noordt et al., "Health Effects of Employment: A Systematic Review of Prospective Studies," *Occupational Environmental Medicine* 71, no. 10 (2014): 730–36.

134 John R. McNeill, *Something New under the Sun* (London: Allen Lane, 2000).

135 The term 'air pollution' here refers to outdoor or 'ambient' air pollution, and not to indoor air pollution which is still an important cause of health problems in developing countries. For quantitative estimates of the burden of disease caused by outdoor air pollution, see GBD 2017 Collaborators, "Global, Regional, and National Comparative Risk Assessment."

Air pollution is not a single thing. Awareness of the health effects was boosted by a number of disastrous events, such as the Great Smog in London in December 1952. Stagnant weather conditions caused a sharp increase in the concentration of air pollutants, causing thousands of deaths. This and other events not only led to first steps in air pollution control, but also to research into the components which actually produced the deleterious health effects. This has, over the years, shown that at least four components are important. These are sulphur dioxide (released during combustion of traditional fuels such as coal), nitrogen oxides (mainly produced by combustion of liquid fuels in motorized vehicles), ozone (produced by the action of sunlight on other air pollutants), and small airborne particles (either emitted directly during combustion of diesel and other fuels, or formed in the atmosphere from gaseous air pollutants).[136]

In Europe, recent trends for air pollution have been favourable, but these declines only occurred after many years of dramatically rising emissions. The very beginnings of man-made air pollution date back to the discovery, hundreds of thousands of years ago, that it was possible to control fire, and to use it for heating and cooking. Indoor air pollution, which already caused health problems in prehistoric times, was replaced by outdoor air pollution as the main risk to human health much more recently, when fossil fuels came to be burned on a massive scale. In the late 19th and early 20th centuries coal combustion in factories and dwellings caused most of the outdoor air pollution, but by the end of the 20th century road traffic had become the largest single source.

Some of these trends can be seen in Figure 21. In Europe as a whole, sulphur dioxide emissions peaked around 1980, but with important differences between West and East. In Northern and North-western Europe, emission reductions already started in the 1970s, when countries began to implement new technologies and switch from coal to gas (the burning of which releases less pollutants than the burning of coal), and were later bound by United Nations protocols that set ceilings for sulphur dioxide emissions. In Central-eastern and Eastern Europe, emissions continued to rise during the 1980s, and only started to fall in the 1990s, first as a result of the economic recession and the closing down of old industries, and later as a result of implementation of new

136 For reviews of the health effects of various air pollutants, see, e.g. Bert Brunekreef and Stephen T. Holgate, "Air Pollution and Health," *Lancet* 360, no. 9341 (2002): 1233–42; World Health Organization, *Health Aspects of Air Pollution*, WHO Regional Office for Europe (Copenhagen, 2004). The evidence was recently updated in World Health Organization, *Review of Evidence on Health Aspects of Air Pollution* (Copenhagen: WHO Regional Office for Europe, 2013).

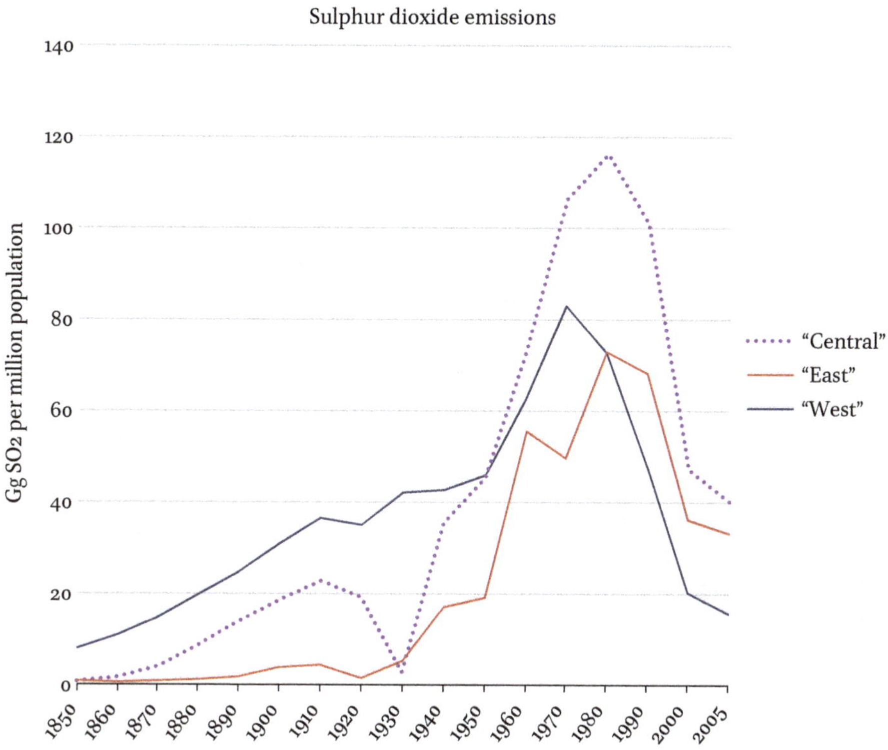

FIGURE 21 Trends in sulphur dioxide emissions in Europe, 1850–2005
Notes: Gg = gigagram = one million kilogram. "West" = Northern, North-western and Southern Europe. "Central" = Central-eastern and South-eastern Europe. "East" = Eastern Europe
SOURCE OF DATA: S.J. SMITH, ET AL. (2011). ANTHROPOGENIC SULFUR DIOXIDE EMISSIONS: 1850–2005. *ATMOSPHERIC CHEMISTRY AND PHYSICS*, 11(3), 1101–16, TABLE 2

technologies and reduction targets agreed as part of accession to the European Union.[137]

Nitrogen oxide emissions peaked somewhat later, around 1990, with again an important role for United Nations protocols and European Union targets. The increase in motorized transport during the 1950s and 1960s led to a huge rise in emissions, which was eventually curbed by technological improvements to vehicles (such as improved combustion and fitting of catalytic converters).

137 For long-term reductions in sulphur dioxide emissions in Europe, see Vigdis Vestreng et al., "Twenty-Five Years of Continuous Sulphur Dioxide Emission Reduction in Europe," *Atmospheric Chemistry and Physics* 7, no. 13 (2007): 3663–81.

As in the case of sulphur dioxide emissions, the turning-point came earlier in the West than in the East. Secular trend data for ozone and particulate matter like those pictured in Figure 21 are not available, but concentration of these pollutants in the atmosphere has probably followed a similar rise-and-fall pattern.[138]

The massive increases in air pollution during most of the 20th century must have had a negative impact on population health, but the exact magnitude of this effect is unknown. Above, we noted in passing that mortality from Chronic Obstructive Pulmonary Disease rose during the 1950s and 1960s in several European countries (Figure 15) – but that this rise was mainly due to smoking. Nevertheless, it is likely that increasing levels of air pollution also contributed to this increase, and also to the increase of cardiovascular diseases and lung cancer in the same period. Likewise, the substantial decline in air pollution in the last decades must have had a positive – but difficult to quantify – impact on population health as well.

While recent trends in air pollutants directly harming human health have thus been favourable, emissions of carbon dioxide have not yet been as effectively curbed by countermeasures, leaving the challenge of climate change mainly to future generations.

---

138 For long-term reductions in nitrogen oxide emissions in Europe, see Vigdis Vestreng et al., "Evolution of NOx Emissions in Europe with Focus on Road Transport Control Measures," *Atmospheric Chemistry and Physics* 9, no. 4 (2009): 1503–20. General overviews of historical trends in emissions can be found in Rachel M. Hoesly et al., "Historical (1750–2014) Anthropogenic Emissions of Reactive Gases and Aerosols," *Geoscientific Model Development* 11 (2018): 369–408; J.-F. Lamarque et al., "Historical (1850–2000) Gridded Anthropogenic and Biomass Burning Emissions of Reactive Gases and Aerosols," *Atmospheric Chemistry and Physics* 10, no. 15 (2010): 7017–39.

CHAPTER 6

Health Problems of Affluent Societies

The health conditions reviewed in this chapter are to some extent characteristic of 'affluent' societies, but this is only true up to a certain point: many of these diseases first rose with rising prosperity in the 20th century, but then started to decline in the second half of the century, despite the fact that prosperity continued to rise. Within high-income societies, they then became concentrated in lower socioeconomic groups, and thus in a sense turned into diseases of poverty. Nevertheless, their rise was in many cases a side-effect of rapid economic growth, which is why we present their secular trends under this heading.

Chronic Diseases

Diseases of the cardiovascular system have spectacularly risen, and then spectacularly declined again, during the 20th century. This was not only a matter of filling the space left by infectious diseases – when people no longer died from infectious diseases, they lived longer, but ultimately had to die from something else – but the rates of cardiovascular disease also increased in real terms in many European countries.

This can clearly be seen in the available mortality data, which for many countries go back to the beginning of the 20th century: not only did the proportion of all deaths attributed to cardiovascular disease increase and then decline again (see Suppl. Figure 5), but absolute levels of cardiovascular disease also first rose and then declined, often dramatically, even after removing the effects of an ageing population. This pattern of 'rise-and-fall' was by no means unique to Europe, but reflects a global phenomenon: with socioeconomic development, mortality from cardiovascular diseases first rises but then declines again.[1]

1 For a world-wide analysis of the association between 'sociodemographic development' and mortality from cardiovascular disease in the period 1990–2015, see Gregory A. Roth et al., "Global, Regional, and National Burden of Cardiovascular Diseases for 10 Causes, 1990 to 2015," *Journal of the American College of Cardiology* 70, no. 1 (2017): 1–25.

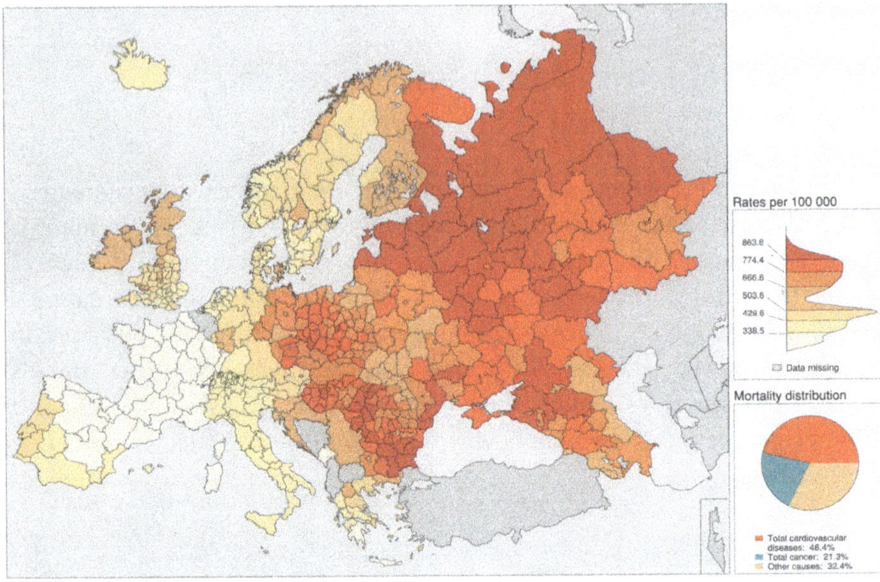

PLATE 14 Map of cardiovascular disease mortality in Europe, 1990
This map shows mortality from cardiovascular diseases by subnational region in almost all European countries, even including a large part of European Russia. Only Belgium (!), Bosnia, Albania, North Macedonia and Turkey were unable to contribute data to the Atlas from which this plate has been reproduced. What we see is dominated by a striking West-East gradient, with generally lower mortality in the West of Europe and higher mortality in the East. National boundaries often produce sharp contrasts in mortality rates, as in the case of Portugal vs. Spain, Germany and Austria vs. Czech Republic and Hungary, and Finland vs. Russia.
WORLD HEALTH ORGANIZATION, ATLAS OF MORTALITY IN EUROPE. SUBNATIONAL PATTERNS, 1980/1981 AND 1990/1991 (COPENHAGEN: WHO EUROPE, 1997), PAGE 77. REPRODUCED WITH PERMISSION

Hiding below these over-all trends, however, are very different trends for the specific diseases that make up the broader group of 'cardiovascular disease'. It includes various forms of heart disease (such as congenital heart disease, chronic rheumatic heart disease, and ischaemic heart disease), cerebrovascular disease, hypertensive disease, aortic aneurysm and many other conditions, all of which have followed their own long-term trends. Thanks to an abundance of epidemiological studies we are relatively well informed about trends and variations in cardiovascular disease (Plate 14). This section will focus on the two diseases that for most of the 20th century have been the most important: ischaemic heart disease and cerebrovascular disease.[2]

2 Currently, more than half of all deaths from cardiovascular disease in Europe are due to ischaemic heart disease, and between one-quarter and one-third to cerebrovascular disease; see Roth et al., "Global, Regional, and National Burden of Cardiovascular Diseases", fig. 4.

Ischaemic Heart Disease

'Ischaemic heart disease' is a disease that has only relatively recently been recognized as a separate disease entity, probably because it was rare before the end of the 19th century. Its current name (as well as synonyms like 'arteriosclerotic heart disease' and 'coronary heart disease') refers to the underlying disease process, i.e., atherosclerosis of the coronary arteries that provide the heart muscle with oxygen. Restriction of the blood flow to the heart muscle may lead to pain during physical exertion (angina pectoris). When combined with coronary thrombosis, as happens when an atherosclerotic plaque ruptures, it may lead to a potentially fatal myocardial infarction.[3]

This understanding of the link between symptoms and underlying disease process has developed slowly between the 1880s and 1920s. This also implies that some of the rise of ischaemic heart disease in the first half of the 20th century probably reflects better recognition. The first clear descriptions of the – then still puzzling – symptoms of angina pectoris date back to the 18th century. The idea that the acute event of what we now call a 'myocardial infarction' was caused by occlusion of the coronary arteries emerged in the last decades of the 19th century, and remained disputed well into the 20th century.[4]

The underlying disease process – atherosclerosis of the coronary arteries – begins early in life, and autopsy studies have shown that the prevalence was already high in several European countries in the first half of the 20th century. These studies also showed that the prevalence temporarily declined during World Wars I and II, suggesting a link between atherosclerosis of the coronary arteries and the abundance or shortage of food.[5]

The rise of ischaemic heart disease led to huge investments in research, particularly in the United States where this 'epidemic' occurred somewhat earlier than in Europe. Research findings have confirmed an important role for dietary

3 See Christian Weber and Heidi Noels, "Atherosclerosis: Current Pathogenesis and Therapeutic Options," *Nature Medicine* 17, no. 11 (2011): 1410–422 for an overview of the current understanding of the pathogenesis of ischaemic heart disease.

4 The first clear description of the suspected link between coronary occlusion and sudden death was given in 1878, and Osler's textbook *The principles and practice of medicine* (1892) briefly referred to what we would now call a myocardial infarction. For the history of the understanding of this disease, see David S. Jones, *Broken Hearts* (Baltimore: Johns Hopkins University Press, 2013); W. Bruce Fye, "The Delayed Diagnosis of Myocardial Infarction: It Took Half a Century!," *Circulation* 72, no. 2 (1985): 262–71.

5 Autopsy trend studies of atherosclerosis in Northern and Western Europe and in the US were summarized in Henschen, *History*, pp. 217–24. A high prevalence of atherosclerosis of the coronary arteries in the first decades of the 20th century, and a lower prevalence in the immediate post-World War II years, was found in an autopsy study from London; see Jerry N. Morris, "Recent History of Coronary Disease," *Lancet* 257, no. 6645 (1951): 1–7.

factors as well as for a number of other risk factors in the aetiology of this disease. The list of established risk factors is quite long. The three most important risk factors are high serum cholesterol, cigarette smoking, and high blood pressure, but diabetes, obesity, lack of physical exercise, low fruit & vegetable consumption, excessive alcohol consumption, depression, job stress, adverse childhood conditions, and genetics also increase the risk of ischaemic heart disease.

This has provided ample opportunities for prevention of ischaemic heart disease, for example by reducing high serum cholesterol (through dietary modification or cholesterol-lowering drugs (statins)), by reducing hypertension (through case finding and treatment with antihypertensive drugs), and by reducing smoking (through smoking cessation advice and support). This has gradually evolved into the adoption of systematic 'cardiovascular disease risk management' by medical professionals, and a growing recognition that this needs to be supported by society-wide measures to reduce saturated fat, trans fatty acids and salt content of foods, to discourage tobacco consumption, and to promote physical exercise.

The growing understanding of the pathogenetic mechanisms underlying ischaemic heart disease has also created ample opportunities for life-saving treatment, both immediately after the acute event of a myocardial infarction and during later stages of the disease. Coronary care units, introduced in the 1970s, were probably not effective in lowering mortality, but thrombolytic therapy and revascularization of the coronary arteries are life-saving. The latter intervention may involve 'coronary artery bypass grafting', or the simpler 'percutaneous coronary intervention' in which a stent is used to re-open an occluded artery. Treatment of the acute event needs to be followed by 'secondary prevention' through similar strategies of risk factor modification as in primary prevention: lifestyle changes, statins, antihypertensive drugs, anticoagulation drugs, …[6]

Trends in ischaemic heart disease mortality in Europe are shown in Figure 22. The country with the longest times-series is England & Wales, where mortality

6 For an overview of the relative importance of the classical risk factors for ischaemic heart disease, see Peter W.F. Wilson et al., "Prediction of Coronary Heart Disease Using Risk Factor Categories," *Circulation* 97, no. 18 (1998): 1837–847. For the effectiveness of secondary prevention, see Finlay A. McAlister et al., "Randomised Trials of Secondary Prevention Programmes in Coronary Heart Disease," *British Medical Journal* 323, no. 7319 (2001): 957–62.

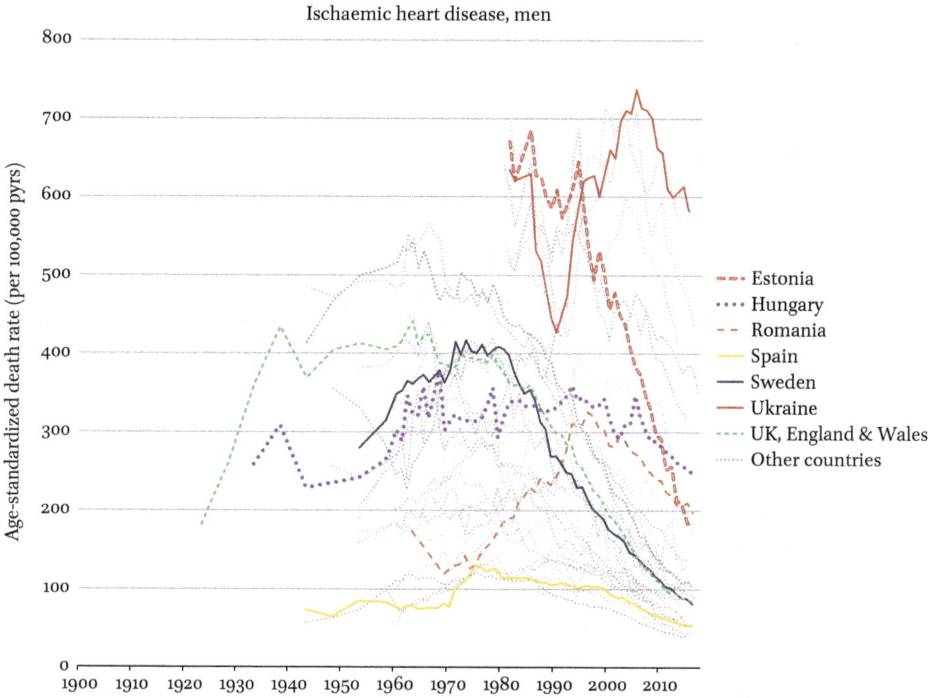

FIGURE 22 Trends in ischaemic heart disease mortality in Europe, 1900–2015
Notes: Quinquennial data before 1960
SOURCE OF DATA: SEE SUPPL. TABLE 1

from ischaemic heart disease can be followed from the 1920s onwards. It shows a rapid rise until the mid-1970s, and a continuous decline thereafter.[7]

Many other European countries also show a clear 'rise-and-fall' pattern, but with important differences in both timing of the peak and level of mortality

7 The rapid rise of ischaemic heart disease mortality in England & Wales in the first half of the 20th century has been well documented, even over a longer period than shown in Figure 22; see Maurice Campbell, "Death Rate from Diseases of the Heart: 1876 to 1959," *British Medical Journal* 2, no. 5356 (1963): 528–35. Time-series of autopsies in London hospitals between 1868 and 1982 also show an increasing prevalence of ischaemic heart disease at death; see Rodney Finlayson, "Ischaemic Heart Disease, Aortic Aneurysms, and Atherosclerosis in the City of London, 1868–1982," *Medical History* 29, no. S5 (1985): 151–68. The temporary decline seen during World War II (Figure 22) may be a coding artefact; see David J. Barker and C. Osmond, "Diet and Coronary Heart Disease in England and Wales During and after the Second World War," *Journal of Epidemiology & Community Health* 40, no. 1 (1986): 37–44.

reached during the peak. In many Northern and Western European countries, ischaemic heart disease mortality peaked somewhat later than in England & Wales, but at similar levels. However, in Southern Europe mortality peaked at much lower levels, whereas ischaemic heart disease mortality in Eastern Europe appears to have followed a 'saw-tooth' trajectory with repeated peaks in the 1980s, 1990s and early 2000s. Despite recent rapid declines, Russia, Ukraine and other countries of the former Soviet Union have the world's highest rates of ischaemic heart disease mortality.[8]

The breath-taking decline of ischaemic heart disease mortality has generated an enormous literature. In the US, the decline started somewhat earlier than in Europe, in the mid-1960s, but at first went unnoticed, and it took quite some time before a certain degree of consensus on the causes of the decline emerged. Even now, 50 years later, the explanation of the decline of ischaemic heart disease mortality throughout the developed world is still somewhat tentative. This is paradoxical because our understanding of the determinants of ischaemic heart disease is much better than that of most other diseases, and because the availability of data on trends in risk factors and treatment patterns is also much more extensive.[9]

Clearly, to explain these trends we need to distinguish between trends in incidence and survival of ischaemic heart disease, but it is important to realize that risk factor trends can influence both incidence and survival, and that medical care does not only influence survival but can also reduce risk factor exposure, for example by lowering serum cholesterol or blood pressure.

The *rise* of ischaemic heart disease mortality must have been due to a rise in incidence, because there is little reason to suspect a rise in case fatality. Although data on risk factor exposure before the 1960s are very limited, it is likely that the rise in incidence in Northern and Western European countries was

8 An analysis of the timing of the peaks in ischaemic heart disease mortality can be found in Masoud Mirzaei et al., "Coronary Heart Disease Epidemics: Not All the Same," *Heart* 95, no. 9 (2009): 740–46. For a comparison between ischaemic heart disease mortality levels in different world regions, see Andrew E. Moran et al., "Temporal Trends in Ischemic Heart Disease Mortality in 21 World Regions, 1980 to 2010," *Circulation* 129, no. 14 (2014): 1483–492.

9 Although the decline of ischaemic heart disease mortality in the US followed improvements in prevention and treatment, the famous Bethesda conference, held in 1978, could not reach conclusions about its causes. It was only later, with the use of quantitative models, that a clearer picture emerged; see David S. Jones and Jeremy A. Greene, "The Contributions of Prevention and Treatment to the Decline in Cardiovascular Mortality," *Health Affairs* 31, no. 10 (2012): 2250–258. The role of risk factor trends and medical care in the decline of cardiovascular disease mortality has been reviewed in Majid Ezzati et al., "Contributions of Risk Factors and Medical Care to Cardiovascular Mortality Trends," *Nature Reviews Cardiology* 12, no. 9 (2015): 508–30.

due to the adoption of an 'affluent' diet rich in saturated fats, to the adoption of a more sedentary way-of-life, and to the rise of cigarette smoking. These changes in risk factor exposure were less strong in Southern Europe, and were compounded by periods of rises-and-falls in excessive alcohol consumption in Eastern Europe, which probably explains some of the regional differences seen in Figure 22.

Because it occurred more recently, we are better informed about factors that may have contributed to the *decline* of ischaemic heart disease mortality. The MONICA study – set up to provide internationally comparable data on ischaemic heart disease incidence, case fatality, mortality and risk factors – showed that between the mid-1980s and mid-1990s declining mortality was the result of both declining incidence and declining case fatality. On average, across the 21 participating countries (many of which are in Europe), declines in incidence contributed two-thirds of the declines in mortality, whereas declines in case fatality contributed one-third.[10]

These declines in incidence and case fatality were due to a combination of favourable risk factor changes, as a result of health promotion programs and cardiovascular risk management, and improvements in medical care. The MONICA study, as well as many national studies, have shown that in many European countries population-level trends in serum cholesterol, smoking (unfortunately, among men only), and blood pressure have been favourable. On the other hand, trends in obesity and smoking among women have been unfavourable, but quantitative analyses have shown that trends in risk factors can indeed partly explain trends in ischaemic heart disease incidence and/or mortality.[11]

On the other hand, improvements in treatment have contributed as well. In-hospital case fatality has declined impressively, probably due to advances in acute care, and in the MONICA study declines in case fatality have been

10 Hugh Tunstall-Pedoe et al., "Contribution of Trends in Survival and Coronary Event Rates to Changes in Coronary Heart Disease Mortality," *Lancet* 353, no. 9164 (1999): 1547–557. Many national studies have been conducted, showing that the relative contribution of incidence and case fatality to mortality decline differed between time-periods and between countries (Ezzati et al., "Contributions").

11 For the results of the MONICA study, see Alun Evans et al., "Trends in Coronary Risk Factors in the WHO MONICA Project," *International Journal of Epidemiology* 30, no. Supplement 1 (2001): S35–S40. More recently, the European Society of Cardiology has compiled and analysed population-based data on ischaemic heart disease and its risk factors; see Adam Timmis et al., "European Society of Cardiology: Cardiovascular Disease Statistics 2017," *European Heart Journal* 39, no. 7 (2017): 508–79. Reduced salt consumption may have contributed to lower blood pressure (Ezzati et al., "Contributions").

strongest in European countries – usually in the Northern and Western part of the region – where the improvements in treatment were strongest.[12]

In general, studies have found that, although improvements in treatment have made important contributions, risk factor changes have contributed more to declines in ischaemic heart disease mortality. Risk factor changes were, however, partly the result of risk factor management within the health care system, so that both medical care and public health can rightly claim to have played an important role in the decline of ischaemic heart disease.[13]

In Chapter 7, we discuss why these trends played out so differently in different European countries.

Cerebrovascular Disease

Cerebrovascular disease is a disease of the brain which is characterized by a sudden and often dramatic failure of neurologic functions, such as paralysis of parts of the body, inability to speak, or loss of consciousness. This frightening event is commonly called 'stroke', and as the official name indicates, it is caused by a problem of the blood vessels of the brain. It occurs in two main forms: 'haemorrhagic stroke' (due to rupture of the wall of a blood vessel, resulting in a blood clot pressing against brain tissue) and 'ischaemic stroke' (due to occlusion of a blood vessel leading to insufficient perfusion of brain tissue). Both forms of cerebrovascular disease have a high case fatality, and when people survive they often suffer from severe disabilities. Currently, ischaemic stroke is more frequent than haemorrhagic stroke, but the reverse was true a century

12 The MONICA study showed that about half of the variation in survival trends was explained by treatment – with more improvement in Western than in Eastern Europe; see Hugh Tunstall-Pedoe et al., "Estimation of Contribution of Changes in Coronary Care to Improving Survival, Event Rates, and Coronary Heart Disease Mortality," *Lancet* 355, no. 9205 (2000): 688–700.

13 The contribution of risk factor changes has been documented both in studies relating population-level trends in risk factors to trends in ischaemic heart disease (Kari Kuulasmaa et al., "Estimation of Contribution of Changes in Classic Risk Factors to Trends in Coronary-Event Rates," *Lancet* 355, no. 9205 (2000): 675–87), and in simulation studies using individual-level data (Tiina Laatikainen et al., "Explaining the Decline in Coronary Heart Disease Mortality in Finland between 1982 and 1997," *American Journal of Epidemiology* 162, no. 8 (2005): 764–73; Belgin Unal, Julia Alison Critchley, and Simon Capewell, "Explaining the Decline in Coronary Heart Disease Mortality in England and Wales between 1981 and 2000," *Circulation* 109, no. 9 (2004): 1101–107). The contributions of risk factor changes and improvements in prevention and treatment may well have differed between time-periods and countries; see Earl S. Ford and Simon Capewell, "Proportion of the Decline in Cardiovascular Mortality Disease Due to Prevention Versus Treatment," *Annual Review of Public Health* 32 (2011): 5–22.

ago, because since then haemorrhagic stroke has declined much more than ischaemic stroke.[14]

The risk factors for cerebrovascular disease have been studied extensively, and are relatively well-known. Hypertension, risk factor number 1, is extremely common: the prevalence of hypertension in European countries typically ranges between 30 and 60% of the adult population. It generally increases with socioeconomic development, probably due to the changes in diet and behaviour that accompany industrialization and urbanization. Hypertension may be due to high salt consumption, low fruits and vegetables consumption, low physical exercise, obesity, excessive alcohol consumption, and/or psychosocial stress, and many of these conditions have become more common during socioeconomic modernization.[15]

Hypertension increases the risk of both types of stroke, but a higher proportion of cases of haemorrhagic stroke is attributable to hypertension, because ischaemic stroke has other important risk factors as well, such as high serum cholesterol and smoking. As hypertension rises with socioeconomic development, the frequency of haemorrhagic stroke may also have risen before starting its 20th century decline, but we have no quantitative data to test this idea.[16]

---

14 This is due to the fact that haemorrhagic stroke has declined more than ischaemic stroke; see Mark O. McCarron, George Davey Smith, and P. McCarron, "Secular Stroke Trends: Early Life Factors and Future Prospects," *Quarterly Journal of Medicine* 99, no. 2 (2006): 117–22.

15 Although there are no historical data on the prevalence of hypertension, circumstantial evidence suggests a rise of hypertension with socioeconomic development. Hypertension is very rare in hunter-gatherers (Trowell and Burkitt, *Western Diseases*), and the Global Burden of Disease study shows that currently the prevalence of hypertension is higher in a number of middle-income countries than in both low- and high-income countries, suggesting an inverted-U-shaped relationship (Mohammad H. Forouzanfar et al., "Global Burden of Hypertension and Systolic Blood Pressure of at Least 110 to 115 Mm Hg, 1990–2015," *Journal of the American Medical Association* 317, no. 2 (2017): 165–82). Estimates of the current prevalence of hypertension in European countries can be found in, e.g., Goodarz Danaei et al., "National, Regional, and Global Trends in Systolic Blood Pressure since 1980," *Lancet* 377, no. 9765 (2011): 568–77.

16 Evidence for a rise of haemorrhagic stroke is circumstantial only. The Global Burden of Disease study shows that the incidence of haemorrhagic stroke is higher in middle-income than in high-income countries, which is compatible with the inverted-U-shaped relationship inferred for hypertension; see Valery L. Feigin et al., "Worldwide Stroke Incidence and Early Case Fatality Reported in 56 Population-Based Studies," *Lancet Neurology* 8, no. 4 (2009): 355–69. The high frequency with which medical treatises on 'apoplexy' – the term under which the disease was known in the past – were published in the 18th century suggests that by then it had become more common; see Pandora Pound, Michael Bury, and Shah Ebrahim, "From Apoplexy to Stroke," *Age and Ageing* 26, no. 5 (1997): 331–37.

Hypertension is a silent killer, because it is usually symptomless and can only be discovered if it is measured using a sphygmomanometer. Before the 1960s hypertension could not be treated, but in the 1960s the first modern drugs for the treatment of hypertension, thiazide diuretics, were introduced. In the 1970s these were followed by beta blockers, and in the 1980s by a whole series of other drugs. Antihypertensive drugs have been shown to not only lower blood pressure, but also to lower the risk of cerebrovascular disease (as well as other complications of hypertension, such as ischaemic heart disease).[17]

As soon as hypertension became amenable to medical intervention, systematic detection of hypertension in otherwise healthy people became a useful thing to do, and recommendations to routinely measure blood pressure in patients consulting their doctors for other reasons, gradually came to be included in clinical practice guidelines around the Western world. However, carrying out these guidelines is far from trivial, and adoption therefore is still incomplete in even the most advanced countries.

Coverage of all people who might have hypertension without knowing it, can only be achieved in primary care. However, not all countries have well-organized primary care services, and even when they have, primary care physicians have not always been willing to incorporate this in their everyday work. Furthermore, antihypertensive drugs need to be available to patients without financial barriers, and patients need to comply with their doctors' advice to take their drugs, sometimes life-long and even if they have side-effects – conditions that haven proven difficult to fulfil. Nevertheless, there has been a gradual increase of the proportion of hypertensives under control, particularly in Northern and Western Europe.[18]

---

17 Blood Pressure Lowering Treatment Trialists' Collaboration, "Effects of Different Blood-Pressure-Lowering Regimens on Major Cardiovascular Events," *Lancet* 362, no. 9395 (2003): 1527–535; Vijaya M. Musini et al., "Pharmacotherapy for Hypertension in the Elderly," *Cochrane Database of Systematic Reviews*, no. 4 (2009): CD000028.

18 For organizational requirements and role of primary care, see, e.g., Liam G. Glynn et al., "Interventions Used to Improve Control of Blood Pressure in Patients with Hypertension," *Cochrane Database of Systematic Reviews*, no. 3 (2010): CD005182. Adherence to modern guidelines for detection and treatment of hypertension has increased over the past decades, at least in North-western Europe; see Stephen Campbell et al., "Quality of Primary Care in England with the Introduction of Pay for Performance," *New England Journal of Medicine* 357, no. 2 (2007): 181–90; Erkki Vartiainen et al., "Thirty-Five-Year Trends in Cardiovascular Risk Factors in Finland," *International Journal of Epidemiology* 39, no. 2 (2009): 504–18. As a result, the number of hypertensives whose blood pressure is under control has increased; see Benjamin A. Steinberg et al., "Nine-Year Trends in Achievement of Risk Factor Goals in the US and European Outpatients with Cardiovascular Disease," *American*

Advances in the treatment of cerebrovascular disease are of even more recent date. Before World War II, supportive care of the acute phase, followed by rehabilitation of bodily functions that had become impaired, was the only option. However, from the 1950s onwards survival after a stroke started to improve. This was probably due to more effective treatment of some of its lethal complications (e.g., pneumonia, which could now be treated with antibiotics), and as a side-effect of more rehabilitation (which reduced the risks of being confined to bed).[19]

It was only in the 1980s and 1990s that causal treatment of the acute event of stroke itself became possible, in the form of thrombolytic therapy for ischaemic stroke, and surgical removal of blood clots for haemorrhagic stroke. Such advanced treatments required highly specialized personnel, and were most effective if delays between the event and the start of treatment were short. Rapid transportation of stroke patients to specialized 'stroke units' therefore became more and more the norm in the 1990s.[20]

What has been the impact of these advances in prevention and treatment on the incidence and mortality of cerebrovascular disease? As usual, only mortality trends can be followed for a longer period, and as shown in Figure 23 mortality from cerebrovascular disease has run a somewhat irregular course since the beginning of the 20th century. This is partly due to the fact that the trends for haemorrhagic stroke and for ischaemic stroke – which cannot be distinguished in routine statistics – have been fundamentally different.

In countries where it has been possible to separate the two using clinical information, e.g., in England & Wales, it has been found that mortality from haemorrhagic stroke has declined since the beginning of the 20th century, whereas mortality from ischaemic stroke has followed a course similar to that of ischaemic heart disease: rising until the 1970s, and then declining. The trend of mortality from cerebrovascular disease in England & Wales thus results from the superposition of two different trends: an epidemic-like pattern of

---

Heart Journal 156, no. 4 (2008): 719–27; Paola Primatesta and Neil R. Poulter, "Improvement in Hypertension Management in England," *Journal of Hypertension* 24, no. 6 (2006): 1187–192.

19 W. Michael Garraway, Jack P. Whisnant, and Ivo Drury, "The Changing Pattern of Survival Following Stroke," *Stroke* 14, no. 5 (1983): 699–703.

20 Systematic reviews have concluded that stroke patients who receive organised inpatient care in a stroke unit are more likely to be alive, independent, and living at home one year after the stroke; see Stroke Unit Trialists' Collaboration, "Organised Inpatient (Stroke Unit) Care for Stroke," *Cochrane Database Systematic Reviews*, no. 9 (2013): CD000197.

ischaemic stroke superimposed on the long-term decline of haemorrhagic stroke.[21]

The tendency for haemorrhagic stroke to decline even before the introduction of antihypertensive treatment in the 1960s is probably due to 'spontaneous' declines in the prevalence of hypertension. These will have occurred as a result of a reduction in the intake of salt, due to less use of salt for food conservation, and also perhaps as a result of an increase in the intake of fresh fruits and vegetables. Studies have shown that in the last decades of the 20th century the prevalence of hypertension has continued to decline in many European countries, probably as a result of further dietary changes combined with better detection and treatment of hypertension.[22]

The 'rise-and-fall' of ischaemic stroke is partly due to the same risk factor trends as played a role in the 'rise-and-fall' of ischaemic heart disease. These include a rising and then declining prevalence of smoking, and a rising and then declining prevalence of high serum cholesterol. Reduced intake of salt, and better detection and treatment of hypertension have contributed to the decline of ischaemic stroke too.[23]

More recently, improvements in the treatment of stroke have contributed to declining mortality from both haemorrhagic and ischaemic stroke, as is clear from studies of trends in incidence and case fatality of stroke in recent decades, which found that both have declined.[24]

---

21 Debbie A. Lawlor et al., "Secular Trends in Mortality by Stroke Subtype in the 20th Century," *Lancet* 360, no. 9348 (2002): 1818–823.

22 That part of the decline in hypertension is due to reduced salt intake, part to improved detection and treatment of hypertension is the conclusion of several studies, including Primatesta and Poulter, "Improvement in Hypertension Management in England"; Emanuela Falaschetti et al., "Continued Improvement in Hypertension Management in England," *Hypertension* 53, no. 3 (2009): 480–86. Declines in stroke mortality have generally been larger in countries with stronger declines in systolic blood pressure; see Martin McKee and Johan P. Mackenbach, "Hypertension," in *Successes and Failures of Health Policy in Europe*, ed. Johan P. Mackenbach and Martin McKee (Maidenhead: Open University Press, 2013).

23 A study from England found that declines in stroke were due partly to reductions in smoking, cholesterol, and blood pressure, partly to increases in treatment with antiplatelet, lipid-lowering, and blood pressure lowering drugs; see Peter M. Rothwell et al., "Change in Stroke Incidence, Mortality, Case-Fatality, Severity, and Risk Factors in Oxfordshire," *Lancet* 363, no. 9425 (2004): 1925–933.

24 The contribution of incidence and case fatality to mortality decline has differed between countries. In Finland declining incidence was more important; see Juhani Sivenius et al., "Continuous 15-Year Decrease in Incidence and Mortality of Stroke in Finland," *Stroke* 35, no. 2 (2004): 420–25. In several other countries declining case fatality was more important; see, e.g., Isabelle Benatru et al., "Stable Stroke Incidence Rates but

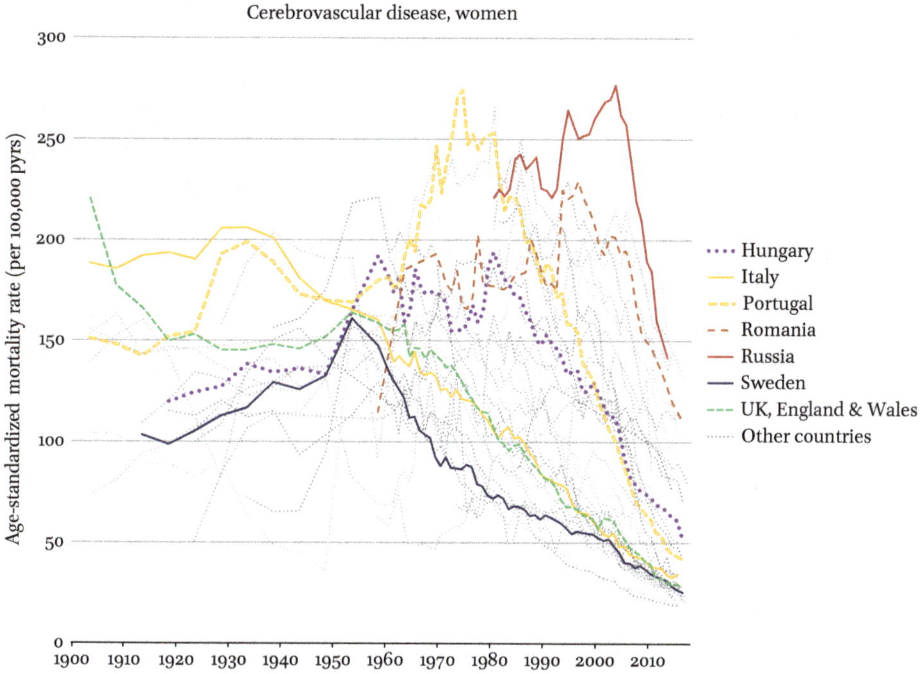

FIGURE 23 Trends in cerebrovascular disease mortality in Europe, 1900–2015
Notes: Quinquennial data before 1960
SOURCE OF DATA: SEE SUPPL. TABLE 1

Let us now return to Figure 23, which covers an unusually long time-range. Because data available in the repository of the World Health Organization do not go further back than 1950, trends in stroke mortality before the 1950s have only rarely been studied.[25]

Trends before World War II were highly variable. Stroke mortality declined in England & Wales, probably reflecting the decline of haemorrhagic stroke mentioned above. However, it increased in many other countries, including Sweden, Italy, Portugal, and Hungary, all marked in the graph. In many countries, this rise continued in the post-war period and led up to a peak in the

Improved Case-Fatality in Dijon, France, from 1985 to 2004," *Stroke* 37, no. 7 (2006): 1674–679; Janika Kõrv, Mai Roose, and Ain-Elmar Kaasik, "Changed Incidence and Case-Fatality Rates of First-Ever Stroke between 1970 and 1993 in Tartu, Estonia," *Stroke* 27, no. 2 (1996): 199–203; Halina Sienkiewicz-Jarosz et al., "Incidence and Case Fatality Rates of First-Ever Stroke," *Neurologia i Neurochirurgia Polska* 45, no. 3 (2011): 207–12.

25 For an overview of trends in stroke mortality, see Masoud Mirzaei et al., "Cerebrovascular Disease in 48 Countries: Secular Trends in Mortality 1950–2005," *Journal Neurology Neurosurgery Psychiatry* 83, no. 2 (2012): 138–45.

1950s or 1960s, which we have earlier identified with the 'epidemic' of ischaemic stroke.

In most countries of Northern, Western and Southern Europe, stroke mortality has declined since the 1960s, with one important exception: Portugal. This country presents one of the most remarkable trends in Figure 23. Portugal already had a high level of stroke mortality before World War II, but experienced a true epidemic after the war, peaking at an exceptionally high level, only to be matched by countries of the former Soviet Union in the 1990s. The timing of this epidemic suggests that ischaemic stroke was the main culprit, but the underlying cause is likely to have been hypertension, because Portugal did not experience a similarly dramatic increase of ischaemic heart disease mortality (see Figure 22).

The Portuguese diet has long been very rich in salt, because foods that were salted for conservation have longer than elsewhere remained an important component of the Portuguese diet. This applies particularly to salted cod – traditional Portuguese cookbooks reputedly contained more recipes for preparing salted cod than there are days in a calendar-year. The fact that a salty diet has lingered on for so much longer in Portugal, is likely due to the fact Portugal has long lagged behind other European countries in social and economic development. It has long remained isolated from international developments under the authoritarian government of António de Oliveira Salazar (governing from 1932 to 1968). Delays in introducing modern methods of hypertension management may also have played a role.[26]

Perhaps even more striking are the trends in Central-eastern and particularly Eastern Europe. In Czechoslovakia, Hungary, Bulgaria, Estonia, and Latvia, stroke mortality peaked in the 1980s, in Romania, Lithuania, and Ukraine in the 1990s, and in Russia and Moldova there was a double peak: a first one in the 1980s and a second, even higher one in the first decade of the 21st century. These high levels and delayed declines of stroke mortality reflect high levels of

26 For a Portuguese study of the high frequency of stroke, see Manuel Correia et al., "Prospective Community-Based Study of Stroke in Northern Portugal," *Stroke* 35, no. 9 (2004): 2048–053. A somewhat speculative analysis of the political background to the delay in 'modernization' of the Portuguese diet can be found in Johan P. Mackenbach, "Bacalhao under the Ponte 25 De Abril: Impressions from Lisbon," *European Journal Public Health* 19, no. 1 (2009): 1. A Portuguese study undertaken in 2003 found that only 11% of those with hypertension were controlled; see Mário Espiga Macedo et al., "Prevalence, Awareness, Treatment and Control of Hypertension in Portugal," *Journal of Hypertension* 23, no. 9 (2005): 1661–666.

hypertension and delayed implementation of hypertension detection and control with modern antihypertensive drugs.[27]

The peaks in stroke mortality in Russia in 1994 and in 2003 resemble those seen for other causes of death (and for total mortality) and coincide with low points in the economy and peaks in excessive alcohol consumption, suggesting that stroke mortality was influenced by either or both of the two. Downturns in the economy may have increased excessive alcohol consumption, and/or may have decreased access to prevention and treatment for hypertension and stroke.[28]

Diabetes Mellitus

Diabetes mellitus is a disease that comes in two forms. Type 1 usually starts in childhood or adolescence, and is probably due to autoimmune destruction of the pancreatic cells that make insulin, a hormone that is needed for glucose metabolism. Type 2 occurs mainly in older adults, and is due to inability of the body to appropriately respond to insulin, which often happens in obesity. Currently, more than 90% of diabetics in Europe have type 2 diabetes.

Both types of diabetes can be fatal, but type 1 used to cause early death in an acute coma, whereas type 2 has a more protracted course and mainly causes death in middle- or old-age through cardiovascular or renal complications. Type 1 needs to be treated with insulin, which was discovered in 1922, whereas type 2 can often also be treated with oral hypoglycaemic drugs, which were developed in the 1950s.[29]

Clinical case-series have shown a strong increase in the survival of diabetes patients, not only due to the treatment of diabetes itself, but also due to prevention and treatment of its complications, such as infection (by means of

27 V. Baláz et al., "Prevalence of Ischaemic Heart Disease Risk Factors in Warsaw and Bratislava. Part 2: Hypertension," *Cor et Vasa* 22, no. 3 (1980): 140–46; L. Mark, A. Katona, and L. Deli, "An Attempt to Evaluate the Risk Factors Related to Coronary Heart Disease in Hungary," *Cor et Vasa* 33, no. 4 (1991): 265–72. In the Soviet Union access to modern antihypertensive drugs such as thiazide diuretics, beta blockers and ACE inhibitors was limited, as was awareness among professionals of the benefits of regular treatment of asymptomatic individuals; see Bayard Roberts et al., "Irregular Treatment of Hypertension in the Former Soviet Union," *Journal Epidemiology Community Health* 66, no. 6 (2012): 482–88.

28 As shown in Andreev et al., "Evolving Pattern" other causes of death amenable to medical intervention fluctuated in a similar way, suggesting that changes in access or quality of health care did play a role.

29 For the development of effective treatments for diabetes, see Chris Feudtner, *Bittersweet* (Chapel Hill & London: University of North Carolina Press, 2004); Awad M. Ahmed, "History of Diabetes Mellitus," *Saudi Medical Journal* 23, no. 4 (2002): 373–78.

antibiotics), cardiovascular disease (by means of cardiovascular risk management) and renal failure (by means of dialysis). Nevertheless, diabetes patients still have higher mortality than non-diabetics.[30]

Unfortunately, both type 1 and type 2 diabetes are on the rise. Not only has increased survival pushed up prevalence, but the incidence of both forms of diabetes has also risen strongly. Diabetes mellitus was already known in antiquity, but was probably rare until the 20th century, when it began to be noted that it was increasingly common, particularly in prosperous and urban areas.[31]

The rising incidence of type 1 diabetes in Europe during recent decades has been extensively documented in epidemiologic studies, and is basically unexplained. The latter also applies to the wide variation in incidence rates between countries. Within Europe, there is a striking North-South gradient, with a more than ten-fold range of variation between Finland, which has record-high rates, and the former Yugoslavia, which has the lowest rates. Both the rising trends and the geographical variations suggest that some aspect of the modern ways of life is involved, but it has so far not been possible to pin-point what this is.[32]

The incidence and prevalence of type 2 diabetes are also rising, but here the explanation is straightforward (Figure 24). Overweight and obesity are the single most important risk factor for type 2 diabetes, and the rise of type 2 diabetes has followed the rise of overweight and obesity. Over the past decades,

30 A famous case-series from the Joslin Clinic in Boston (USA) shows continuous reductions in mortality of diabetes patients between 1897 and 1961, with some acceleration of mortality decline among younger patients in the 1920s; see Herbert H. Marks, "Longevity and Mortality of Diabetics," *American Journal of Public Health and the Nations Health* 55, no. 3 (1965): 416–23. In Denmark, survival of diabetes type 1 patients treated in a central hospital improved considerably between 1933 and 1972; see K. Borch-Johnsen, S. Kreiner, and T. Deckert, "Mortality of Type 1 (Insulin-Dependent) Diabetes Mellitus in Denmark," *Diabetologia* 29, no. 11 (1986): 767–72. Survival has continued to improve in the last decades of the 20th century; see Charbel Abi Khalil et al., "Cause-Specific Mortality in Diabetes: Recent Changes in Trend Mortality," *European Journal of Preventive Cardiology* 19, no. 3 (2012): 374–81.

31 For a short history of diabetes before the 1950s, see Henschen, *History*, p. 195–99. Trends of type 1 diabetes during the 20th century were reviewed in Edwin A.M. Gale, "The Rise of Childhood Type 1 Diabetes in the 20th Century," *Diabetes* 51, no. 12 (2002): 3353–361.

32 For rising incidence and between-country variations in Europe, see Eurodiab ACE Study Group, "Variation and Trends in Incidence of Childhood Diabetes in Europe," *Lancet* 355, no. 9207 (2000): 873–76; J. Tuomilehto et al., "Record-High Incidence of Type I (Insulin-Dependent) Diabetes Mellitus in Finnish Children," *Diabetologia* 42, no. 6 (1999): 655–60; Christopher C. Patterson et al., "Incidence Trends for Childhood Type 1 Diabetes in Europe During 1989–2003 and Predicted New Cases 2005–20," *Lancet* 373, no. 9680 (2009): 2027–033.

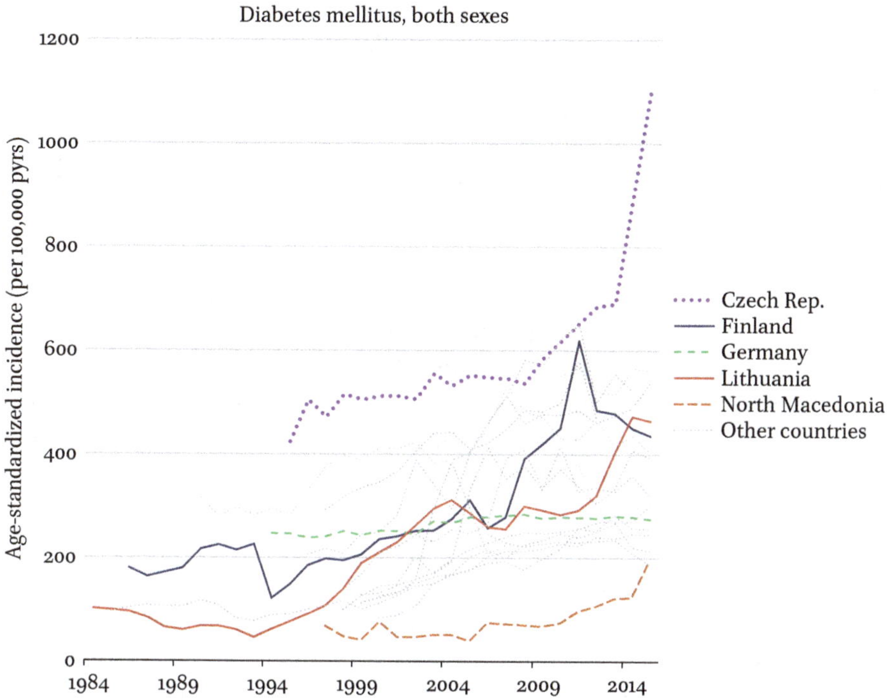

FIGURE 24 Trends in diabetes mellitus incidence in Europe, 1984–2015
Notes: Number of patients with newly diagnosed diabetes during the given calendar year as estimated from registrations of health care utilization
SOURCE OF DATA: EUROPEAN HEALTH FOR ALL DATABASE (WWW.GATEWAY.EURO.WHO.INT, ACCESSED 04/10/19)

the prevalence of overweight and obesity have increased everywhere in Europe, although there are signs in some countries that the epidemic is levelling off among adolescents.[33]

Within Europe, both the prevalence of obesity and that of diabetes vary considerably between countries. Obesity is relatively less prevalent in the Nordic countries, the Netherlands, France, and the Baltic countries, and more prevalent in the South, Central-east and the United Kingdom. The latter

33 For a review of the epidemiology of type 2 diabetes, which is somewhat more complex than suggested here, see Lei Chen, Dianna J. Magliano, and Paul Z. Zimmet, "The Worldwide Epidemiology of Type 2 Diabetes Mellitus – Present and Future Perspectives," *Nature Reviews Endocrinology* 8, no. 4 (2012): 228–36. For recent trends in overweight and obesity, see Benjamin Rokholm, Jennifer L. Baker, and Thorkild I.A. Sørensen, "The Levelling Off of the Obesity Epidemic since the Year 1999," *Obesity Reviews* 11, no. 12 (2010): 835–46.

country seems to act like a bridge to the United States, where the prevalence of obesity is even higher. The prevalence of diabetes follows roughly the same pattern.[34]

Long-term trends in diabetes mortality are somewhat chaotic (see Suppl. Figure 15). Certification and coding of diabetes as a cause of death have undergone many changes over time, and also differ between countries, so we should exercise caution in interpreting these trends. Nevertheless, some interesting patterns can be discerned. For example, despite the introduction of insulin in the early 1920s, a reduction in mortality from diabetes during the 1920s is not always apparent, which suggests that the effect was more limited at the population-level than suggested by clinical reports.

On the other hand, in many European countries diabetes mortality did decline strongly in the 1940s, reflecting the often noted decrease in the incidence of diabetes during the war, as a result of more restrictive food supplies. This decline also occurred in Spain, which went through a period of food scarcity after its Civil War (1936–1939).[35]

However, in the early 1950s diabetes mortality started to rise again, and reached a peak in many Northern and Western European countries in the 1970s or 1980s. These will mainly have been deaths from the long-term cardiovascular complications of diabetes, as suggested by the fact that this peak in diabetes mortality coincided with the peak in ischaemic heart disease mortality. The subsequent decline in diabetes mortality is probably due to advances in the prevention and treatment of cardiovascular disease among diabetes patients.

Stomach, Colorectal, Breast, Prostate Cancer

During the 20th century, cancer has become a much more important cause of death, not only as a percentage of all deaths, but also in absolute terms. This increase in cancer death rates was partly the result of increasing life expectancy, due to which people survived to older ages at which cancer is more frequent. Yet, this is not the whole story: we also see a strong increase when the

34 For between-country differences in the prevalence of obesity, based on nationally representative surveys with measurements of height and weight, see Anne Berghöfer et al., "Obesity Prevalence from a European Perspective: A Systematic Review," *BMC Public Health* 8, no. 1 (2008): 200. For differences in the prevalence of diabetes, see NCD Risk Factor Collaboration, "Worldwide Trends in Diabetes since 1980," *Lancet* 387, no. 10027 (2016): 1513–530.

35 See Gale, "The Rise of Childhood Type 1 Diabetes." For declining incidence of diabetes during World War II in the Netherlands, see J. Hermanides et al., "Lagere Incidentie van Diabetes Mellitus Type 2 bij Verandering van Leefstijl," *Nederlands Tijdschrift voor Geneeskunde* 152, no. 44 (2008): 2415–417.

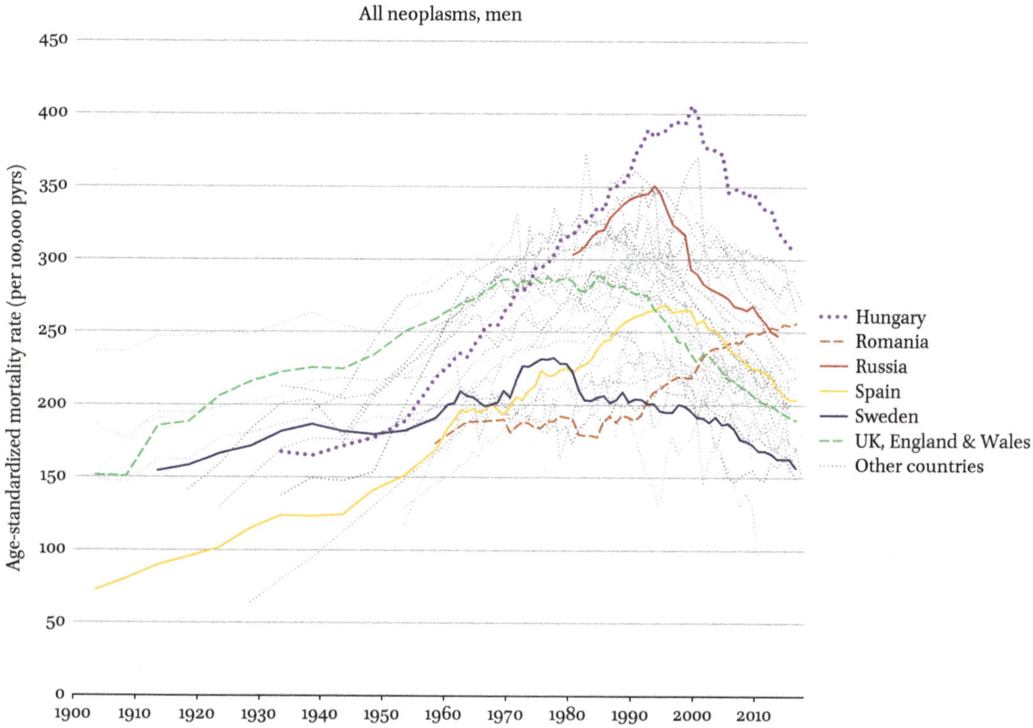

FIGURE 25 Trends in cancer mortality in Europe, 1900–2015
Notes: Quinquennial data before 1960
SOURCE OF DATA: SEE SUPPL. TABLE 1

effect of aging is removed, as in Figure 25. The age-standardized mortality rates from all cancers combined have risen dramatically in most European countries. They peaked somewhere between the 1970s and early 2000s, and then started to decline again, with large variations between countries.

Cancer registries with which trends in the occurrence of new cases of cancer can be followed, were created much later than cause-of-death statistics. Nevertheless, as we have seen in Chapter 2, cancer registries show rising incidence rates of cancer since whenever cancer registrations were established. This suggests that behind the rise of cancer mortality was a general rise of cancer incidence – although increased recognition likely also played a role, particularly of cancers located deeper within the body.[36]

36 There has been a long debate about whether the increase in cancer incidence and cancer mortality was real, or an artefact of better recognition, due to greater access to care and better diagnostic methods. The conclusion that a substantial part of the increase was real,

When the rising frequency of cancer was first noted by contemporaries, at the end of the 19th century, cancer was certainly not a new disease. Millennia-old medical treatises had already described cancer. Still, cancer must long have remained less common, and the increasing frequency of cancer gave rise to many speculations about its causes. Cancer clearly seemed to be a 'disease of civilization': the price one paid for the on-going changes in society, which brought both good and bad things. The suspected causes of cancer ranged from environmental pollution to repressed emotions, and from degenerate morals to the increased survival of people with a hereditary predisposition to cancer.[37]

Currently, cancer is understood as a 'genetic' disease, in the sense that its 'pathologic onset' is a change in cellular DNA that leads to uncontrolled cell growth. More specifically, cancer is believed to arise from mutations in the DNA of tissue-specific stem cells. These are undifferentiated cells that are present in small numbers in all organs, and that constantly multiply to produce the new differentiated cells necessary for tissue maintenance and repair. Cancer-producing mutations may occur as a result of exposure to 'mutagenic' factors such as radiation, carcinogenic substances and – perhaps surprisingly – sex hormones, or as a result of random errors during the replication of these cells' DNA when they divide.[38]

---

is based on several arguments. Increases were not only seen for cancers in which diagnostic techniques had improved but also for cancers in which they had not. Also, for many common cancers, increases in incidence or mortality can be explained from increasing exposure to well-known causes such as tobacco smoking. For an overview of these discussions, see Robert N. Proctor, *Cancer Wars* (New York: Basic Books, 1995), Chapter 1.

37 For a general history of cancer, of how it was understood, and of how prevention and treatment developed over time, see Siddhartha Mukherjee, *The Emperor of All Maladies* (New York etc.: Scribner, 2010). A more politically oriented history of cancer can be found in Proctor, *Cancer Wars*. The putative link between cancer and psychological or cultural factors made cancer a metaphor for personal failings, and a source of guilt and shame, as famously described in Susan Sontag, *Illness as Metaphor* (New York: Farrar, Straus & Giroux, 1978).

38 Two types of mutations are thought to be required for normal cells to become cancer cells: mutations that activate an 'oncogene' (i.e., a gene that promotes cell proliferation) and mutations that de-activate 'tumour-suppressor genes' (genes that limit cell proliferation). There is controversy about the relative importance of exposure to mutagenic factors versus that of random replication errors, with some oncologists arguing that random replication errors account for the large majority of cancers; see Cristian Tomasetti and Bert Vogelstein, "Variation in Cancer Risk among Tissues Can Be Explained by the Number of Stem Cell Divisions," *Science* 347, no. 6217 (2015): 78–81; Cristian Tomasetti, Lu Li, and Bert Vogelstein, "Stem Cell Divisions, Somatic Mutations, Cancer Etiology, and Cancer Prevention," *Science* 355, no. 6331 (2017): 1330–334. However, others argue that random replication errors contribute only 10–30% of lifetime cancer risk; see Song Wu et al.,

Any increase in the occurrence of cancer must therefore be the result of an increase in the exposure to mutagenic factors, and as we will see below trends in many common cancers can indeed be understood in this way. However, the fact that the risks of cancer in so many different organs, and linked to so many different exposures, went up during the 20th century raises a further and deeper question. Is there a common factor underlying all these changes? Why has there been a general rise of cancer – and not of many other diseases that afflict the human body – during this stage of human development? If a vague reference to 'civilization' does no longer satisfy us, what else could it be?

One possibility is that the rise of cancer is due to a generalized increase in exposure to a much wider range of chemical substances than our ancestors were exposed to. Our industries have increased the production of almost everything, in almost infinite chemical variation, bringing prosperity but also exposing workers and consumers to more carcinogens. Environmental pollution increased the inhalation and ingestion of carcinogenic substances by everyone in the population. However, other sources of carcinogens were probably more important. Increased agricultural production has allowed us to eat more and to live on a less monotonous diet, exposing us to a larger variety and to larger quantities of natural carcinogens. The rise of cigarette smoking and excessive alcohol consumption can also be seen as obvious – and quantitatively very important – examples of this generalized increase in exposure to a wider range of chemical substances.[39]

Yet, the rise of these 'unfavourable exchanges with the environment' is unlikely to be the whole explanation. Think of breast cancer, which as we will see below has risen as a result of changes in reproductive behaviour, which have increased exposure of breast tissue to oestrogen. Although this change was mainly driven by changes in fertility behaviour, which could be regarded as changes in how women interacted with their environment, it has little to do with increased exposure to chemical substances. It is inevitable to also invoke 'design failures' when we want to explain the generalized rise of cancer during

"Substantial Contribution of Extrinsic Risk Factors to Cancer Development," *Nature* 529, no. 7584 (2016): 43–7. In view of the large variations in cancer risk between populations and over time, the latter position seems much more credible.

39 This question has been discussed extensively, not only in the late 19th and early 20th centuries, but also more recently. During the 1960s and 1970s, there were wide-spread suspicions that the rise of cancer was due to an increase of industrially produced chemical pollutants (see Proctor, *Cancer Wars*, Chapter 3). These ideas were refuted by Doll and Peto's 1981 report, mentioned above, which showed that most cancers were due to behaviourally mediated factors (diet, tobacco, alcohol, sexual behaviour, …) (Doll and Peto, "Causes").

the 20th century. Humans appear to be highly vulnerable to a disturbance of the biological system that regulates cell proliferation. Many different exposures, to both external and internal agents, can cause a break-down of this system, suggesting that it is just not robust enough. To be more precise: evolution has apparently not selected us for fitness in an environment in which this system comes under attack so frequently.[40]

After this general introduction, let's now look at the secular trends for a few specific cancers, focusing on some of the most important ones. The trend for all cancers combined that we saw in Figure 25, actually hides some striking differences between cancers originating in different organs.

Stomach cancer is one the few cancers for which mortality already declined in North-western Europe before World War II (see Suppl. Figure 16). It is not really possible to identify the starting-point of this decline, although in some of these countries, such as Norway, stomach cancer mortality appears to have peaked around 1920. For Southern European countries, the trends can be followed since the 1930s or 1940s, and show a peak in the 1950s for Italy, the 1960s for Spain and Greece, and the 1970s for Portugal. In other European regions, stomach cancer mortality declined from the moment trend data are available, but suggest a considerable delay as compared to North-western Europe, particularly in Eastern Europe. All-in-all, it seems likely that the long-term trend for stomach cancer has followed a 'rise-and-fall' pattern, with a peak somewhere between the last decades of the 19th century and the 1970s.[41]

The decline of stomach cancer has been called 'an unplanned triumph', and it is certainly true that the decline cannot be attributed to any planned interventions. Current insights into the aetiology of stomach cancer suggest that the secular decline is due to a combination of two factors. The first factor is a

40 This 'design failure' was already briefly mentioned in Chapter 3, when we discussed the difficulty of our organism to deal effectively with 'entropy' (random errors in DNA replication). Our organism is also imperfect in dealing with non-random errors in DNA, such as those due to mutagenic factors. Most of these errors are removed in time, but a tiny fraction escapes and causes cancer. This 'design imperfection' has not disappeared during our evolution, probably because a higher degree of perfection was not necessary for our genetic material to be propagated from one generation to the next: most cancers kill after we have reproduced (Kirkwood, *Time*).

41 There are many studies documenting the secular decline of stomach cancer mortality, e.g., Levi et al., "Cancer Mortality in Europe." For a recent update, see Karim-Kos et al., "Recent Trends." For an up-to-date overview of the epidemiology of stomach cancer, see Catherine De Martel and Julie Parsonnet, "Stomach Cancer," in *Cancer Epidemiology and Prevention (Fourth Edition)*, ed. Michael Thun et al. (Oxford etc.: Oxford University Press, 2017). I have not found literature on a possible rise of stomach cancer before the 20th century.

declining prevalence of *Helicobacter pylori* infection. Infection with this micro-organism is not only involved in the aetiology of peptic ulcer (see Chapter 5), but also in that of a large majority of cases of stomach cancer. It is not exactly known how this infection causes cancer. One of the possible pathways is that, as in other chronic infections leading to cancer, the bacteria form nitrosamines from other nitrous compounds present in food. Nitrosamines are potent carcinogenic substances which are present in some foods, but can also be produced within the body. Over the 20th century, the prevalence of *Helicobacter pylori* infection has gradually declined, as a result of increased hygiene and smaller families.[42]

The second factor contributing to the decline of stomach cancer is changes in diet. Epidemiologic studies have shown that consumption of salted and pickled foods increases the risk of stomach cancer, whereas consumption of fruits decreases this risk. This is probably because salted and pickled foods contain nitrosamines, whereas fruits contain anti-oxidants which are thought to protect against DNA damage. Over the 20th century, the consumption of the first has declined considerably, whereas consumption of the second has increased. Both changes were made possible by the introduction of refrigeration, which reduced the use of salt for food preservation and facilitated year-round transport and storage of fresh produce. Along the same lines, a historical increase in the intake of salted and pickled foods may then explain the rise of stomach cancer in previous time-periods.[43]

---

42 The decline of stomach cancer thus shares some of its causes with the decline of peptic ulcer (through reduced infection with *Helicobacter pylori*). The expression "unplanned triumph" was used in Christopher P. Howson, Tomohiko Hiyama, and Ernst L. Wynder, "The Decline in Gastric Cancer: Epidemiology of an Unplanned Triumph," *Epidemiologic Reviews* 8, no. 1 (1986): 1–27. For the role of a declining prevalence of *Helicobacter pylori* infection, see, e.g., M. Blanca Piazuelo, Meira Epplein, and Pelayo Correa, "Gastric Cancer: An Infectious Disease," *Infectious Disease Clinics* 24, no. 4 (2010): 853–69. On the role of nitrosamines, see Paula Jakszyn and Carlos Alberto González, "Nitrosamine and Related Food Intake and Gastric and Oesophageal Cancer Risk," *World Journal of Gastroenterology* 12, no. 27 (2006): 4296–303.

43 An interesting study looking at the role of the refrigerator in reducing the risk of stomach cancer (in South Korea, which has modernized more recently than most European countries) is Boyoung Park et al., "Ecological Study for Refrigerator Use, Salt, Vegetable, and Fruit Intakes, and Gastric Cancer," *Cancer Causes & Control* 22, no. 11 (2011): 1497–503. *Helicobacter pylori* has accompanied humans on their journey out of Africa, and is found in all human populations around the world. However, the European variants of the micro-organism have mutations that make it particularly virulent; see Nuri Kodaman et al., "Human and Helicobacter Pylori Coevolution Shapes the Risk of Gastric Disease," *Proceedings of the National Academy of Sciences* 111, no. 4 (2014): 1455–460.

In contrast to stomach cancer, most other cancers have had rising incidence trends from the first moment of cancer registration in the 1950s or 1960s. These range from cancer of the oesophagus to non-Hodgkin's lymphoma and from laryngeal cancer to malignant melanoma of the skin. For some of these cancers recent trends have reversed, showing that the familiar 'rise-and-fall' pattern also manifests itself for these diseases. It is probably fair to say that – in contrast to the decline of stomach cancer – these favourable trends are mostly a result of deliberate efforts to reduce the risk of cancer and/or to reduce its case fatality.

Over the past half century, the incidence of *colorectal cancer* has increased in many European countries, probably as a consequence of a rise of several of its main risk factors, including a diet low in fibre and rich in red and/or processed meat, and a sedentary lifestyle and obesity. Current understanding of colorectal cancer suggests that these risk factors work as follows, illustrating how complex 'unfavourable exchanges with the environment' can be. Like salted and pickled foods, processed meat is an exogenous source of nitrosamines, but the other factors involved in the rise of colorectal cancer promote exposure to endogenously produced carcinogens. Intestinal bacteria, essential for digestion, produce carcinogens from compounds naturally present in food. Both fibre and physical activity increase bowel motility, thereby reducing transit time and shortening the duration of exposure to carcinogenic faecal contents. Finally, obesity leads to increased secretion of insulin, which promotes cell proliferation.[44]

Whereas colorectal cancer incidence has recently stabilized (at a high level) in some countries in North-western Europe, it is still rising in other parts of Europe. Mortality from colorectal cancer, however, is declining in many countries after reaching a peak somewhere between the 1970s and early 2000s (see Suppl. Figure 17). The decline is mainly due to increased survival as a result of more effective treatment, plus (in some North-western European countries) a favourable effect on disease incidence from mass screening for pre-cancerous polyps.[45]

Mortality from *breast cancer* has also started to decline in many countries, after decades of continuous increase which probably started in the late 19th century (Figure 26). Like in the case of colorectal cancer, the rising mortality

44 For the current understanding of colorectal cancer, see Kana Wu et al., "Cancers of the Colon and Rectum," in *Cancer Epidemiology and Prevention* (*Fourth Edition*), ed. Michael Thun et al. (Oxford etc.: Oxford University Press, 2017).

45 Karim-Kos et al., "Recent Trends"; Wu et al., "Cancers of the Colon and Rectum"; Carlo La Vecchia et al., "Cancer Mortality in Europe, 2000–2004, and an Overview of Trends since 1975," *Annals of Oncology* 21, no. 6 (2009): 1323–360.

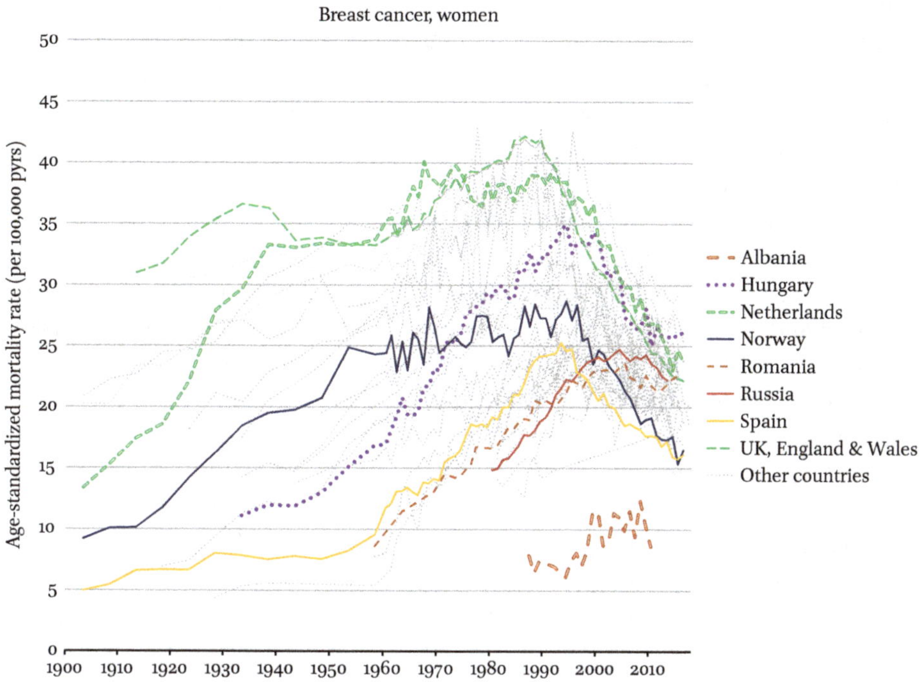

FIGURE 26 Trends in breast cancer mortality in Europe, 1900–2015
Notes: Quinquennial data before 1960
SOURCE OF DATA: SEE SUPPL. TABLE 1

from breast cancer during most of the 20th century was due to a rising incidence, which in its turn was due to a rising prevalence of several of breast cancer's main risk factors. These include reproductive factors (young age at menarche, no or few children, older age at first birth, low breast-feeding, older age at menopause) as well as some other factors (e.g., obesity, alcohol use and hormone replacement therapy). Here again, we have a disease that is a direct consequence of the modern way of life, but in a way that defies easy attribution to 'unfavourable exchanges with the environment'.

Current understanding of breast cancer aetiology suggests that the crucial factor is exposure of breast tissue to oestrogen. This sex hormone, whose production rises and falls during each menstrual cycle, promotes cell growth in the breast and other reproductive organs, which is important for reproduction but also increases the risk of uncontrolled cell proliferation. The reproductive factors mentioned above are all determinants of the number of menstrual cycles women have during their life-time. For example, women bearing no or few children have more menstrual cycles than women with more children, because menstrual cycles stop during pregnancy. Also, fat tissue produces oestrogen, which probably explains the association between obesity and breast cancer.[46]

Fortunately, mortality has started to decline as a result of improvements in treatment (resulting in increased survival) and introduction of mass screening for early stages of breast cancer (resulting in – paradoxically – a further increase in incidence).[47]

Mortality from *prostate cancer* also shows a striking 'rise-and-fall' pattern, with rises starting before World War II (see Suppl. Figure 18). Although prostate cancer is very frequent, its aetiology is not well understood. Many environmental and lifestyle factors have been investigated, but none shows a consistent relationship with the risk of prostate cancer. Like other cancers, prostate cancer has genetic determinants, but these cannot explain its rapid rise in incidence and mortality over most of the 20th century. Improved detection most likely plays a role, aided (in the last decades) by the introduction of a blood test for Prostate Specific Antigen (PSA). Nevertheless, mortality has recently started to decline in many European countries, probably as a result of earlier detection and improved treatment.[48]

For many more cancers, trends in mortality have partly become uncoupled from trends in incidence. This was due to sometimes substantial, but more often modest, improvements in survival. These improvements in survival have been won in a hard-fought and expensive battle which has explicitly been called a 'war on cancer', announced by US President Richard Nixon in 1971. Political mobilization over the threat of cancer led to huge investments in research over the following decades, both in the US and Europe. This has led to great strides in the understanding of cancer, and to advances in treatment which – from a public health perspective – have been rather underwhelming.[49]

---

46 For the current understanding of breast cancer, see Louise A. Brinton, Mia M. Gaudet, and Gretchen L. Gierach, "Breast Cancer," in *Cancer Epidemiology and Prevention (Fourth Edition)*, ed. Michael Thun et al. (Oxford etc.: Oxford University Press, 2017).

47 La Vecchia et al., "Cancer Mortality"; Brinton et al., "Breast Cancer"; Karim-Kos et al., "Recent Trends."

48 Karim-Kos et al., "Recent Trends"; La Vecchia et al., "Cancer Mortality"; Catherine M. Tangen, Marian L. Neuhouser, and Janet L. Stanford, "Prostate Cancer," in *Cancer Epidemiology and Prevention (Fourth Edition)*, ed. Michael Thun et al. (Oxford etc.: Oxford University Press, 2017).

49 See Proctor, *Cancer Wars* for the history of the war against cancer. Too slow increases in cancer survival rates fuelled criticisms of the 'war on cancer'; see John C. Bailar III and Elaine M. Smith, "Progress against Cancer?," *New England Journal of Medicine* 314, no. 19 (1986): 1226–232; John C. Bailar and Heather L. Gornik, "Cancer Undefeated," *New England Journal of Medicine* 336, no. 22 (1997): 1569–574.

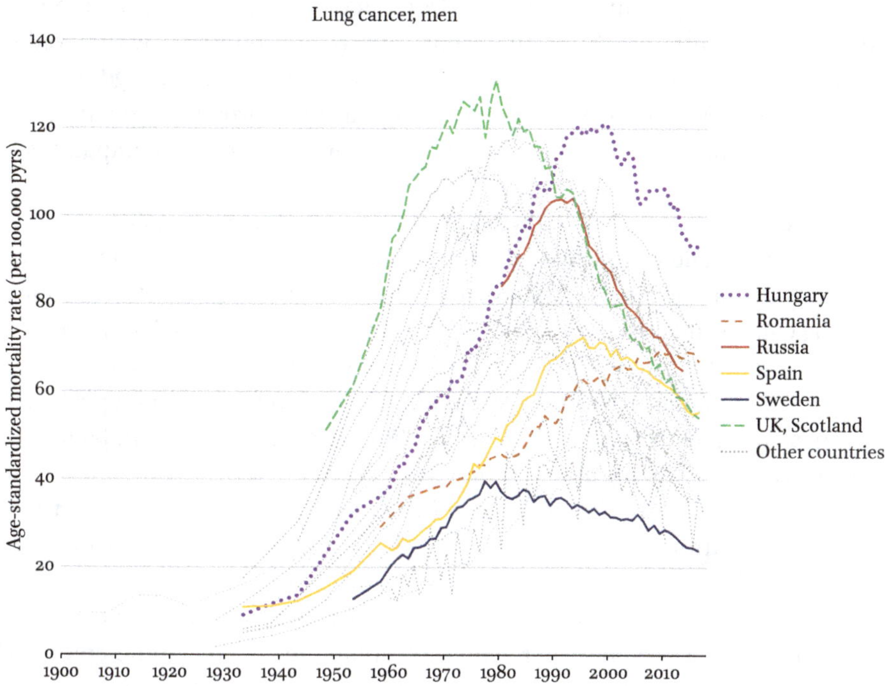

FIGURE 27 Trends in lung cancer mortality in Europe, 1900–2015
Notes: Quinquennial data before 1960
SOURCE OF DATA: SEE SUPPL. TABLE 1

Lung Cancer

Trends in lung cancer will be discussed in more detail, because these are almost completely determined by trends in smoking behaviour, which also determine trends in many other health outcomes. As survival from lung cancer used to be very poor, trends in incidence and mortality are very similar, and as trends in lung cancer mortality are available for more countries over a longer period of time, these are illustrated in Figure 27. Exceptionally, trends for men and women are very different (see Suppl. Figure 19).

Among men, we see a very striking pattern of 'rise and-fall' in nearly all European countries, but with enormous differences between countries in timing and height of the peak. Lung cancer mortality rates peaked in the mid- to late-1970s in the United Kingdom, and in the early 1990s in countries like Spain and Hungary. Whereas Sweden's lung cancer mortality peaked at around 40 deaths per 100,000, Scotland's peaked at 130 deaths per 100,000.

Among women, the general pattern is that of a dramatic increase in lung cancer mortality rates. Only few countries have already reached their peak in the early 2000s, e.g., United Kingdom, Denmark, Sweden. Here again, levels of lung cancer mortality differ enormously between countries, with Sweden peaking at a much lower level than Denmark or the United Kingdom. And whereas lung cancer mortality rates among Eastern European men are comparatively high, rates among Eastern European women are still comparatively low.[50]

Cigarette smoking is the main risk factor for lung cancer mortality, accounting for between 80 and 90% of all cases. Cigarette smoke contains a bewildering array of carcinogens, including nitrosamines but also many others. Trends in lung cancer thus mainly reflect population histories of smoking, with a delay of 20–30 years. Survey data on self-reported smoking and tobacco sales data indeed show similar patterns of 'rise-and-fall'. Smoking among men peaked in the 1950s in many Northern and Western European countries, and later elsewhere, whereas smoking among women is still on the rise in many countries in Southern and Eastern Europe. Tobacco sales peaked in the 1970s in Northern and Western Europe, and in the 1980s, 1990s or even later in Southern and Eastern Europe.[51]

This pattern of 'rise-and-fall' – of both smoking and lung cancer – has understandably been characterized as an 'epidemic'. The 'cigarette epidemic' follows a characteristic pattern that has been compared to the diffusion of innovations. It starts among 'early adopters', who tend to be men and people in higher social classes, and then becomes mainstream, being gradually adopted by women and people in lower social classes as well. When the health risks become widely known and smoking loses its power of social distinction, it is renounced first by the same people who were 'early adopters', i.e., men and higher social classes. This produces a similar pattern of socially differentiated 'rise-and-fall' for lung cancer mortality, but with a few decades delay.[52]

---

50 Detailed analyses of recent trends in lung cancer in European countries can be found in, e.g., P. Brennan and Issy Bray, "Recent Trends and Future Directions for Lung Cancer Mortality in Europe," *British Journal of Cancer* 87, no. 1 (2002): 43–8; J. Ferlay et al., "Cancer Incidence and Mortality Patterns in Europe," *European Journal of Cancer* 103 (2018): 356–87; Karim-Kos et al., "Recent Trends."

51 Trends in smoking behaviour in Europe can be followed in the WHO Health for All Database (https://gateway.euro.who.int/en/datasets/european-health-for-all-database/). Trends in tobacco sales can be found in Barbara Forey et al., *International Smoking Statistics* (Oxford etc.: Oxford University Press, 2009).

52 The concept of the 'tobacco epidemic' was introduced by Alan D. Lopez, Neil E. Collishaw, and Tapani Piha, "A Descriptive Model of the Cigarette Epidemic in Developed Countries," *Tobacco Control* 3, no. 3 (1994): 242–47. It was later somewhat refined in Michael J. Thun et al., "Stages of the Cigarette Epidemic on Entering Its Second Century," *Tobacco Control* 21, no. 2 (2012): 96–101. While this concept helps to recognize regularities in trends

Indirectly, trends in lung cancer tell us much about the role of smoking in determining trends and variations in over-all population health. In countries where peak lung cancer mortality rates among men have been very high, such as the United Kingdom, the Netherlands and Hungary, total smoking-attributable mortality has also been very high, accounting for more than 30% of male all-cause mortality in peak-years. In most other countries, smoking-attributable mortality peaked between 20 and 30% of all-cause mortality, which of course is still very high. The main exception is Sweden where it was never more than 12%.[53]

The 'cigarette epidemic' has a long history. Tobacco was brought from the Americas to Europe in the 16th century, and was at first mostly used as snuff and in pipes. It was only after the invention of 'cigarettes' in the 1840s and a machine for the industrial production of cigarettes in the 1880s, that cigarette smoking became a mass habit in some countries in the early decades of the 20th century. As smoking is still prevalent and smoking-attributable mortality is still high, even in countries where the 'cigarette epidemic' started, this is clearly a very slow epidemic that takes more than a century to play out.

There are at least three reasons for this. First, nicotine is a strongly addictive substance, and after young people have taken up smoking, many of them continue smoking during their lives. This also explains why smoking and lung cancer trends manifest themselves as birth-cohort phenomena. Because replacement of generations takes time, the epidemic takes many decades to unfold. Second, there is a long delay between exposure to tobacco smoke and some of its major health effects, particularly lung cancer, other cancers, and COPD, putting decades between the peak in smoking and the peak in lung cancer. Third, the policy response to smoking and its health effects has been slow. Sadly, decades have passed between the demonstration of the harmful effects of smoking and the implementation of systematic tobacco control measures. This was partly due to active resistance by the tobacco industry, partly due to reluctance

of smoking and lung cancer, one should not be misled to think that the decline of smoking automatically follows its rise, like the decline of infectious diseases follows their rise when the number of susceptibles becomes too low to sustain agent's spread.

53 At least two methods have been developed to derive the quantitative contribution of smoking to total mortality from the level of lung cancer mortality: Richard Peto et al., "Mortality from Tobacco in Developed Countries: Indirect Estimation from National Vital Statistics," *Lancet* 339, no. 8804 (1992): 1268–278; Samuel H. Preston, Dana A. Glei, and John R. Wilmoth, "A New Method for Estimating Smoking-Attributable Mortality in High-Income Countries," *International Journal of Epidemiology* 39, no. 2 (2009): 430–38. The estimates presented here come from Thun et al., "Stages." One explanation for the exceptionally low rates of smoking, and low proportions of smoking-attributable deaths, in Sweden is the wide-spread use of 'snus' (see Chapter 7).

on the part of public authorities to interfere with behaviour that was perceived to be an individual choice.[54]

In order to more fully understand the 'cigarette epidemic', we must distinguish between 'supply' and 'demand'. Like in the case of other consumption products, the rise in cigarette use was both a matter of supply responding to demand, and demand responding to supply. The tobacco industry has been highly effective in promoting cigarette use, e.g., by clever advertising campaigns, by raising nicotine content and adding compounds that help to tolerate tobacco smoke in the lungs, and by developing "light cigarettes" when ordinary cigarettes were shown to have harmful effects on health. The tobacco industry has also often tried to delay government action against smoking, by hiding internal information on the harmful effects of smoking, by spreading misinformation, and by lobbying Ministers and parliaments.

While this is all true and highly objectionable, we should not close our eyes to the fact that there is also a demand-side. Nicotine has psychogenic effects which are appreciated by tobacco users. When it reaches the brain it acts as a stimulant, improves mood and concentration, and gives a feeling of relaxation and decreased stress. These are all temporary effects, and withdrawal of nicotine increases anxiety, thereby creating dependence. Yet, these psychogenic effects must have had an important function in European societies for smoking to become so wide-spread. One plausible explanation is that smoking helped to relieve stress and frustration in times of rapid economic and social change – and, in contrast with other forms of mood regulation, such as alcohol consumption, could be combined with a high pace of work.

Cigarette smoking was also a cultural phenomenon: it came to symbolize all kinds of positive things – often cleverly reinforced by the marketing strategies of the tobacco industry – which increased its appeal among potential consumers. Cigarette smoking came to be perceived as a sign of 'masculinity', perhaps because smoking became popular among soldiers, first in the Crimean war and

54 Histories of smoking, the discovery of its harmful effects, and the development of anti-smoking policies can be found in, e.g., Richard Doll, "Tobacco: A Medical History," *Journal of Urban Health* 76, no. 3 (1999): 289–313; Arthur W. Musk and Nicholas H. De Klerk, "History of Tobacco and Health," *Respirology* 8, no. 3 (2003): 286–90; Robert N. Proctor, "The History of the Discovery of the Cigarette–Lung Cancer Link," *Tobacco Control* 21, no. 2 (2012): 87–91. Extensive histories, focusing on the pernicious role of the tobacco industry, particularly in the US, can be found in Robert N. Proctor, *Golden Holocaust* (Berkeley etc.: Univ of California Press, 2011); Allan M. Brandt, *The Cigarette Century* (New York: Basic Books, 2007). A specifically British, and somewhat more benign, history is Virginia Berridge, *Marketing Health: Smoking and the Discourse of Public Health in Britain, 1945–2000* (Oxford etc.: Oxford University Press, 2007).

later in World Wars I and II, during which cigarettes were distributed among soldiers in their rations. Originally, cigarette smoking was seen as unsuitable for women, because it signalled promiscuity, but when smoking among women became more acceptable, it came to symbolize 'emancipation', which strongly increased its appeal among women. More generally, cigarette smoking signalled 'modernity', which propelled it through European populations in parallel with socioeconomic modernization.[55]

Fortunately, in view of its disastrous health effects, the rise in smoking was followed by a fall, at least among men, and hopefully soon also among women. This decline started when the harmful effects of smoking became more widely known, and this again was a long process. Rising rates of lung cancer were already noticed by pathologists and surgeons around the turn of the 20th century. Suspicions that this rise was due to the increasing popularity of cigarette smoking were quite common in the medical profession in the 1930s, but still competed with alternative hypotheses.

The first epidemiological evidence for a connection between smoking and lung cancer came from case-control studies, the first of which was published in 1939 by a medical doctor working in Nazi Germany, later followed by a series of American and British case-control studies published in 1950. A few years later, the results were confirmed in a series of prospective cohort studies, again in the United States and the United Kingdom. Animal experiments, cellular pathology studies, and chemical studies of the compounds present in tobacco smoke completed the picture, and by the mid-1950s there was no longer room for reasonable doubt about the link between smoking and lung cancer.[56]

---

55 See, for example, Matthew Hilton, *Smoking in British Popular Culture 1800–2000* (Manchester: Manchester University Press, 2000); Virginia Berridge, *Demons: Our Changing Attitudes to Alcohol, Tobacco, and Drugs* (Oxford etc.: Oxford University Press, 2013). The shifting social significance of cigarette smoking can be followed in popular and highbrow culture through the ages; see Sander L. Gilman and Xun Zhou, *Smoke: A Global History of Smoking* (London: Reaktion Books, 2004).

56 The Nazis were preoccupied with smoking, long before the Allies were. The leaders of the Third Reich had very strict non-smoking policies including bans on smoking and extensive health education campaigns. In some of these the non-smoking Führer was used as an example for the German people, and anti-tobacco activists pointed out that while Churchill, Stalin and Roosevelt were all smokers, the three fascist leaders in Europe, Hitler, Mussolini and Franco, were non-smokers. The Nazis considered tobacco smoke a 'genetic poison', which would lead to a degeneration of the Aryan race; see Weindling, *Health, Race and German Politics*; Robert N. Proctor, *The Nazi War on Cancer* (Princeton: Princeton University Press, 2000). For the history of the discovery of the link between smoking and lung cancer generally, see Proctor, "History."

Based on the available evidence the American Surgeon General ultimately concluded – in 1964 – that the link was "causal." At that time only two diseases could definitely be linked to smoking, namely lung cancer and COPD, but now we know that more than 30 diseases can be caused by smoking. Until recently it was believed that, as a result of the higher frequency of all these different diseases, the over-all mortality rate among life-long smokers is twice as high as that among life-long non-smokers. This would imply that half of all life-long smokers eventually die from the consequences of their tobacco use. However, recent studies have indicated that the relative risk is not 2 but 3, which implies that two-thirds of life-long smokers are killed by their smoking habit.[57]

Anti-smoking action by public authorities, health care professionals, and voluntary organizations started in a health education mode, in which smokers were persuaded to stop smoking, and non-smokers were advised against taking up smoking. We now know that such campaigns have limited effectiveness, particularly among people in lower socioeconomic groups. Nevertheless, smoking already declined substantially (among men) in many countries in Northern and Western Europe between their peak rates in the 1950s/1960s and the 1990s, when more systematic 'tobacco control' policies started to take shape. The current standard for tobacco control policies, the 'MPOWER' package of the World Health Organization, was defined in 2008, in order to help countries adhere to the 2003 Framework Convention on Tobacco Control. This is a convention to which almost 200 countries world-wide have signed up.[58]

Implementation of these measures has taken time in all European countries, but more so in some than in others. This is shown in regular monitoring reports which now cover the period 2004–2016. In general, the Nordic countries, the United Kingdom and Ireland have been most active, and far ahead of other countries in implementation of tobacco control measures, whereas the German-speaking countries of Western Europe (Germany, Austria, Switzerland, Luxembourg) lag surprisingly far behind. Southern European countries have also become quite active, and there is some recent catch-up in countries

57 The estimate of 2 comes from the famous British Doctors Study (Richard Doll et al., "Mortality in Relation to Smoking: 50 Years' Observations on Male British Doctors," *British Medical Journal* 328, no. 7455 (2004): 1519–528). The estimate of 3 comes from the American Cancer Prevention Studies (Michael J. Thun et al., "50-Year Trends in Smoking-Related Mortality in the United States," *New England Journal of Medicine* 368, no. 4 (2013): 351–64).

58 This package consists of: M = monitoring; P = protecting people from tobacco smoke; O: offering assistance to smokers to help them quit; W: warning about the dangers of tobacco use; E = enforcing bans on advertising, promotion and sponsorship; R = raising tobacco taxes.

in South-eastern and Eastern Europe, which started their anti-smoking policies much later than most Western European countries. Despite considerable progress, and despite an increasingly important role of the European Union in harmonizing and strengthening tobacco control measures in its member states, there is still a huge gap between ideal and reality in many European countries.[59]

While the effectiveness of the tobacco control measures included in the MPOWER package has been demonstrated, it is unlikely that they have already contributed to the trends in lung cancer mortality seen in Figure 27. For example, most peaks in lung cancer mortality pre-date systematic tobacco control efforts by many years. However, there is a much shorter delay between smoking and some other health outcomes, such as ischaemic heart disease, and studies have shown that, for example, restrictions on smoking in public places have led to almost immediate reductions in the incidence of ischaemic heart disease.[60]

So what explains the patterns seen Figure 27? Northern and Western European countries had early smoking epidemics, both among men and among women. As these were also the European countries which were early modernizers in many other respects, the obvious explanation is that earlier uptake of smoking was a side-effect of their earlier economic, social and cultural modernization. This applies to men in these countries, and also to women, because these countries' higher levels of gender equality have facilitated an early take-up of smoking among women.[61]

These were also the countries where smoking started to decline early. Although part of this may reflect a decline of fashion, and a loss of the opportunities for 'social distinction' that smoking originally offered, this decline certainly occurred partly in response to the message that smoking was dangerous. Because the evidence was originally published in the United States and the United Kingdom, this message had little difficulty of reaching health care professionals and lay audiences in Northern and Western Europe.

---

59 I am referring to a series of reports in which European countries are ranked on the 'Tobacco Control Scale'. The most recent report was published in 2017 (Luk Joossens and Martin Raw, *The Tobacco Control Scale 2016 in Europe* (Brussels: Association of the European Cancer Leagues, 2017)).

60 For a general review of tobacco control efforts and their effect on smoking rates in Europe, see Laura Currie and Anna B. Gilmore, "Tobacco," in *Successes and Failures of Health Policy in Europe*, ed. Johan P. Mackenbach and Martin McKee (Maidenhead: Open University Press, 2013).

61 However, see Fred C. Pampel, "Cigarette Diffusion and Sex Differences in Smoking," *Journal of Health and Social Behavior* 42, no. 4 (2001): 388–404, for a different view.

The later timing of the smoking epidemic in Southern, Central-Eastern and Eastern Europe has a largely similar, but symmetrically opposed explanation. The history of smoking in communist Europe, however, has some specific aspects that are worth briefly dwelling on. In most of these countries (with the exception of, e.g., Czechoslovakia and Hungary where men already took up smoking before World War II), the wide-spread uptake of smoking started when they were under communist regimes.

Although the wide-spread use of cigarettes is usually associated with commercial enterprise – and now with 'Big Tobacco', i.e., a handful of powerful multinational companies – cigarette production by state-run enterprises in communist countries was centrally planned to accommodate growing consumer demand. Cigarettes were cheap, smoking rates reached very high levels, and as we have seen in Figure 27, lung cancer mortality rates among men soared. Although anti-smoking campaigns were mounted, these were generally ineffective due to lack of trust in the government and lack of enforcement.

After the fall of communism, Western tobacco companies started aggressive marketing campaigns and made huge investments in building up a commercial tobacco sector in Central-eastern Europe and the former Soviet Union. This contributed to a stabilisation or even increase (creating a double peak) in smoking rates among men, and an increase in smoking rates among women. As a result, Russian, Belarussian, and Ukrainian men had some of the highest smoking rates of Europe in the 1990s and 2000s.[62]

Finally, when we step back from the tragic story of smoking and its health effects in the 20th century, and try to place this in the broader perspective of the generally favourable trends in population health in Europe over several centuries, the obvious question to ask is: was this an 'accident of history'? Or is there a deeper link between the massive progress made in the 18th, 19th and

62 For trends in smoking in Central-eastern Europe and the Soviet Union, see Antonin K. Kubik et al., "Patterns of Cigarette Sales and Lung Cancer Mortality in Some Central and Eastern European Countries," *Cancer* 75, no. 10 (1995): 2452–460; Richard Cooper, "Smoking in the Soviet Union," *British Medical Journal* 285, no. 6341 (1982): 549–51. For trends after 1990, and the role of the tobacco industry in promoting smoking in Central-eastern Europe and the former Soviet Union, see Witold Zatonski et al., "Tobacco Smoking in Countries of the European Union," *Annals of Agricultural and Environmental Medicine* 19, no. 2 (2012): 181–92; Bayard Roberts et al., "Changes in Smoking Prevalence in 8 Countries of the Former Soviet Union between 2001 and 2010," *American Journal of Public Health* 102, no. 7 (2012): 1320–328; Martin McKee et al., "Patterns of Smoking in Russia," *Tobacco Control* 7, no. 1 (1998): 22–6; Anna B. Gilmore and Martin McKee, "Tobacco and Transition: An Overview of Industry Investments, Impact and Influence in the Former Soviet Union," *Tobacco Control* 13, no. 2 (2004): 136–42.

20th centuries, and the setbacks caused by smoking, which made the latter more than a simple 'accident'?

As we have alluded to on several occasions above, the rise of smoking occurred in response to changes in economic and sociocultural conditions which were also involved in the improvements in European population health. As a luxury product, smoking became affordable when economic growth led to rising average incomes, and became a symbol of luxury (and many things else) with which people could distinguish themselves. Also, mass consumption was made possible by the industrial production and aggressive promotion of cigarettes – an economic mode that also brought many useful and even healthy products to consumers. Probably, smoking also satisfied psychological needs that arose with the profound social changes accompanying industrialization and urbanization.

While this suggests that the setbacks caused by smoking were certainly more than a simple 'accident', similarly fatal epidemics did not occur with other consumer products. Economic growth brought thousands of products (foods, drinks, household appliances, means of transport, ...) within reach of European consumers, but none of these were as lethal as smoking. That widespread diffusion occurred with a fatal and addictive product like cigarettes, long before its pernicious effects were known, may therefore be seen as a tragic 'accident', but that sales continued after the early 1960s was a crime.

Liver Cirrhosis

Alcohol consumption, particularly in higher doses, is a risk factor for many fatal and non-fatal health problems. Acute intoxication is a risk factor for injuries, both accidental and non-accidental, and for cardiovascular disease, whereas chronic heavy drinking is a risk factor for liver cirrhosis, various forms of cancer, and again cardiovascular disease. There is also a lot of psychiatric co-morbidity.[63]

A quick sketch of the history of alcohol-related health problems must start from the fact that beer was already brewed in prehistory, and wine was already made in the third millennium BCE. Despite the fact that the social and health problems associated with excessive drinking must also be very old, alcohol consumption is still widely accepted in most European cultures, probably because of its tension-reducing properties and indispensable role as a social lubricant.

63 For a recent overview of the many alcohol-related health problems, see World Health Organization, *Global Status Report on Alcohol and Health 2018* (Geneva: WHO, 2018).

As in the case of tobacco in a later period, mass production of alcoholic drinks like beer and spirits, together with the social changes associated with industrialization and urbanization, played an important role in the rise of drunkenness and other alcohol-related problems in the 18th and 19th centuries. For example, industrial production of distilled spirits led to a 'gin epidemic' in England in the 18th century, and the resulting social problems made the British government adopt increasingly strict 'Gin Acts' which limited points of sale and raised taxes, and in the end reduced consumption to lower levels.

Although epidemiological data for the 19th century are not available, anecdotal evidence testifies to the high prevalence of drunkenness in this period, particularly in the lower social classes. That alcohol-related problems were wide-spread is also suggested by the rise of the 'temperance movement'. This civic movement advocated government intervention against excessive alcohol consumption, sometimes successfully.

The 'temperance movement' was concentrated in English-speaking and Northern European countries, perhaps because of an underlying cultural link with Protestantism. It led to Prohibition of the production and sale of alcohol in the 1920s in the United States, and to less severe but ultimately more effective countermeasures in the 1920s and 1930s in the Nordic countries. These have, however, more recently been relaxed as a result of integration into the European Union.[64]

Alcohol consumption declined – in the few North-western European countries for which we have data – since the last decades of the 19th century, probably in response to this increased regulation of alcohol sales and greater awareness of alcohol problems. It reached a low point in the 1950s, but then started to increase again, as a result of rising prosperity and relaxation of cultural restrictions on alcohol consumption (just like restraints on other forms of need-satisfying behaviour were loosened in this period). In Central-Eastern and Eastern Europe, wide-spread dissatisfaction and 'anomie' during the years of

64 On Britain's 18th century 'gin epidemic', see Jessica Warner et al., "Can Legislation Prevent Debauchery? Mother Gin and Public Health in 18th-Century England," *American Journal of Public Health* 91, no. 3 (2001): 375–84. For the history of the 'temperance movement' in Britain, see Brian Harrison, *Drink and the Victorians* (London: Faber and Faber, 1971). Differences between European countries in 'temperance cultures' have been analysed in Harry G. Levine, "Temperance Cultures: Alcohol as a Problem in Nordic and English-Speaking Cultures," in *The Nature of Alcohol and Drug Related Problems*, ed. M. Lader, G. Edwards, and D.C. Drummond (New York, 1993).

economic and political stagnation, and insecurity in the turbulent years after the end of communism, also played an important role.[65]

As in the case of smoking and the tobacco industry, the aggressive marketing strategies of the alcohol industry have also contributed to the persistence of problematically high levels of alcohol consumption, as well as to the rise in alcohol consumption in Central-eastern and Eastern Europe in the 1990s.[66]

The only alcohol-related health problem for which long-term trends can be assessed is mortality from liver cirrhosis (Figure 28). Possibly, liver cirrhosis mortality rose during the 19th century and then declined in the first half of the 20th century, but only the latter trend can be seen in the few countries for which we have early data. Liver cirrhosis mortality increased sharply again since the 1950s, and then peaked at hugely varying points in time: in the 1970s in France, Spain, Italy and Sweden, in the 1990s in Hungary and Romania, and in the early 2000s in the United Kingdom and Finland.[67]

The recently favourable trends in the Mediterranean countries have been attributed to a tightening of alcohol control policies, whereas the (until recently) unfavourable trends in Central-Eastern and Eastern Europe and in the United Kingdom have been attributed to a combination of increased affordability of alcohol and relaxation of alcohol control policies.[68]

Trends of mortality from other alcohol-related conditions than liver cirrhosis, for which comparable data are available over a more recent period only, have been studied less often. Within Europe, mortality from alcoholic psychosis, alcohol poisoning and alcohol dependence appears to have a different

65 For a more extensive discussion of the role of excessive alcohol consumption in the fluctuating mortality rates in Russia and other former parts of the Soviet Union, see Chapter 7.

66 See, e.g., David H. Jernigan et al., "Alcohol Marketing and Youth Alcohol Consumption," *Addiction* 112, no. Suppl. 1 (2017): 7–20; David H. Jernigan, "The Global Alcohol Industry: An Overview," *Addiction* 104, no. Suppl. 1 (2009): 6–12.

67 On trends in liver cirrhosis mortality in Europe, see Cristina Bosetti et al., "Worldwide Mortality from Cirrhosis: An Update to 2002," *Journal of Hepatology* 46, no. 5 (2007): 827–39; Witold A. Zatoński et al., "Liver Cirrhosis Mortality in Europe, with Special Attention to Central and Eastern Europe," *European Addiction Research* 16, no. 4 (2010): 193–201. The extraordinarily high peak of liver cirrhosis mortality in Hungary is partly an artefact. Because alcoholic liver cirrhosis was common in Hungary, it was easy to assign liver cirrhosis as a cause of death when the cause of death was not known with certainty. This practice changed in the 1990s, and this, together with the implementation of alcohol control policies, led to the reversal in the Hungarian liver cirrhosis trend seen in Figure 28; see Peter Józan, "Main Features of Epidemiological Development in Hungary after the Second World War," *Hungarian Statistical Review* 86, no. 12 (2008): 1–78.

68 Peter Anderson, "Alcohol," in *Successes and Failures of Health Policy in Europe*, ed. Johan P. Mackenbach and Martin McKee (Maidenhead: Open University Press, 2013).

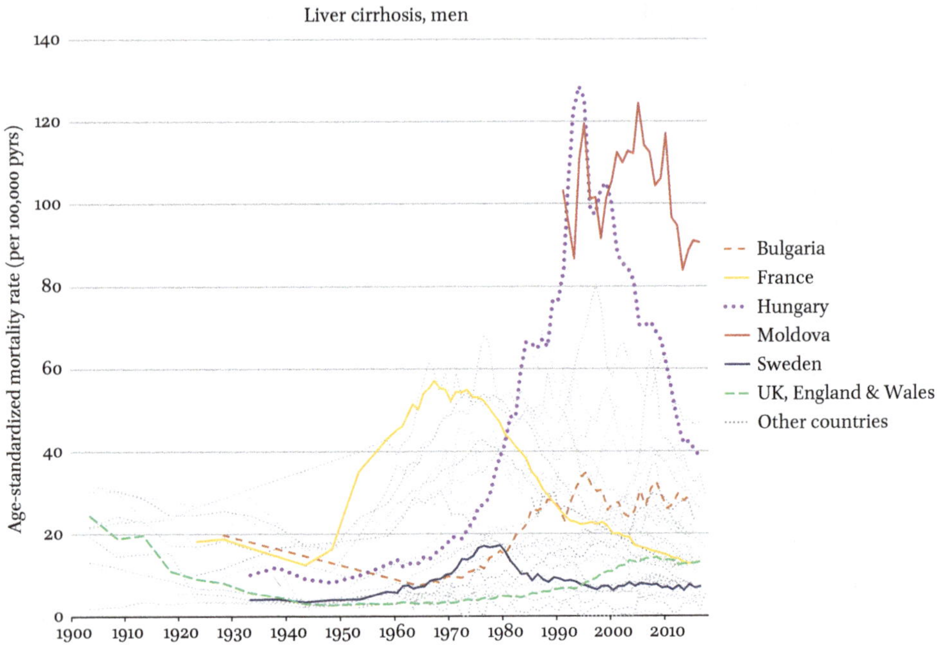

FIGURE 28 Trends in liver cirrhosis mortality in Europe, 1900–2015
Notes: Quinquennial data before 1960
SOURCE OF DATA: SEE SUPPL. TABLE 1

geographical pattern as compared to mortality from liver cirrhosis, with relatively high rates in the Nordic countries and in Eastern Europe. This has been attributed to a style of drinking characterized by non-daily drinking and frequent intoxication. Mortality from these intoxication-related conditions has been rising in many European countries, again pointing to the fact that alcohol-related health problems are far from being under control.[69]

Dementia

The declines in cause-specific mortality that we have seen in the previous sections have shifted the mean age of death upwards, and it is easy to understand that the share of diseases typical of very old age has increased. Some early authors, writing in the late 1970s when this had only just begun, even warned for a "pandemic of mental disorders and disabilities."

69 Mats Ramstedt, "Alcohol-Related Mortality in 15 European Countries in the Postwar Period," *European Journal of Population/Revue Européenne de Démographie* 18, no. 4 (2002): 307–23.

As we have seen in Chapter 2, it is indeed true that, even after taking into account changes in age-distribution of the population, the share of some diseases of old age in total mortality has increased in many European countries. Mental and neurological diseases are among the very small number of causes of death for which trends in mortality have been upwards instead of downwards over the past decades. This should not be exaggerated, as the average share of these conditions in total mortality in Europe is still below 5%, but it already exceeds 10% among women in several countries.

'Dementia', a group of brain diseases causing a decline in the ability to think and remember, is an important component of this broader category. It includes Alzheimer's disease (which accounts for more than half of all cases, and whose cause is unknown) and vascular dementia (which accounts for about a quarter of all cases, and which is caused by problems in the blood supply of the brain, such as small ischaemic strokes)(Plate 15).

Dementias are now among the top-10 (men) or even top-5 (women) of most frequent causes of death in several European countries, as a result of rapid rises in age-adjusted mortality. Mortality from motor neuron diseases (such as amyotrophic lateral sclerosis (ALS)) has also risen, but reports on trends in mortality from Parkinson's disease, multiple sclerosis and epilepsy have not shown consistent trends up or down.[70]

It is only since about 1980 that Alzheimer's disease and other dementias can clearly be identified in cause-of-death statistics (see Suppl. Figure 20). Since then, dementia mortality has increased strongly in many Northern and Western European countries, but remained low in South-eastern and Eastern Europe. Finland has extremely high, and continuously rising, levels of dementia mortality throughout the last decades: the difference now is more than 50-fold between Finland and Bulgaria.

70 For warnings of a "pandemic of mental disorders and disabilities," see M. Kramer, "The Rising Pandemic of Mental Disorders and Associated Chronic Diseases and Disabilities," *Acta Psychiatrica Scandinavica* 62, no. Suppl. 285 (1980): 282–97; Ernest M. Gruenberg, "Epidemiology of Senile Dementia," *Advances in Neurology* 19 (1978): 437–57. The rise of dementia as a cause of death in Europe has been described in Vidar Hjellvik et al., "Dementia in the National Cause of Death Registry in Norway 1969–2010," *Norsk Epidemiologi* 22, no. 2 (2012): 217–24; Mackenbach et al., "Rise of Mortality." On trends in Parkinson's disease, multiple sclerosis, and epilepsy, see, e.g., Aidan Neligan et al., "Temporal Trends in the Mortality of People with Epilepsy," *Epilepsia* 51, no. 11 (2010): 2241–246; Michael J. Goldacre et al., "Trends in Death Certification for Multiple Sclerosis, Motor Neuron Disease, Parkinson's Disease and Epilepsy," *Journal of Neurology* 257, no. 5 (2010): 706–15; Colin W. Pritchard, David S. Baldwin, and Andrew G. Mayers, "Changing Patterns of Adult Neurological Deaths in the Major Western World Countries," *Public Health* 118, no. 4 (2004): 268–83.

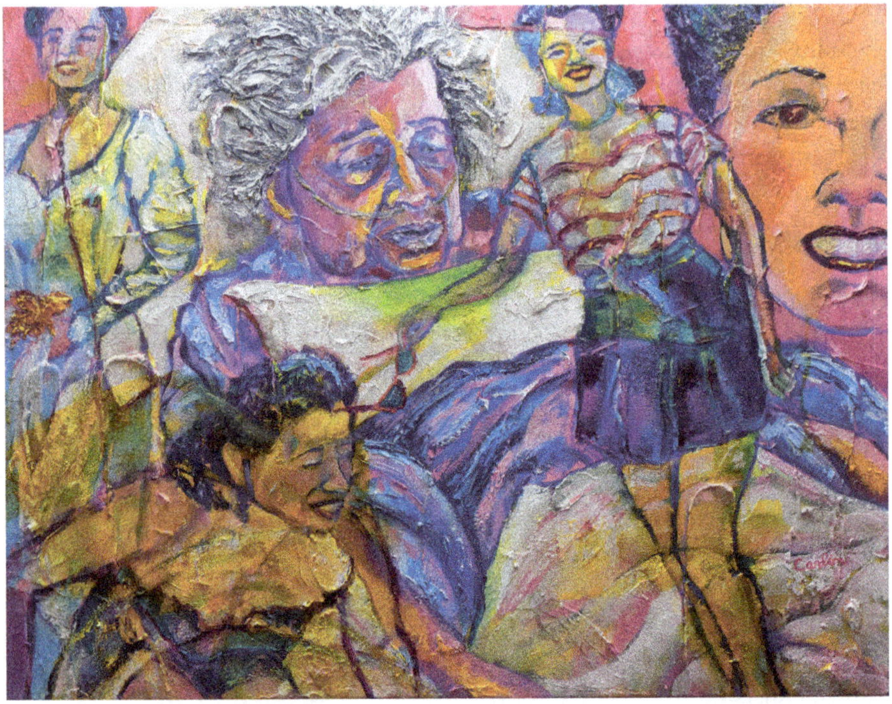

PLATE 15 "I was really something." Painting of a woman dying from Alzheimer's, 2015
According to the artist, Judith Carlin, this is a "painting of a woman dying from Alzheimer's remembering when she was young and beautiful and healthy." This tangled painting conveys the confusion of dementia patients – a confusion mirrored by modern societies' mixed feelings about the price we pay for our increased life expectancy
HTTPS://COMMONS.WIKIMEDIA.ORG/WIKI/CATEGORY:ALZHEIMER%27S_DISEASE#/MEDIA/FILE:I_WAS_REALLY_SOMETHING.JPG (CC BY SA 4.0; ACCESSED 18/10/2019)

Are these striking trends and variations real, or an artefact of trends and variations in cause-of-death classification? Studies of time-trends in the incidence or prevalence of dementia over longer time-periods are scarce. A recent review suggests, however, that the age-adjusted incidence of dementia has been declining in several European countries, perhaps as a result of improvements in cardiovascular risk factors. The latter have been shown to increase the risk of both Alzheimer's and vascular dementia.

It is unlikely, therefore, that the increase in mortality from dementia represents an increase in incidence of the disease. As it is also unlikely that survival of patients with dementia has declined substantially – on the contrary: the evidence suggests that survival has been improving – this leaves improved recognition, diagnosis, certification and/or coding as the most likely explanation for the increase in mortality from dementia.[71]

This can be understood as follows. Dementia is less straightforward as a cause of death than, say, stroke or colorectal cancer. On the one hand, it does increase the risk of dying: the risk of dying among dementia patients is two or three times higher than that of people of the same age without dementia. On the other hand, the immediate cause of death of patients with dementia is often pneumonia or cardiovascular disease, and as a result dementia is not always mentioned on death certificates or coded as the underlying cause of death.[72]

This implies that there is a lot of scope for changes and variations in physicians' and statisticians' attitudes to affect the level of registered mortality from dementia. For example, recognition of dementia's role in causing patients' deaths is likely to have increased, particularly after other causes of death had gradually been eliminated. Nevertheless, even if the observed rise in dementia mortality is to a large extent artefactual, and if better recognition partly explains the higher rates in Northern and Western Europe, we are still left with a reality in which dementia has become a very important cause of death – and an even more important cause of disability.

Depression

If secular trends in dementia are difficult to measure, try mental illness! We are much better in monitoring health conditions that are on the decline, than in monitoring trends in diseases that are not, or not yet, declining. Like so many other things this is not a coincidence, because the existence of an effective monitoring machinery often reflects past attention to the problem by health care professionals and health policy-makers, and thus correlates with past investments in disease control. As an example of what we know and do not know about secular trends in mental illness, we will have a look at depression.

---

71 For a review of trends in incidence, prevalence and survival in dementia, see Martin Prince et al., "Recent Global Trends in the Prevalence and Incidence of Dementia, and Survival with Dementia," *Alzheimer's Research & Therapy* 8, no. 1 (2016): 23.

72 For the risk of dying with dementia, see Uta Guehne, Steffi Riedel-Heller, and Matthias C. Angermeyer, "Mortality in Dementia," *Neuroepidemiology* 25, no. 3 (2005): 153–62, for the immediate causes of death in patients dying with dementia, see Janet Keene et al., "Death and Dementia," *International Journal Geriatric Psychiatry* 16, no. 10 (2001): 969–74, and for changes in coding, see Office for National Statistics, *Results from the ICD-10 V2010 Bridge Coding Study*, Statistical Bulletin, (Newport: Office for National Statistics, 2011).

Depression, a disorder of mood of which the aetiology is not well understood, is one of the most common mental disorders, and even one of the most common health conditions over-all. According to the Global Burden of Disease study, depressive disorders are currently the number 3 most important cause of years-with-disability world-wide, after low back pain and headache. Apart from causing disability, depression is also an important risk factor for other health problems, including cardiovascular disease. Furthermore, about half of all suicides occur among people suffering from depression.

The cross-national World Mental Health Survey has recently collected data on the prevalence of 'major depressive disorder' (MDD), a sub-form of depression characterized by at least two weeks of serious symptoms in a row. The proportion of respondents who had experienced at least one such episode in the previous 12 months ranged between 3% in Italy and Germany and 6% in France. Although the measurement of depression was carefully harmonized between countries, we unfortunately do not know whether these differences are real or not.[73]

Awareness that depression is a major health problem is relatively recent, and only a few countries world-wide have data collection systems for monitoring trends in the incidence or prevalence of depression, e.g., in the form of periodic surveys using psychiatric screening instruments. In most cases, these have opened a 10 to 20 year time-window on recent trends in depression. This is hardly sufficient to qualify as a view on the history of depression, and even if we could extrapolate the results backwards in time this would not help much, because the trends found in these studies are inconsistent. Over the last decades, some European studies have found an increase in depression, others have found either a decrease or a stable rate.[74]

---

73 On the specific diagnostic criteria for Major Depressive Disorder, and the current understanding of its aetiology, see Christian Otte et al., "Major Depressive Disorder," *Nature Reviews Disease primers* 2 (2016): 16065. For the most recent Global Burden of Disease estimates, see GBD 2017 Collaborators, "Global, Regional, and National Incidence, Prevalence, and Years Lived." The comparative results of the World Mental Health Survey were summarized in Ronald C. Kessler and Evelyn J. Bromet, "The Epidemiology of Depression across Cultures," *Annual Review of Public Health* 34 (2013): 119–38.

74 Studies concluding on an increase include Cross-National Colaborative Group, "The Changing Rate of Major Depresion: Cross-National Comparisons," *Journal of the American Medical Association* 268 (1992): 3098–105; Hans W. Jeuring et al., "Secular Trends in the Prevalence of Major and Subthreshold Depression among 55–64-Year Olds over 20 Years," *Psychological Medicine* 48, no. 11 (2018): 1824–34; Eric Fombonne, "Increased Rates of Depression," *Acta Psychiatrica Scandinavica* 90, no. 3 (1994): 145–56. Stable rates were found in Ron de Graaf et al., "Prevalence of Mental Disorders and Trends from 1996 to 2009," *Social Psychiatry and Psychiatric Epidemiology* 47, no. 2 (2012): 203–13. A decline was found

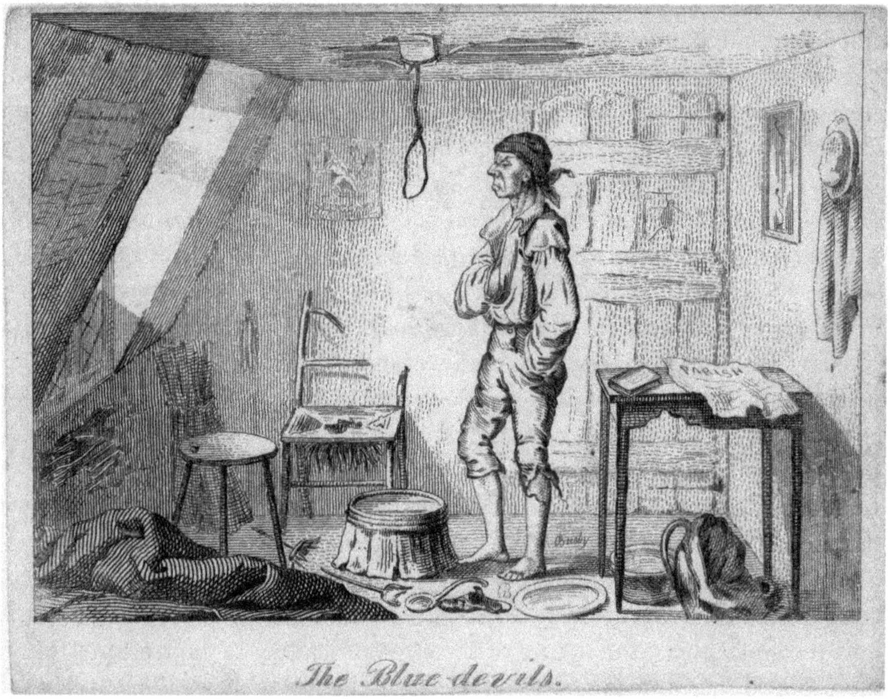

PLATE 16 A poor depressed man prepares to hang himself, 1826
A man suffering from the "blue devils," i.e., the demons that were believed to cause melancholia, looks at a noose attached to a roof-beam. On the table is a notice from the "Parish": possibly a tax-demand or a summons to the workhouse. This illustration shows that melancholia was not limited to the upper classes.
ETCHING BY T.L. BUSBY, CA. 1826. WELLCOME COLLECTION (CC BY)

Although it is impossible to compare depression's current prevalence with figures for previous historical periods, it is certain that depression is not a new disease (Plate 16). Patients with symptoms that we would now label 'depression' have been described in antiquity, but the term that has long been used to designate the condition was 'melancholia'. Very severe case histories have been published in the 17th and 18th centuries, perhaps suggesting that the disorder had become more common then, particularly among the educated classes.

Melancholia was a somewhat fluent concept, however, and even in the late 19th century, when modern psychiatry was born, classifications of different types of depression were very different from how the disorder and its sub-forms

in Cecilia Mattisson et al., "First Incidence Depression in the Lundby Study," *Journal of Affective Disorders* 87, no. 2–3 (2005): 151–60.

are understood today. The modern classification according to the Diagnostic and Statistical Manual of Mental Disorders (DSM) is entirely symptom-based. This avoids potentially false assumptions about aetiology, but has led to an increased recognition of milder forms of depression which qualify for treatment, mostly in the form of pharmaceutical drugs.[75]

For a naïve observer, it is difficult to understand that modern, prosperous societies have such high rates of depression. Important environmental correlates are childhood trauma, absence of a partner, experience of negative life events, financial or social problems, and low socioeconomic position. One would expect exposure to many of these environmental factors to have diminished over time, together with so many other unfavourable life circumstances. After all, in the 18th and 19th centuries, the risk of childhood neglect, loss of loved ones through death, and loss of shelter, work and income was far higher than in the early 21st century.[76]

In order to explain this paradox we must therefore dig a bit deeper. Modern theories of depression, while still recognizing the importance of these environmental factors, have become considerably more complex, integrating biological, psychological and social factors, often in an evolutionary framework. It is now recognized that the nature of the stressor leading to depression is often more subtle than previously assumed: attachment loss, social defeat, loss of prestige, subordination, … Vulnerable people may respond to such stressors by depression, which can be seen as an originally adaptive response inherited from humans' long evolution. When we lose out against others, depression makes us avoid further conflict, and when we are frustrated in our ambitions, depression protects us against continuing to pursue unrealistic goals.

These subtler forms of stress are probably not less common now than they were in previous centuries, which may help to explain the persistence of depression. For example, human competition is still overwhelmingly present, if not in the form of competition for material security then in the form of competition for prestige and being seen as attractive and useful to others. The same

75 A general history of the concept of depression through the ages, with an analysis of how changes in the understanding of the disorder translated into changes in classification, is Clark Lawlor, *From Melancholia to Prozac* (Oxford etc.: Oxford University Press 2012). Although the increased 'medicalization' of mild symptoms of depression may be criticized, it may also have contributed to the decline of suicide (see one of the following sections).

76 A classical study of the "social origins of depression" distinguished between provoking factors (such as the loss of one's job), symptom-formation factors (such as having experienced a previous episode) and vulnerability factors (such as early loss of one's mother); see George W. Brown and Tirril Harris, *Social Origins of Depression* (London: Tavistock Publications, 1978).

applies to real and perceived inequalities in social rank, which translate into steep social inequalities in the prevalence of depression.[77]

A more general explanation, which does not only apply to depression but to many more forms of mental illness, is that during the second half of the 20th century European societies have become 'knowledge economies', in which people no longer work with their hands but with their heads. Jobs in the expanding service sector require flexibility, self-management and adaptability, and a higher level of cognitive, social, and emotional skills than jobs in the shrinking agricultural or industrial sectors. In such a society mental ill-health is a serious barrier to individual success, and will therefore more readily be recognized and more often lead to seeking care.[78]

Injuries

Road Traffic Injuries

Prominent among the "man-made diseases" rising during Omran's epidemiologic transition were road traffic injuries. These indeed increased impressively during the decades preceding the publication of his landmark paper, mainly due to the rise of the automobile (Figure 29).[79]

---

77 For a recent integrative theory of depression, see Paul Gilbert, *Depression: The Evolution of Powerlessness* (London: Routledge, 1992). For evolutionary theories of depression, see Randolph M. Nesse, "Is Depression an Adaptation?," *Archives of General Psychiatry* 57, no. 1 (2000): 14–20; Paul Gilbert and Steven Allan, "The Role of Defeat and Entrapment (Arrested Flight) in Depression: An Exploration of an Evolutionary View," *Psychological Medicine* 28, no. 3 (1998): 585–98; for a critical assessment of these theories, see Edward H. Hagen, "Evolutionary Theories of Depression: A Critical Review," *Canadian Journal of Psychiatry* 56, no. 12 (2011): 716–26. A recent review of empirical evidence for the "social rank theory of depression" is Karen Wetherall, Kathryn A. Robb, and Rory C. O'Connor, "Social Rank Theory of Depression," *Journal of Affective Disorders* 246 (2019): 300–19.

78 The importance of "mental capital" has been argued in, e.g., John Beddington et al., "The Mental Wealth of Nations," *Nature* 455, no. 7216 (2008): 1057–060. A thorough analysis of the changed nature of work and the importance of mental health for job performance in service economies can be found in Rifka Maria Weehuizen, "Mental Capital" (PhD Maastricht University, 2008).

79 Omran, "Epidemiologic Transition" lists road traffic injuries as "man-made," but many more factors are involved. "Road traffic injuries can be constructed as the result of individual misbehaviour, corporate irresponsibility, lack of administrative regulation or control, insufficient public maintenance and medical services, misguided transportation arrangements, [...] or just bad luck" (Iris Borowy, "Road Traffic Injuries: Social Change and Development," *Medical History* 57, no. 1 (2013): 108–38, p. 111).

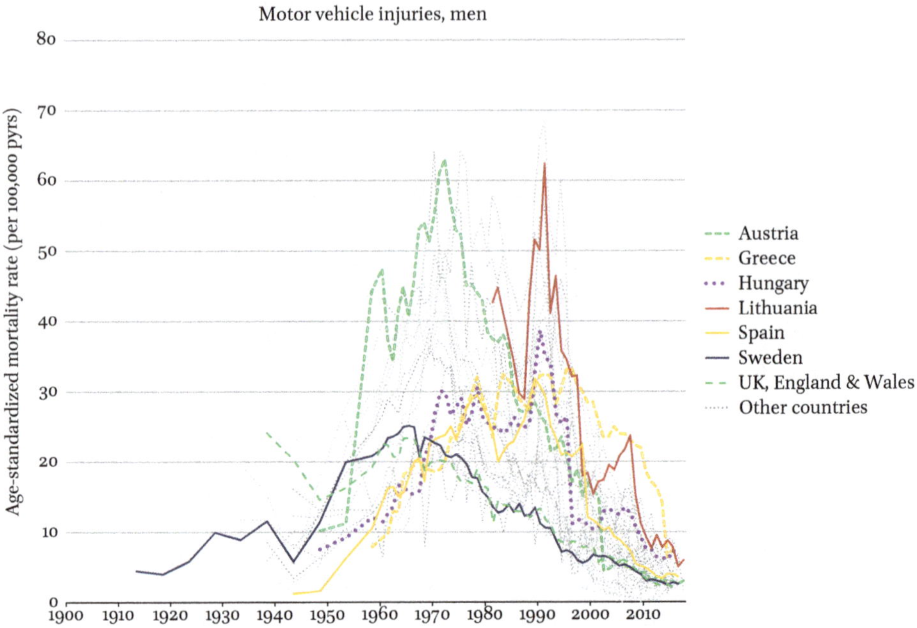

FIGURE 29 Trends in motor vehicle injury mortality in Europe, 1900–2015
Note: Mortality among motor vehicle occupants. Quinquennial data before 1960
SOURCE OF DATA: SEE SUPPL. TABLE 1

In Europe as a whole, deaths among road traffic participants occur predominantly among motor vehicle occupants (53%), followed by pedestrians (28%), riders of motorized two-wheelers (8%), and cyclists (2%). The distribution differs importantly between countries, depending on the most frequently used modes of transport. For example, in the Netherlands motor vehicle occupants and cyclists each account for about a third of all deaths. Nonetheless, because many deaths among pedestrians and cyclists are actually caused by collisions with motor vehicles, these, and particularly private passenger cars, are the main culprit everywhere.[80]

The modern automobile was developed in Europe, but first became part of everyday life in the United States during the early decades of the 20th century, after cheaper versions like the Model-T Ford had been developed. In the 1930s, Britain was the first European country where automobiles became more widespread, and other Western European countries followed during the post-War

80 World Health Organization, *European Status Report on Road Safety* (Copenhagen: WHO Regional Office for Europe, 2009).

economic boom of the 1950s and 1960s. Currently, the number of passenger cars per 1000 population is around 500 in Europe as a whole, and varies between 200 in Moldova and 700 in Iceland.

Behind the Iron Curtain the growth of car ownership followed more slowly, partly because the possession of a such a 'mobile private space' was seen to be in conflict with communist ideology. Yet, consumer demand ultimately trumped ideology, as illustrated by automobile production in the Soviet Union. After World War II car production in the Soviet Union grew rapidly, and while trucks were at first produced in much larger numbers than automobiles, passenger car production overtook truck production in the early 1970s.[81]

Like the cigarette, the automobile developed a highly positive image which increased its appeal to consumers. It was (and is) not only a miracle of technology, but also stood for a modern way of life characterized by freedom of movement and a high level of comfort. Although the automobile's image was tainted when air pollution became a major concern in the 1970s, and perhaps even more so when carbon dioxide emissions and climate change became an issue more recently, it is easy to understand why the automobile became so popular. It does not only satisfy modern man's seemingly insatiable desire for mobility, but is also a source of self-esteem.[82]

But, unfortunately, cars kill. They kill like horses killed their riders and bystanders in previous centuries, and like trains killed their passengers in the 19th century, but the death toll of cars in the 20th century has been innumerably higher. The first deaths due to motor vehicles occurred in Britain in 1896, and as Britain was ahead of other European countries in its rate of motorization, motor vehicle injury mortality already reached high levels in the 1930s and peaked in the early 1940s. This was followed by a temporary decline in later years of World War II and the immediate post-war period, due to restrictions in fuel. Although there was a second peak in the early 1960s, the debates sparked by the peak in the early 1940s led to an early emphasis on road traffic safety,

81 For the social history of the automobile, and how it became seen as a source of health damage, see Borowy, "Road Traffic Injuries." The history of automobile production and ownership in the Soviet Union has been documented in Lewis H. Siegelbaum, *Cars for Comrades* (Ithaca: Cornell University Press, 2008).

82 In a Scottish study, car ownership was found to be independently associated with longevity and better health – an effect that appeared to go partly through the higher self-esteem of car owners; see Sally Macintyre et al., "Do Housing Tenure and Car Access Predict Health Because They Are Simply Markers of Income or Self Esteem?," *Journal of Epidemiology & Community Health* 52, no. 10 (1998): 657–64. Another study found that travelling by car conferred more self-esteem than travelling by public transport; see Anne Ellaway et al., "In the Driving Seat," *Transportation Research Part F: Traffic Psychology and Behaviour* 6, no. 3 (2003): 217–31.

which ensured that Britain never reached the high levels of motor vehicle injury mortality seen in other European countries.[83]

As Figure 29 shows, few other countries shared in the relatively favourable trends in Britain, which peaked at a rate about one third of that reached in some other European countries. Nevertheless, a similar pattern of 'rise-and-fall' can be seen everywhere. Motor vehicle injury mortality peaked in the late 1960s or 1970s in most countries in Northern and Western Europe, somewhat later in Southern Europe, and in the 1990s in most countries in Central-eastern and Eastern Europe.

In order to understand these trends, we need to keep in mind that, arithmetically, motor vehicle injury mortality equals injury incidence times case fatality, and that injury incidence equals injuries per kilometre travelled, times total kilometres travelled. Trends in mortality are thus determined by three different underlying trends: kilometres travelled, injuries per kilometre, and deaths per injury. Generally speaking, the rise in motor vehicle injury mortality seen before its peak is due to an increase in kilometres travelled, whereas the decline seen after the peak is due to a decline in both injuries per kilometre and deaths per injury.[84]

This decline in the likelihood of sustaining injury while travelling, and in the likelihood of dying after sustaining an injury, is a major achievement which can largely be attributed to the road safety policies which European countries (and the European Union) have undertaken. During the 1950s and 1960s, the increasing toll of road traffic casualties came to be recognized as an 'epidemic' which needed to be approached like any other epidemic: based on a systematic analysis of its determinants and with an emphasis on 'passive safety measures', which did not necessitate active behaviour change in fallible traffic participants.[85]

83 The rise in road traffic injury mortality in Britain in 1939, 1940, and 1941 was partly due to the 'Black Out', i.e., restrictions on road lighting to protect Britain from German bombardments. This led to debates about whom to blame, but resulted in an early consensus that improving road safety was necessary; see Bill Luckin, "War on the Roads: Traffic Accidents and Social Tension in Britain, 1939–45," in *Accidents in History*, ed. R. Cooter and B. Luckin (Amsterdam & Atlanta: Editions Rodopi, 1997).

84 For an example of an analysis along these lines, see Eduard F. van Beeck, C.W. Looman, and Johan P. Mackenbach, "Mortality Due to Unintentional Injuries in the Netherlands, 1950–1995," *Public Health Reports* 113, no. 5 (1998): 427–39. Although the decline of motor vehicle injury mortality in Western Europe is due to a decline of both the injury per kilometre and case fatality rate, the oil crisis of the early 1970s helped by causing a temporary stabilization of the rise in kilometres travelled.

85 The history of the public health approach to road traffic injuries can be traced in Leslie G. Norman, *Road Traffic Accidents: Epidemiology, Control, and Prevention* (Geneva: World

The development of effective policies to improve road traffic safety crystallized in a consensus that legislation, regulation, enforcement, engineering and education are all needed to create both safer road behaviour and improve the safety of vehicles and roads. Key areas for preventive interventions include controlling speed, stopping driving when under the influence of alcohol, enforcing use of safety equipment such as seat-belts, improving vehicle crash protection, and making roads safer for vehicles and vulnerable road users. Case fatality could be reduced by improving trauma care, e.g., by ensuring the quick arrival of emergency response teams and by optimizing the organization of trauma services.[86]

Implementation of these policies has been gradual, starting early in Britain, with Sweden and the Netherlands also in the forefront in the 1960s and 1970s, and with countries in the rest of Europe following later, and sometimes much later. Road traffic safety policies have been a major determinant of trends in road traffic mortality, with declines in mortality often following implementation of one of the measures mentioned above.[87]

From the late 1960s onwards, many countries in Northern and Western Europe have continued to stack one road traffic safety policy upon another, which led to a spectacular decline in road traffic injury deaths, albeit it more so among motor vehicle occupants than among more vulnerable road users (Figure 29). In Southern European countries, which had experienced a somewhat delayed 'epidemic' of road traffic deaths, the turning-point came later. In the case of Spain, Portugal and Greece this was helped by adherence to the European Union. This required harmonization with European road traffic safety regulations, and provided road infrastructure investment funds.

Health Organization, 1962). This approach would later be elaborated in the so-called Haddon matrix; see William Haddon, "Options for the Prevention of Motor Vehicle Crash Injury," *Israel Journal of Medical Sciences* 16, no. 1 (1980): 45–65.

86 This consensus, as well as the underlying scientific evidence, has been summarized in Margie Peden et al., *World Report on Road Traffic Injury Prevention* (Geneva: World Health Organization, 2004) and in Dinesh Sethi, *Injuries and Violence in Europe: Why They Matter and What Can Be Done* (Copenhagen WHO Regional Office Europe, 2006).

87 Autonomous influences have probably also played a role in the decline of road traffic injury mortality, such as learning effects among car drivers, but these were enhanced by road safety education efforts. Similarly, improvements in car design have also been important, but stricter safety requirements imposed by the European Commission have accelerated that process. For implementation of road traffic safety policies across Europe, see Dovile Adminaite et al., *Ranking EU Progress on Road Safety* (Brussels: European Transport Safety Council, 2018). For their impact on road traffic mortality, see Dinesh Sethi and Franco Mitis, "Road Traffic Injuries," in *Successes and Failures of Health Policy in Europe*, ed. Johan P. Mackenbach and Martin McKee (Maidenhead: Open University Press).

In Central-eastern, South-eastern and Eastern Europe, the collapse of the communist regimes was followed by a period of economic and social disruption, when both cars and alcohol flooded the market. This resulted in soaring rates of road traffic injury deaths. In the case of the (former) Soviet Union, cycles of increasing and decreasing alcohol consumption also strongly affected the trends. This is illustrated by the dip in motor vehicle injury mortality during Mikhail Gorbachev's anti-alcohol campaign in the mid-1980s, and several renewed rises and declines in the 1990s and early 2000s. The response to this calamity has been slow, but recent trends suggest that these countries are finally bringing this public health problem under control.[88]

These declines show that, although economic growth often goes together with rising road traffic injury mortality, declines can follow when effective countermeasures are taken – and these are of course more easily affordable with continued economic growth. Indeed, analyses of the world-wide association between national income and road traffic injury mortality show a striking reversal of the association between the two around the level that many Western European countries reached in the 1970s. When national income goes up, road traffic injury mortality rises too, but only up to a certain point after which it declines again.[89]

Suicide

The term 'suicide' was not used before the 1650s, but taking one's own life has occurred at all times in human history. This is shown by the examples of depressive King Saul (ca. 1100 BCE), who killed himself after being defeated by the Philistines, and Stoic philosopher Seneca (ca. 4 BCE–65 CE), who saw suicide as a road to freedom and killed himself when he was accused of plotting against

88 For the slow policy response, see Martin McKee et al., "Health Policy-Making in Central and Eastern Europe: Lessons from the Inaction on Injuries?," *Health Policy and Planning* 15, no. 3 (2000): 263–69. On cycles in alcohol consumption and cycles in injury mortality in Russia, see Vladimir M. Shkolnikov, France Meslé, and Jacques Vallin, "Recent Trends in Life Expectancy and Causes of Death in Russia, 1970–1993," in *Premature Death in the New Independent States*, ed. J.A. Bobadilla, C.A. Costello, and F. Mitchell (Washington (DC): National Academies Press, 1997). For an analysis of recent anti-alcohol campaigns and decline of road traffic injury deaths in Russia, see William A. Pridemore et al., "The Impact of a National Alcohol Policy on Deaths Due to Transport Accidents in Russia," *Addiction* 108, no. 12 (2013): 2112–118.

89 Eduard F. van Beeck, Gerard J.J. Borsboom, and Johan P. Mackenbach, "Economic Development and Traffic Accident Mortality in the Industrialized World, 1962–1990," *International Journal of Epidemiology* 29, no. 3 (2000): 503–09; Elizabeth Kopits and Maureen Cropper, "Traffic Fatalities and Economic Growth," *Accident Analysis and Prevention* 37 (2005): 169–78.

Roman emperor Nero. However, from the late 17th century the frequency of recorded suicides started to rise, first in England, later in other Western European countries, and still later in other parts of the subcontinent.[90]

National data on suicide only started to be collected in the 18th and early 19th centuries, and show a dramatically rising long-term trend, interrupted by temporary declines and epidemic peaks (Figure 30). Sweden was the first country to collect nation-wide statistics on suicide, to be followed by a number of other Northern and Western European countries. Despite strong fluctuations many of these countries experienced a large net increase in suicide rates until some point in the second half of the 20th century, after which the trend reversed.[91]

Very high rates of suicide were temporarily recorded in the Nordic countries, for example by Denmark in the 1850s and by Finland in the 1930s, and in German-speaking countries, for example by Austria and Germany in the 1930s. Although England's long-term trend of suicide is roughly similar to that of other Northern and Western European countries, its suicide rate never reached very high levels. The same is true for the Netherlands.

In Southern, Central-eastern, South-eastern and Eastern Europe, suicide rates generally started to rise later, i.e., in the second half of the 19th century or in the first decades of the 20th century. Despite this general increase, suicide rates remained comparatively low in Italy, Spain, Portugal and Greece. On the other hand, suicide rates in Hungary, Russia and several other countries rose explosively during the 20th century and reached extremely high levels before starting to decline more recently.

Covering a very long time-span, Figure 30 clearly brings out an over-all trend of 'rise-and-fall', but there were many temporary interruptions of the long-term trend, such as the peak in suicide mortality that several countries experienced in the 1930s. Below the surface of a single 'rise-and-fall', suicide in England has followed a trend of multiple smaller 'rises-and-falls'. For example, it

90 For the early history of suicide, see Georges Minois, *Histoire du Suicide* (Paris: Fayard, 1995). Based on the London Bills of Mortality, Barbagli, *Farewell* sees the rise of suicide starting in the 1680s. Both authors conclude that the rise in the frequency of recorded suicides reflected a real rise in the occurrence of suicide. The rise of suicide in England was well known among contemporaries elsewhere, who called it 'the English Malady'.

91 Currently, there are two main sources of information on suicide: cause-of-death statistics (based on registration by physicians) and judicial statistics (based on an evaluation of unnatural causes of death by the prosecutor or similar judicial authority). The reliability of suicide registration data is far from perfect, for example due to taboos on suicide leading to under-registration. Although the data in Figure 30 therefore need to be taken with a grain of salt, the larger changes and variations are likely to be valid. See Barbagli, *Farewell*, p. 313–14, for a short note on suicide registration.

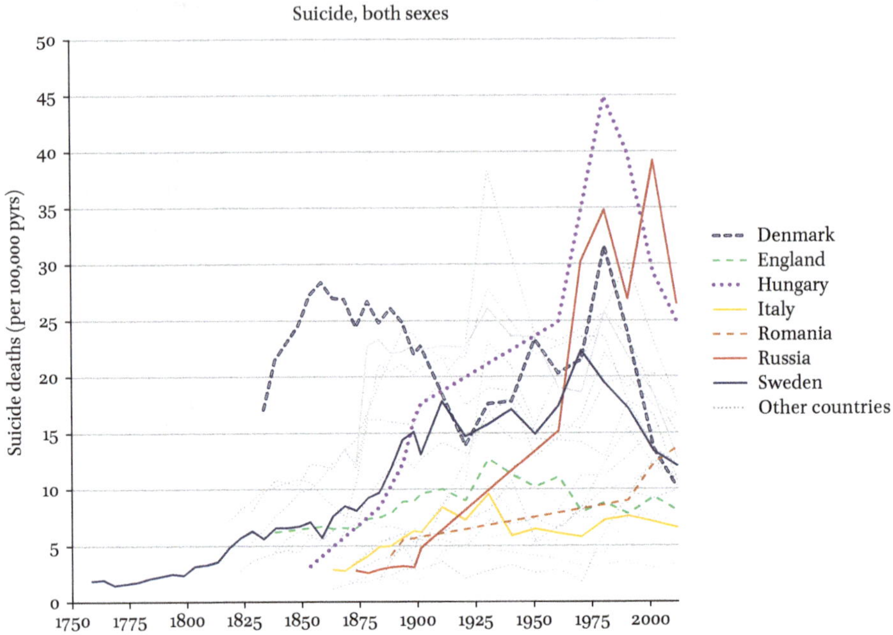

FIGURE 30 Trends in suicide in Europe, 1750–2010
Notes: Quinquennial or decadal data
SOURCE OF DATA: MARZIO BARBAGLI. *FAREWELL TO THE WORLD: A HISTORY OF SUICIDE*. CAMBRIDGE & MALDEN: POLITY PRESS, 2015, TABLE A.1–A.4

peaked in 1905, dipped during World War I, peaked again at a higher level during the Great Depression of the 1930s, dipped in World War II, rose again slightly in the 1950s, etc.[92]

Detailed year-by-year analyses of single countries have shown that dramatic political events have sometimes been accompanied by equally dramatic rises of suicide mortality, as in the case of the defeat of France in the Franco-Prussian War in 1871, the occupation of the Netherlands by Germany in 1940, and the repression of the Hungarian uprising by the Soviet Union in 1956. On the other hand, as mentioned above for England, suicide rates often declined during

92 See Kyla Thomas and David Gunnell, "Suicide in England and Wales 1861–2007: A Time-Trends Analysis," *International Journal of Epidemiology* 39, no. 6 (2010): 1464–475 for an analysis of long-term trends in suicide in England and Wales. Figure 30 does not show that trends sometimes differ between men and women, and between younger and older people (see, e.g., David J. Gunnell et al., "Why Are Suicide Rates Rising in Young Men but Falling in the Elderly?," *Social Science & Medicine* 57, no. 4 (2003): 595–611).

war-time, particularly among men, perhaps as a result of strengthened national unity.[93]

What explains these secular trends? There is an enormous literature on the determinants of suicide as an individual act, but what primarily concerns us here are the determinants of suicide rates as a collective phenomenon. This perspective was first systematically elaborated by French sociologist Émile Durkheim (1858–1917), who argued that the frequency of suicide in a society reflects its degree of 'social integration'.

Social integration is dependent on the number and strength of ties that bind individuals to various social groups, and that protect against suicide by providing support and by regulating behaviour. According to Durkheim the suicide rate will be low when the degree of integration is high, whereas the suicide rate will rise during times of rapid social change. Then, ties are loosened and a situation of temporary or permanent 'anomie' arises, for example when people migrate from rural areas to larger cities.[94]

When compared with the long-term trends of suicide in Europe (Figure 30), Durkheim's theory does indeed appear to have some explanatory power. As mentioned above, the decline of suicide in war may be an effect of increased social integration. Loss of social integration, as a result of industrialization and urbanization, can probably explain some of the rise of suicide in Western and Northern Europe during the 19th century, and in other parts of Europe during the 20th century.[95]

The further rise of suicide in communist countries after World War II may be due to a further increase in 'anomie' as a result of profound societal changes, combined with a rise of excessive alcohol consumption which reduces behavioural inhibition and thereby lowers the threshold for committing

93 On the effects of political events and wars on suicide, see Chesnais, *Histoire* and Barbagli, *Farewell*. Cornelis S. Kruijt, *Zelfmoord: Statistisch-Sociologische Verkenningen* (Assen Van Gorcum, 1960), Chapter 4 analysed the effect of the German occupation on suicide in the Netherlands.

94 Durkheim's study was published in 1897, and reflected the increasing concern all around Western Europe with rising suicide rates (Emile Durkheim, *Suicide: Étude de Sociologie* (Paris: Félix Alcan, 1897)). Durkheim noted that the (seemingly) individual act of suicide gave rise to remarkably stable rates of suicide at the aggregate level. While this is true in the short run, Figure 30 shows that this is not really true in the longer run. For a modern re-think of Durkheim's 'social integration', see Lisa F. Berkman et al., "From Social Integration to Health: Durkheim in the New Millennium," *Social Science & Medicine* 51, no. 6 (2000): 843–57.

95 The rise of suicide in Denmark and Norway in the first half of the 19th century is not due to industrialization and urbanization, but to brutal agrarian reforms; see Kruijt, *Zelfmoord*, p. 29.

suicide. After the collapse of the Soviet Union in 1991, rates of suicide rose even further, partly as a result of the severe economic crisis that accompanied the rapid transformation of a communist into a capitalist society.[96]

But loss of social integration is certainly not the whole story. The rise of suicide started long before the take-off of industrialization and urbanization: as we have seen above, it started in England as early as the 1680s and in Sweden as early as the late 18th century. The most likely explanation, extensively documented in contemporary writings and changes in formal procedures surrounding suicide, is that suicide started to rise as a result of cultural changes. In the Middle Ages and early modern period, suicide used to be strictly forbidden and severely sanctioned for religious reasons, but this changed under the influence of the Enlightenment and the gradual recognition that suicidal tendencies often reflected mental disorders such as melancholia.[97]

That loss of social integration is not the only important determinant of long-term trends in suicide is also clear from the rise of suicide during economic crises. Suicide rose not only during the economic crisis in former communist countries during the 1990s, but during all the major economic crises of the 20th century, including the Great Depression after the 1929 financial crisis, and the Great Recession after the 2008 financial crisis. This rise occurs particularly among young and middle-aged men and among the unemployed, and is likely due to despair among those who lose their jobs, incomes, feelings of self-worth, etc. Although loss of social integration may also play a role, this is only one of the social-psychological mechanisms involved in the rise of suicide during unemployment.[98]

While the factors described so far – social integration, political upheavals, cultural restrictions, economic despair – all to a greater or lesser extent reflect the nature of a society, two other factors have a more incidental character, but can nevertheless profoundly modify the relationship between the nature of society and the frequency of suicide.

The first of these is access to the means of committing suicide. A well-known example is the declining incidence of suicide by gassing in the 1960s in

96 See Barbagli, *Farewell* and Chesnais, *Histoire* for an interpretation of long-term trends in suicide in Central-eastern and Eastern Europe.

97 These cultural changes have been documented in Minois, *Histoire* and Barbagli, *Farewell*. On the medicalization of suicide and its role in making suicide acceptable, see Michael MacDonald, "The Medicalization of Suicide in England: Laymen, Physicians, and Cultural Change, 1500–1870," *Milbank Quarterly* 67, no. Suppl. 1 (1989): 69–91.

98 Barbagli, *Farewell*; Chesnais, *Histoire*. For an analysis of the effects of the 2008 financial crisis, see Shu-Sen Chang et al., "Impact of 2008 Global Economic Crisis on Suicide: Time Trend Study in 54 Countries," *British Medical Journal* 347 (2013): f5239.

England, when domestic gas produced from coal, which had a high content in carbon monoxide, was replaced by non-poisonous natural gas. As this was not compensated by a rise in other methods of suicide, total incidence of suicide also declined, illustrating that a simple change in the means available for suicide can fundamentally affect the frequency with which people kill themselves.[99]

The second factor that may modify the relationship between society's underlying tendency for suicide and the actual rate at which suicide occurs, is the availability of effective mental health care. The recent decline of suicide that has been observed across Europe (Figure 30) is unlikely to be explained by increased social integration. It is probably at least partly attributable to increased access to mental health care, increased use of anti-depressants, increased awareness of the risk of suicide among mental health care professionals, more wide-spread implementation of suicide prevention programs, and more effective treatment of pain from somatic conditions.[100]

Clearly then, suicide trends do not have a simple explanation. The rise of suicide appears to be explained by a combination of economic, sociocultural and psychological 'modernization' of society, but the influence of these societal factors is strongly modified by other factors. This also implies that suicide is not a reliable indicator of population mental health.[101]

A New Plague

AIDS

AIDS (Acquired Immuno-Deficiency Syndrome) came as a shock. In the 1960s and 1970s, large-scale mortality from infectious diseases seemed to have become a thing of the past, at least in high-income countries, and then a new

99 Norman Kreitman, "The Coal Gas Story. United Kingdom Suicide Rates, 1960–71," *Journal of Epidemiology & Community Health* 30, no. 2 (1976): 86–93; Thomas and Gunnell, "Suicide in England and Wales."

100 For a general analysis, see Barbagli, *Farewell*, For the role of anti-depressants, see Svein Reseland, Isabelle Bray, and David Gunnell, "Relationship between Antidepressant Sales and Secular Trends in Suicide Rates in the Nordic Countries," *British Journal of Psychiatry* 188, no. 4 (2006): 354–58. For the role of suicide prevention programs, see Bruce Singh and Rachel Jenkins, "Suicide Prevention Strategies: An International Perspective," *International Review of Psychiatry* 12, no. 1 (2000): 7–14.

101 This is also clear from the fact that 'parasuicide' ('unsuccessful' suicide attempts), while being much more frequent than suicide, has a completely different epidemiology; see David J. Gunnell, "The Epidemiology of Suicide," *International Review of Psychiatry* 12, no. 1 (2000): 21–6.

epidemic disease arrived which threatened to become as deadly as the plague. And so it did – world-wide, the annual number of AIDS deaths currently is around 1 million, and the total death toll since the early 1980s is around 35 million.[102]

Most of these deaths have occurred in Sub-Saharan Africa, and the epidemic has been less severe in Europe, but it still caused large numbers of deaths, in a curiously bimodal pattern (Figure 31). Trends in mortality can be followed from 1983, when the International Classification of Diseases was provisionally adapted to include this new disease amongst its codes. Many countries in Northern, Western, and Southern Europe had a peak of AIDS mortality in the early 1990s, but there were enormous differences in peak level. Spain and Portugal stand out with much higher peak levels than other countries. Many countries in Eastern Europe had a high peak of AIDS mortality around 2010, and in some countries, such as Russia, mortality is still increasing as judged on the basis of the latest available data.

The first cases of AIDS were reported in 1981 in the United States, but it soon turned out that the first European cases had occurred at about the same time, i.e., in 1979 or 1980. Later, studies of stored blood and tissue samples uncovered many earlier cases, that had already occurred in the 1940s and 1950s but had gone unrecognized. It is now thought that sporadic cases of AIDS have probably occurred in Africa since the beginning of the 20th century, and that the disease was already wide-spread in parts of Africa during the 1970s and 1980s.[103]

The infectious agent that caused AIDS was discovered very rapidly, in 1983, by teams of American and French researchers. The *Human Immunodeficiency Virus* (HIV) comes in two types, HIV-1 and HIV-2, and both probably evolved

102 Statistics on HIV and AIDS are collected and published by UNAIDS (http://www.unaids.org/en/resources/fact-sheet), the World Health Organization (https://www.who.int/gho/hiv/en/), and the European Centre for Disease Prevention and Control European Centers for Disease Control, *HIV/AIDS Surveillance in Europe: 2017 Data* (Copenhagen: World Health Organization, 2018).

103 The first historian to publish a detailed and well-informed history of AIDS (already in 1989!) was Mirko Grmek; see Mirko D. Grmek, *Histoire du Sida* (Paris: Payot, 1989). Since then, many more pieces of evidence on the origins and early spread of AIDS have surfaced. For an overview of the history of AIDS in Africa, see John Iliffe, *The African AIDS Epidemic: A History* (Athens: Ohio University Press, 2006). Genetic analyses of the virus as found in stored blood samples of early patients suggest that the epidemic spread from Africa to the Caribbean in the 1960s, and from there to (first) New York and (then) San Francisco in the 1970s; see Michael Worobey et al., "1970s and 'Patient 0' HIV-1 Genomes Illuminate Early HIV/AIDS History in North America," *Nature* 539, no. 7627 (2016): 98–101.

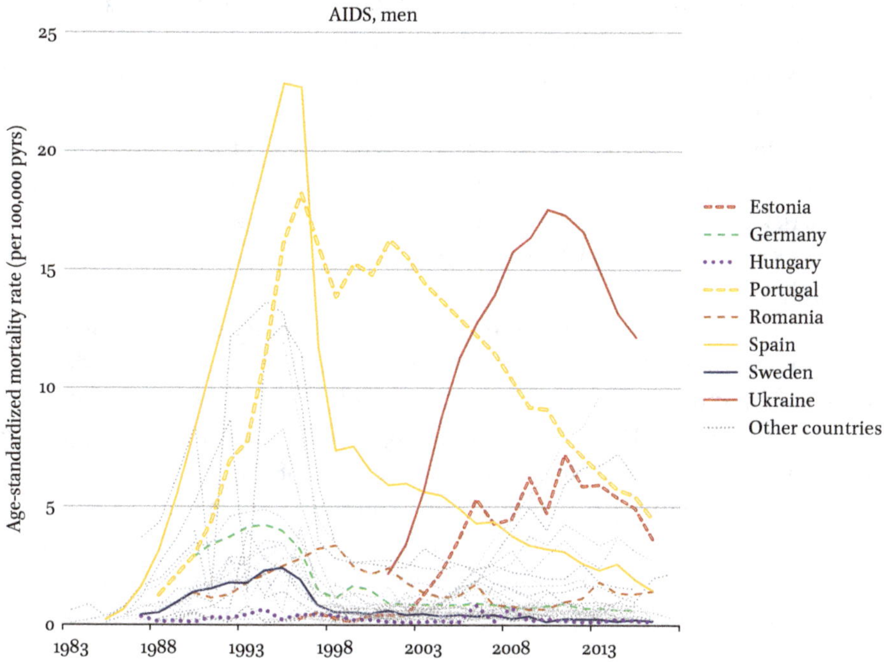

FIGURE 31 Trends in AIDS mortality in Europe, 1983–2017
SOURCE OF DATA: SEE SUPPL. TABLE 1

from similar viruses in chimpanzees and monkeys in Africa, from which they transferred to humans in the early 20th century. HIV-infection did not spread widely beyond Africa at the time, and gave rise to a world-wide epidemic only when conditions arose that promoted its spread, at first within the global gay community.

Increased tourism and international travel were one important condition fostering the spread of HIV. Sexual liberation and gay emancipation were another, intensifying sexual relations and increasing the number of sexual contacts. Medical developments also played a role: the increased use of blood products made it possible for the virus to spread to patients needing blood transfusions, and the wide availability of disposable injection needles made it possible for the virus to spread to intravenous drug users.

The world-wide AIDS epidemic started among gay men, and HIV transmission between men-who-have-sex-with-men still accounts for 21% of all cases in Europe as a whole. With 40% this is still the most important mode of transmission in Western Europe. Nevertheless, over time other modes of HIV transmission have become more important, and in Europe as a whole the most common mode now is heterosexual sex (49%), whereas intravenous drug use accounts for 13% and transmission between mother and child for 1%.[104]

Before the advent of effective drug treatment, the disease itself was almost as frightening as plague, cholera and tuberculosis had been in the past. HIV infection interferes with the immune system, increasing the risk of tuberculosis and other infections (such as *Pneumocystis carinii pneumonia*), and increasing the risk of tumours that are extremely rare in people without HIV infection (such as Kaposi's sarcoma). When these complications occurred, AIDS used to be highly fatal.

However, the public response to AIDS in North America and Western Europe was extremely rapid. American and European governments made large investments in research, and these soon paid off in the development of effective drug treatment. The first effective drug, zidovudine (AZT), was approved by the American Federal Drug Administration in 1987, but did only suppress the virus for a relatively short time. The real breakthrough was the introduction in 1996 of highly active antiretroviral therapy (HAART), a combination of different antiviral agents. These treatments have drastically reduced case fatality, and contributed to the precipitous decline of AIDS mortality in the second half of the 1990s.[105]

Simultaneously, effective prevention strategies were developed, at first focusing on the promotion of 'safe sex' practices among gay men. Because homosexuality was not yet accepted in all sectors of society, a subtle approach was needed, and there were large differences between European countries in the extent to which they were able to develop and implement prevention programs that were both effective and acceptable. Countries in Northern and Western Europe were generally much more successful than the culturally more conservative countries in the rest of Europe.[106]

---

104 European Centers for Disease Control, *HIV/AIDS Surveillance.*

105 Yet, people in Europe still die from AIDS in large numbers; see R.D. Simmons et al., "Ten-Year Mortality Trends among Persons Diagnosed with HIV Infection in England and Wales," *HIV Medicine* 14, no. 10 (2013): 596–604; Valerie Delpech and J. Lundgren, "Death from AIDS Is Preventable, So Why Are People Still Dying of AIDS in Europe?," *Eurosurveillance* 19, no. 47 (2014): 20973.

106 Virginia Berridge and Philip Strong, eds., *AIDS and Contemporary History* (Cambridge etc.: Cambridge University Press, 1993); Virginia Berridge, "AIDS in the UK: The Making of Policy, 1981–1994," in *Sex, State and Society: Comparative Perspectives on the History of Sexuality*, ed. Lars-Göran Tedebrand (Umeå: Nyheternas tryckeri, 1996); Bernd Rechel, "HIV/AIDS in the Countries of the Former Soviet Union," *Central European Journal of Public Health* 18, no. 2 (2010): 110–15; Carlos Alvarez-Dardet and I Hernandez Aguado, "AIDS in Spain: Lessons Learned from a Public Health Disaster," *Journal of Epidemiology and Community Health* 48, no. 4 (1994): 331–32.

It is not easy to assess the effects of these prevention programs, because national trends in incidence of HIV infection can only be followed from a relatively recent point in time onwards, after diagnosis of HIV diagnosis had become notifiable or other registration systems had been installed. Since 2008, the incidence of HIV infection still appears to be increasing in Europe as a whole, but to be declining in several Western European countries, which may partly reflect the impact of prevention programs.[107]

While the epidemic rise of HIV infection, and then the impact of treatment and prevention, help to understand the general pattern of 'rise-and-fall' of AIDS mortality, it does not immediately explain the enormous variations between countries. One important clue is that the highest peaks of AIDS mortality occurred in countries in which the virus was spread by intravenous drug users, from whom it also spread into the heterosexual population. This applies to Spain and Portugal, and also to Eastern European countries.

Intravenous drug users are a group that is very difficult to reach by prevention campaigns, including secondary prevention aimed at early detection of HIV-infection. As a result HIV-infection is often detected at a late stage in which treatment is less effective. The massive epidemics of HIV infection and AIDS mortality seen in Spain and Portugal are due to the fact that, due to cultural and religious conservatism, harm reduction strategies (methadone treatment, needle exchange, …) were unacceptable when the epidemic broke out.[108]

Similar explanations apply to Eastern European countries where massive epidemics of HIV infection and AIDS mortality have occurred: Estonia, Ukraine, Russia, Moldova. Intravenous drug use generally arrived in these countries after the collapse of the Soviet Union, coinciding with the economic and social crisis during the 1990s. In addition to the cultural barriers just mentioned,

---

107 European Centers for Disease Control, *HIV/AIDS Surveillance*.

108 For the same reasons, campaigns to promote 'safe sex' among homosexuals were also less feasible. On Spain, see Alvarez-Dardet and Aguado, "AIDS in Spain"; Marta Torrens et al., "Methadone Maintenance Treatment in Spain," *Bulletin of the World Health Organization* 91 (2013): 136–41. The introduction of harm reduction strategies among intravenous drug users was delayed in Spain, but the AIDS epidemic caused a shift in attitudes in the 1990s, which made methadone maintenance treatment more acceptable; see Torrens et al., "Methadone." On Portugal, see Paula Santana and Helena Nogueira, "AIDS/HIV Mortality in Portugal in the 90s," *Revista Portuguesa de Saúde Pública*, no. 1 (2005): 57–68. On Greece, see Anastasia Pharris et al., "Human Immunodeficiency Virus in Injecting Drug Users in Europe," *Eurosurveillance* 16, no. 48 (2011): 20032.

a failure of national health systems to cope with such an unusual threat also played a role.[109]

109 On AIDS in all countries of the former Soviet Union as a whole, see Rechel, "HIV/AIDS in the Countries of the Former Soviet Union." On Russia specifically, see Elena Tkatchenko-Schmidt et al., "Why Do Health Systems Matter?," *Health Policy and Planning* 25, no. 4 (2010): 283–91. On Estonia specifically, see Kaja-Triin Laisaar et al., "Estonia at the Threshold of the Fourth Decade of the AIDS Era in Europe," *AIDS Research and Human Retroviruses* 27, no. 8 (2011): 841–51.

PART 3

Synthesis and Outlook

CHAPTER 7

Why?

Scientific explanations come in many different forms, and can be roughly classified in two types: explanations of 'how' certain things occur, and explanations of 'why' they occur. In the previous chapters, we have mainly focused on the 'how', but have already started to address some 'why'-type questions, for example when we related the rise of public hygiene to the Enlightenment, and the reversal in the trends of syphilis to the sexual revolution of the 1960s. But in this chapter we will do this in a more systematic way, along two lines. We will first try to understand why, over the past three centuries, European population health has improved so much. Is it possible to identify a 'prime mover'? After that, we will use a few special cases – countries that did remarkably well, or remarkably badly – to understand why the European experience has been so diverse. How did economic, political and sociocultural factors combine to produce this diversity? For example, is there a deeper explanation for the consistently good performance of the Swedes, and the consistently bad performance of the Russians?[1]

Why Did European Population Health Improve?

The Rise and Fall of Disease

The trends of most diseases reviewed in this book have followed a 'rise-and-fall' pattern. Most diseases which were common at one point in time were much less frequent in previous centuries. As we have noted above in Chapters 2 and 3, this clearly suggests an exogenous or environmental origin. Equally remarkable is the fact that most diseases have at some point in their history started to decline, which suggests that humans have usually succeeded in counteracting whatever caused the previous rise.[2]

1 For a lucid account of the difference between "how" and "why" questions in science, see Ernst Mayr, "Cause and Effect in Biology," *Science* 134, no. 3489 (1961): 1501–506. Mayr points out that the everyday word "why" is ambiguous, because it means both "how come" and "what for." It is the first that concerns us here, i.e., "what was the process that over time led to the phenomenon," and not the second, "what purpose does the phenomenon have."

2 This book has reviewed the histories of 'only' 40 diseases, but a pattern of 'rise-and-fall' also applies to many other diseases that were not covered, such as most other infectious diseases,

The time-scale at which such a pattern of 'rise-and-fall' manifested itself varied between several millennia (as in the case of infectious diseases which became endemic after the Neolithic or first agricultural revolution, and only were pushed back during the 20th century) and two decades (as in the case of the AIDS epidemic in which incidence started to rise in the early 1980s and already started to decline in the 1990s and early 2000s). In the long run, delays between rise and decline have become shorter, with the case of AIDS being an extremely successful example, suggesting that collective human action to reduce the incidence (or case fatality) of disease has become more effective over time.

That 'rise-and-fall' is the usual time-pattern in which diseases afflict human populations must have a deeper explanation. Why have, in the course of human history, so many diseases emerged? Why have, on the other hand and with shorter or longer delay, most of these diseases become less common again, or at least become less lethal? And is there a causal link between the disappearance of one disease and the emergence of another?

The history of specific diseases shows that the emergence of new diseases is often linked to changes in human behaviour. These can bring existing health risks from elsewhere (as in long-distance trade that resulted in a "confluence of disease pools"), or enhance existing health risks (as in the case of increasing population density), or create entirely new health risks (as in the case of introduction of industrial modes of production). The fundamental cause here is that improving their living conditions often requires humans to undertake activities beyond earlier boundaries on their behaviour, and sometimes allows them to indulge in new forms of behaviour, which are only later shown to be health-damaging.[3]

Fortunately, the history of specific diseases also shows that after some time they often retreat or become less severe. This is sometimes the result of the self-limiting character of a disease (as in the case of some infectious diseases which over time have become less lethal), but more often a side-effect of human development. Human development is associated with reductions in health risks, because better living conditions on balance and unintentionally reduce health risks, and – equally importantly – create the means for intentionally reducing health risks. That human development is associated with a

most other cancers, gout, many skin diseases, psychotropic drug use disorders, dental caries, occupational injuries, etc.; see Kiple, *World History*, various chapters.

3 That, through human history, contact between previously separated civilisations led to a "confluence of disease pools" was proposed by William McNeill; see William H. McNeill, *Plagues and Peoples* (New York: Anchor Press/Doubleday, 1976).

net reduction of health risks must at least partly be due to the fact that humans have a strong drive to avoid disease and death, and thus tend to steer their development into the direction of health improvement.

That human history is littered not only with rises followed by declines, but also with declines of one set of diseases followed by rises of another set of diseases, is not a coincidence either. Disappearance of one set of diseases may be followed by the emergence of another set of diseases due to various mechanisms. There may be mutual antagonism of the micro-organisms or vectors involved. There may be increased survival to an age at which these other diseases strike. Or changes in behaviour or living conditions that help to avoid one disease give rise to another, as in the case of diseases of poverty being replaced by diseases of affluence.[4]

In any case, trends in 'aggregate' population health are the net result of rises and falls of many specific health outcomes. Over time, rises and falls of specific health risks occur continuously, and improvements in 'aggregate' population health can only occur when declines of health risks exceed the concurrent increases. The improvement of 'aggregate' population health over the past three centuries can therefore also be seen as the result of a favourable change in the balance between 'rising' and 'falling' diseases.

The Role of Human Agency

In Chapter 1, when we introduced the debate about the role of public health and medical care in the long-term decline of mortality, we proposed a five-point scale for the degree of intentionality of population health improvements. This scale goes from entirely 'spontaneous' to completely 'intentional', with several shades of grey in-between. Where on this scale should the factors involved in the more than 30 'falls' of disease reviewed in the previous chapters be placed?

Entirely spontaneous improvements, resulting from changes in living conditions that happened without any human involvement, have been rare, and most of these cases are also disputed. Some of the 'health problems of pre-industrial societies' may have diminished spontaneously. It has been suggested that the end of the 'Little Ice Age' contributed to a reduction in the frequency

4 Recognizing the mutual dependence of diseases on each other, directly or indirectly, Grmek has coined the term 'pathocenosis': "the qualitatively and quantitatively defined group of pathological states present in a given population at a given time"; see Mirko D. Grmek, "Préliminaires d'une Étude Historique des Maladies," *Annales. Histoire, sciences sociales* 24, no. 6 (1969): 1473–483.

or severity of hunger, and that a change in rat populations contributed to the attenuation of plague epidemics. It has also been suggested that spontaneous declines in virulence contributed to the decline of smallpox.

Similarly, declines in virulence may have contributed to the decline of some 'health problems of industrializing societies', particularly tuberculosis and various streptococcal infections. On the other hand, we have found no examples of (putatively) spontaneous declines in the 'health problems of affluent societies'. Spontaneous changes are difficult to prove or disprove, but even if they have occurred their contribution to over-all mortality decline can only have been modest, in view of the small number of health conditions in which they may have played a (partial) role.

Changes in human behaviour or man-made changes in living conditions which simply occurred, and were not pursued for reasons directly or indirectly related to health – our lightest shade of grey – have also sometimes made a contribution. Some cultural changes should probably be classified in this category. It is likely that the 'civilizing process' led to the adoption of more hygienic habits for reasons completely unrelated to health. Similarly, the decline of cigarette smoking may partly reflect a reversal of the symbolic value of smoking for 'social distinction', which might also have occurred if the health risks of smoking had not been discovered.

Other examples are changes in food conservation methods, which led to a reduction of the salt content of food, and the shift from an industrial to a service economy, which reduced exposure to hazardous work. However, while some of these changes may have contributed to population health improvement, at least as many have contributed to (temporary) health deteriorations, and it would be difficult to defend the idea that the net effect of all these changes has been positive.

Changes in human behaviour or man-made changes in living conditions which were actively pursued, but for reasons only indirectly related to health, may well form a much larger category than the previous two. Famine, one of the main 'health problems of pre-industrial societies' and an important cause of large-scale epidemics, has disappeared as a result of the (second) agricultural revolution. Although Europeans have probably never aimed for higher harvest yields in order to reduce their risk of infectious disease, their active drive to eliminate hunger did nevertheless have that effect.

Several 'health problems of industrializing societies' declined as a result of fertility control. Again, Europeans did not limit their family size in order to reduce the risk of infection, but mainly for reasons that are only indirectly related to health, such as greater family welfare and increased educational opportunities for their children (and perhaps to reduce the burden of multiple pregnancies to women). Nevertheless, smaller families did contribute to a decline of infectious disease mortality. Improvements in living standards as a result of economic growth did not fall out of a blue sky, but were actively pursued, and although this was not primarily for health-related reasons they did contribute importantly to population health improvements.

The fourth category, changes in human behaviour or living conditions which were achieved by public health interventions have also been very important in the decline of many diseases. Among the 'health problems of pre-industrial societies', these contributed to the decline of famine (public grain-stores and famine relief), plague (various measures of epidemic containment), smallpox (vaccination campaigns), typhus (promotion of personal hygiene and vector control) and malaria (irrigation of marshes and vector control).

Among the 'health problems of industrializing societies', respiratory infections declined partly as a result of improvements in housing which were pursued, not only to provide people with more comfortable lodgings, but also as part of public health policies. Sanitation measures succeeded in eliminating cholera and other diarrheal diseases. Regulation of prostitution contributed to the decline of syphilis, and pasteurization of milk to the decline of intestinal infections. Public health measures were essential in the decline of pellagra, rickets and goitre, and even more so in the decline of the pneumoconioses.

More recently, public health interventions have continued to make important contributions to the decline of 'health problems of affluent societies'. Tobacco and alcohol control measures have contributed to the decline of ischaemic heart disease, lung cancer and liver cirrhosis, screening programs to the decline of breast cancer mortality, and road traffic safety measures to the decline of road traffic injury.

However, over time the relative importance of individual patient care has also grown strongly. Medical care already made a contribution to the decline of malaria (quinine), and its contributions became more substantial towards the decline of many 'health problems of industrializing societies'. This included the decline of tuberculosis, syphilis, childhood infections, pneumonia, nutrient deficiencies, peptic ulcer and appendicitis (surgery, antibiotics, antisera, substitution therapy, ...). Medical care even was the dominant factor in the decline of maternal and late foetal mortality (obstetric care).

Finally, as we have seen in the previous chapters, the recent declines in cardiovascular disease, cancer and several other 'health problems of affluent societies' would have been impossible without improvements in prevention and treatment of these conditions. As mentioned in Chapter 3, it has been estimated that health care interventions have contributed up to one half of the increases in life expectancy at birth over the past decades.

It seems, then, that we can safely conclude that the improvement of population health over the past three centuries is mostly due to 'human agency', and even to 'intentional human agency' (the third, fourth and fifth positions of our scale of intentionality).

The Role of Public Health and Medical Care

Table 2 is an attempt to summarize the above, and to more specifically apportion credit for population health improvements in Europe to public health and medical care. It includes the same health conditions as Table 1, with the exclusion of those which even in North-western Europe have not (yet) gone in decline (diabetes, depression, dementia). It combines an overview of the contributions of public health and medical care to each health condition, with an estimate of the contribution of each health condition to total mortality decline.[5]

Before we look at the contents of this table, it is important to note some of its limitations. First of all, it is the result of what is often euphemistically called a 'heroic' exercise. Quantitative estimates of the effect of public health and medical care on the decline of specific diseases are scarce, and in many cases the percentage contribution of specific diseases to total mortality decline is rather uncertain. This is why the data are presented in a semi-quantitative mode, using symbols to indicate broad outcome ranges. It is all we have – better than nothing, but far from ideal.

A second limitation is that the contributions to over-all health improvement only include the contributions to mortality decline, thus ignoring effects on the health of the living population. It may well be that the contribution towards mortality decline of, for example, medical care is different from that towards morbidity decline – but we don't know. Furthermore, the health conditions in the table (i.e., the specific health conditions reviewed in this book) only represent about two-thirds of total mortality in the 19th and 20th centuries. The rest is taken up by other specific conditions (e.g., acute bronchitis, other heart diseases, Chronic Obstructive Pulmonary Disease, other accidents, …) and by ill-defined causes of death.

5 Similar analyses have previously been done for England & Wales, but only for the period up to 1970; see, e.g., McKeown, *Rise of Population*. See Woods, *Demography*, table 8.7 for a more sophisticated approach than the one used in Table 2.

The main benefit of Table 2 is that it allows us to identify the diseases that were important for mortality decline in different 'stages' of the epidemiologic transition, and then to again try to compare the relative importance of public health and medical care. Although contributions to mortality decline could not be calculated for the first stage, in which the 'health problems of pre-industrialized societies' were tackled, the table clearly shows that public health was far more important in this stage than medical care.

TABLE 2 Estimated contributions of public health and medical care to mortality decline

		Causes of declining incidence and/or mortality[a]			Contribution to total mortality decline[c]	
Group	Health problem	All other changes	Public health	Medical care[b]	ca. 1870–1950[d]	ca. 1970–2015[e]
Health problems of pre-industrial societies	War	+++++			[crisis]	.
	Homicide	+++++			+	+
	Famine	++++	+		[crisis]	.
	Plague	+	++++		.	.
	Smallpox	+	++++		++	.
	Typhus	+	++++		[crisis]	.
	Malaria	++	++	+	++	.
Health problems of industrializing societies	Cholera, intestinal infections	+	++++		++++	++
	Respiratory tuberculosis	++	++	+	++++	++
	Syphilis	+	++	++	+	+
	Childhood infections[f]	++	++	+	++++	+
	Pneumonia	++	+	++	+++	+++
	Influenza	++	+	++	[crisis]	++
	Puerperal fever	+		++++	+	.
	Infant mortality[g]	[++]	[++]	[+]	[+++++]	[+++]
	Still-births[h]	+		++++	-	-
	Pellagra	++	++	+	++	.
	Rickets	++	++	+	.	.
	Goitre	+	+++	+	.	.
	Peptic ulcer	++		+++	-	+
	Appendicitis	++		+++	+	+
	Pneumoconiosis	+	++++		-	.
	Stomach cancer	+++++			++	+++

TABLE 2 Estimated contributions of public health and medical care to mortality decline (*cont.*)

Group	Health problem	Causes of declining incidence and/or mortality[a]			Contribution to total mortality decline[c]	
		All other changes	Public health	Medical care[b]	ca. 1870–1950[d]	ca. 1970–2015[e]
Health problems of affluent societies	Ischaemic heart disease		++	+++	*rise*	+++++
	Cerebrovascular disease	+	+	+++	++	++++
	Colorectal cancer[i]		+	++++	*rise*	*rise*
	Breast cancer		++	+++	*rise*	+
	Prostate cancer[i]			+++++?	*rise*	*rise*
	Lung cancer[i]	+	++++		*rise*	*rise*
	Liver cirrhosis	+	++++		+	+
	Road traffic injuries	+	+++	+	*rise*	++
	Suicide	++?	+?	++?	*rise*	++
	AIDS	+	++	++	-	[crisis]

a Estimated relative contribution to disease-specific decline (sum over all three columns = +++++; source: see text)
b This includes preventive interventions given as part of medical care
c Contribution to total mortality decline

-	Unknown, inestimable or inapplicable
[crisis]	Substantial contribution, but inestimable because of strong fluctuations
.	<0.1%
+	0.1–1%
++	1–5%
+++	5–10%
++++	10–25%
+++++	>25%

d Based on various datasources, see Suppl. Table 8
e Based on WHO Mortality Database, see Suppl. Table 9
f Scarlet fever, whooping cough, measles, diphtheria
g Specific causes of infant mortality include other causes mentioned in the table
h Still-births are not included in countries' mortality rates; contribution to mortality decline undetermined
i Mortality from these diseases is declining in some parts of Europe only

Notes: This is a 'semi-quantitative' summary of the explanatory insights reviewed in Chapters 4–6 (first three columns), combined with quantitative analyses for two stages of mortality decline (last two columns). For each health condition, 5 points (indicated by '+') were allocated to three different causes of incidence or mortality decline: public health, medical care, and 'other changes'. The latter included completely 'spontaneous' changes, as well as unintentional and intentional changes in human behaviour outside the health system. In contrast to Table 1, this table covers all of Europe.

In the second stage, represented in the table by the 1870–1950 period, a few infectious diseases dominated European mortality decline. Intestinal infections, tuberculosis, and four childhood infections each accounted for between 10 and 25% of total mortality decline. For the decline of these diseases, public health interventions were considerably more important than improvements in medical care, although medical care also made a contribution.

In the third stage, represented by the 1960–2015 period, ischaemic heart disease dominated European mortality decline, accounting for more than 25% of total mortality decline. Cerebrovascular disease comes second in importance, and is (surprisingly) followed by three conditions that already declined in the second stage: pneumonia, infant mortality, and stomach cancer. Both public health measures and medical care were important in the decline of these conditions. There was less evidence for a contribution of 'other changes' in this period as compared to the previous two stages.

These results show that, over time, medical care has become much more important for mortality decline, but that over the three centuries covered by this book public health has been the most important of the two. This is all the more likely when we take into account that mortality decline in the second stage, in which public health was clearly more important than medical care, was considerably greater than in the third stage. Between 1870 and 1950, mortality declined from ca. 2500 to ca. 1100 deaths per 100,000 in Europe as a whole. Between 1960 and 2015, age-standardized mortality declined from ca. 1200 to ca. 600 per 100,000 – still a considerable decline, but less (in absolute terms) than in the earlier period.

The Rise of the West: *Was There a 'Prime Mover'?*

Why did the increase of life expectancy, and many other improvements in population health, start in Europe (and its offshoots in North America and Oceania), and why did it, within Europe, start in the North-west? And was there a 'prime mover', i.e., a single factor present in North-western Europe that can be held responsible for the whole train of changes that produced these health improvements?

This is a question that – for a similar phenomenon, namely economic growth – has been discussed extensively in the historical literature. The title of this section, *The Rise of the West,* refers to a book by historian William McNeill, in which he tries to explain how over the past few centuries Western civilization gradually achieved global dominance. Why 'the West' took such an enormous economic lead over the rest of the world, has occupied historical sociologists, economic historians, as well as comparative political scientists. A brief review of the answers given to this question provides a good starting-point for a discussion of why 'the West' also took the lead in population health.[6]

Most authors agree that, somewhere in the deepest layers of causality, physical geography must have played a role. North-western Europe has a moderate climate which keeps tropical parasites away, and which produces abundant rainfall throughout the year that allows agriculture without large-scale irrigation – a technical solution which has elsewhere in the world allowed extractive social hierarchies to emerge. It also lies far away from the Eurasian steppes from which nomads could come to periodically destroy whatever had been built up.

Furthermore, it has many small river valleys which fostered the emergence of small and competing political units, instead of one all-powerful centre of power, and it has a long coast-line which made it easy to transport goods and people. Under its surface also lie abundant stores of coal. Within Europe, North-western Europe gained the upper hand when trans-Atlantic trade could be developed, because they were in a better position than countries bordering on the Mediterranean.[7]

But the complete story is, of course, considerably more complex than a simple sum of the hard facts of physical geography. For the fact that the Industrial Revolution started in North-western Europe, to be more precise: in England, economic historians have offered several explanations, in addition to proximity of trans-Atlantic trade routes. (The latter provided higher levels of prosperity from the 16th century onwards, and therefore facilitated many other developments.)[8]

A first stream of analysis has emphasized the role of institutions. Political decentralization, with many smaller political units and the early rise of

6 William H. McNeill, *The Rise of the West* (Chicago etc.: University of Chicago Press, 1963). A balanced summary is given in Daniel Chirot, "The Rise of the West," *American Sociological Review* 50, no. 2 (1985): 181–95. An analysis emphasizing the role of coal and colonies in 'the Great divergence' between Europe and East Asia is Kenneth Pomeranz, *The Great Divergence* (Princeton & Oxford: Princeton University Press, 2000). Recent books have tried to answer this question again (e.g., Ian Morris, *Why the West Rules – for Now* (London: Profile Books, 2010); Niall Ferguson, *Civilization: The West and the Rest* (London: Allen Lane, 2011)).

7 Jared Diamond has argued that geographical factors have also determined why Eurasia (not only North-western Europe) has long been ahead of Africa and the Americas. The Neolithic revolution occurred much earlier on the Eurasian continent than in Africa or the Americas, because the first happens to have more domesticable plants and animals, and because it lies along a West-East axis which makes it easier for plants and animals from one part of the continent to be used in another; see Jared M. Diamond, *Guns, Germs, and Steel* (New York: W.W. Norton & Company, 1997).

8 For a discussion of the explanations given, see Joel Mokyr and Hans-Joachim Voth, "Understanding Growth in Europe, 1700–1870: Theory and Evidence," in *Cambridge Economic History of Europe. Volume 1: 1700–1870*, ed. Stephen Broadberry and Kenneth H. O'Rourke (Cambridge etc.: Cambridge University Press, 2010).

independent towns, has long been a feature of North-western Europe. The resulting competition may have promoted innovation and the development of economic and cultural liberalism. The adoption of 'constraints on the executive', i.e., curtailing the power of monarchs and others who could seize property and thereby discourage private enterprise, probably also played a role. For example, after the Glorious Revolution (1688), which increased the powers of parliament and the common law-courts, English kings could no longer expropriate the gains of private initiative. This was in contrast to the more powerful kings and princes on the continent, and may partly explain the early take-off of the Industrial Revolution in Britain.

After 1700 there was a strong increase in the involvement of European governments in the economy, with tax reforms, legislative changes and investments in infrastructure promoting economic growth. This again happened earlier and more forcefully in North-western Europe, where 'mercantilism' was popular, than in Southern, South-eastern and Eastern Europe. The question then remains, of course, why these institutional changes happened earlier in North-western Europe than elsewhere – a question that physical geography cannot completely answer.[9]

Another stream of analysis has emphasized technological change as an important determinant of the transition to modern economic growth. A revolution in agricultural methods, based on rational experimentation, preceded the Industrial Revolution in the 17th century in England (and in the Dutch Republic). The increase in agricultural productivity subsequently freed labour for industrial production, and led to financial profits which allowed investments in industry. Also, some of the early breakthroughs in manufacturing, such as the invention and further development of the steam engine in the 18th century, and many of the later advances in industrial production methods had never been possible without the scientific advances of the 17th and 18th centuries.

However, although technological changes were necessary to realise growth in economic productivity, many of the breakthroughs in manufacturing in the 18th and 19th centuries were not based on scientific breakthroughs, but on advances in the application of lower-grade knowledge, e.g., by better communication and collaboration. Changes in the organisation of knowledge gathering and diffusion, by creating learned societies and re-organizing universities, also played a role. All these advances in science and technology and their

9 One of the main proponents of the institutional determinants of economic development is American economist Daron Acemoğlu, who has argued that variation in economic performance among Atlantic trading nations is explained by the fact that countries with non-absolutist institutions, such as England, experienced faster growth; see Daron Acemoğlu, Simon Johnson, and James Robinson, "The Rise of Europe: Atlantic Trade, Institutional Change, and Economic Growth," *American Economic Review* 95, no. 3 (2005): 546–79.

diffusion are certainly proximal causes of economic growth, but this again raises the question why these early advances occurred in North-western Europe and not elsewhere.[10]

A third stream of analysis has focused on 'human capital', in the form of literacy, numeracy, and other economically useful human abilities. There is evidence that relatively high levels of literacy preceded the transition to modern economic growth in North-western Europe (cf. Figure 8). This suggests that this factor facilitated several of the other changes mentioned above, including institutional change (because educated people are more likely to strive for democracy) and technological change (because educated people are better in inventing and applying new modes of agricultural and industrial production). The gradual rise of levels of education may also have stimulated the acquisition of more general skills, such as discipline, punctuality, respect and 'industriousness'. But why was North-western Europe more literate to start with?[11]

Economic historians have not agreed on one general explanation for the start of modern economic growth and its spread across Europe. Most of them seem to agree that the explanation lies in the beneficial interaction ('co-evolution') of many different factors, between which important feedback loops have operated. For example, growth-promoting institutions are more likely in a literate society, but economic growth will also allow investments in education which further promote literacy. The explanation also appears to be context-dependent, with different countries following different paths to a similar end result. Such variation in explanatory pathways is to be expected when the ultimate outcome, prosperity, is partly determined by goal-oriented human agency: when one pathway to growth was impossible or did not work, European countries tried another one.[12]

---

10 On the role of technological change, see Joel Mokyr, *The Gifts of Athena* (Princeton: Princeton University Press, 2002).

11 Numeracy, i.e., the ability to count, may also have been important, and levels of numeracy were already higher too in North-western Europe before economic take-off. An important proponent of the idea that literacy and numeracy have played a decisive role in economic take-off is German economic historian Joerg Baten (see, e.g., Joerg Baten, ed., *A History of the Global Economy* (Cambridge etc.: Cambridge University Press, 2016)).

12 This idea of 'co-evolution' has been embraced by many historians, not only to explain economic growth but historical developments more generally. For example, Bayly writes that "historical development [in the period 1780–1914] seems to have been determined by a complex parallelogram of forces constituted by economic changes, ideological constructions, and mechanisms of the state" (see Christopher A. Bayly, "The Birth of the Modern World, 1780–1914," (Oxford: Blackwell, 2004)., p. 7). Variation in pathways to economic growth between European countries has been documented in Broadberry and O'Rourke,

As I am not an economic historian, I am reluctant to propose a 'prime mover' of economic growth. Nevertheless, reading this literature it is almost inevitable to point to developments in the realm of 'thinking' as the '*nec plus ultra*' of explaining the start of modern economic growth, or – to return to the main topic of this section – improvements in population health. It seems to me that an increase in rational thinking is a common factor that underlies the institutional changes, the technological changes and the changes in literacy and levels of education.

In a long process that accelerated in the pre-modern period, during the Renaissance and Reformation, the people of North-western Europe developed a more rational outlook to life, which was less clouded by tradition and superstition. This led to the 'Age of Reason' in the 17th century and the 'Age of Enlightenment' in the 18th century, and along the way these changes in 'thinking' resulted in the changes mentioned above that promoted economic growth as well as improvements in population health.

That this happened in North-western Europe may have been conditioned by geographical and long-standing cultural factors, but what changed was the way of thinking, and this occurred in an autonomous process in which one step logically followed another. If it can be shown that the sun does not circle around the earth, as previously assumed, but that the earth revolves around the sun, many other received wisdoms may be false as well. If it can be shown that the reasoning on which the absolute power of monarchs rests is false, we can also start to think that all men are equal. If it can be shown that some city districts have much higher mortality rates than others, we may begin to believe that some deaths can be prevented.[13]

Why Did Some Countries Rush Ahead or Lag Behind?

As has been abundantly illustrated throughout this book, there have been large variations between European countries in the 'rise-and-fall' of diseases, but it is difficult to get a clear picture of these differences in chapters organized on a disease-by-disease basis. We will therefore now reassemble some of the information on a country-by-country basis, to discover why some countries were

---

Cambridge Economic History of Modern Europe. Volume 1; Broadberry and O'Rourke, *Cambridge Economic History of Modern Europe: Volume 2*.

13 I borrowed the idea that developments in 'rational thinking' can be seen as an independent determinant of human development from Pinker, *The Better Angels of Our Nature*, Chapter 4.

consistently ahead of others, or consistently stayed behind, or changed their relative positions over time. Since space does not permit us to do this exhaustively, we will sample a few remarkable countries that allow us to highlight the most interesting, or most puzzling, findings.

These countries were identified by inspecting – again – some Preston-curves. As will be remembered from Chapter 3, it was not until the first decades of the 20th century that a positive relationship between national income and life expectancy emerged. However, Sweden, Norway and Denmark already had higher-than-average life expectancy in the last decades of the 19th century, and Sweden persisted in having a high life expectancy throughout the 20th century, also relative to its rapidly rising national income. Norway and particularly Denmark performed less well, and we will therefore focus on the 'Swedish advantage'.

Another country that did remarkably well, but over a much shorter period, is the Netherlands. It had below average life expectancy in the 1870s (among the few European countries that already collected mortality data), but rapidly moved ahead of most other countries to achieve a much higher life expectancy than predicted by its national income from the 1920s to the 1960s. Thereafter, the Netherlands lost its championship. Why did the Dutch not manage to keep up with the Swedes?

The Mediterranean countries also followed remarkable trajectories. Over the course of the 20th century, Spain, Portugal, Italy and Greece switched from being in the rear-guard to being front-runners in life expectancy. For example, Spain had lower life expectancy than predicted by its national income in the first half of the 20th century, but this changed into higher-than-predicted from the 1960s onwards. Life expectancy among Spanish women recently even surpassed that among Swedish women. Can these trends, and those for other Mediterranean countries, be understood from their economic, political and sociocultural history?

South-eastern Europe also contains a few big surprises. Many countries in this part of the subcontinent have struggled to keep up with other European countries, both economically and health-wise. However, Albania, despite a history of underdevelopment under Turkish rule, and despite severe repression under communist rule, managed to have higher life expectancy than countries with a similar national income since the 1980s. The Albanian experience will therefore be highlighted in a separate section, together with (former) Yugoslavia.

Finally, during the second half of the 20th century (data for the first half are often lacking) countries of the former Soviet Union have performed much worse than accounted for by their lower-than-average national incomes. This applies to Russia, which we will discuss in detail, but also to Belarus and Ukraine, and to the Baltic states, although the latter are on a trajectory of rapid health improvements, particularly in the case of Estonia. The consistently bad performance of Russia suggests the existence of long-standing factors in Russian society that hinder the catch-up movement made by many other European countries – do Russians not value life to the extent that other Europeans do?

Northern Lights: the Swedish Advantage

In this book, Sweden has often been used as a bench-mark for other countries. This was partly because of the convenience of having a country with data on population health going back to the 18th century, but mostly because of Sweden's consistently better performance in population health than almost all other European countries.

Many examples of this extraordinary performance have been shown in previous chapters. In the early 19th century, Sweden was an early adopter of large-scale and compulsory smallpox vaccination. In the latter part of the 19th and first half of the 20th century, it was early and exceptionally successful in reducing infant and maternal mortality. Throughout the 20th century, Sweden's recruits grew in height in advance of those of many other countries. And in the second half of the 20th century, Sweden was early and successful in bringing down ischaemic heart disease and motor vehicle injury mortality. This has not gone unnoticed, and there is a relatively large English-language literature on the history of population health in Sweden, with Swedish experts trying to explain to the outside world how this has been possible.[14]

Sweden started to have ambitions for the health of its population in the 18th century, under the influence of the Enlightenment and mercantilism. In Sweden these ambitions may have arisen more acutely than in other countries, because it had lost its large empire in the Great Northern War, and had become aware that its small population size was a liability. Population registers were established in the 1720s, and parish priests were ordered to regularly report the number of births and deaths, as well as the size and composition of the population they served (Plate 17). In order to compile and analyse these data, *Tabellverket*, the predecessor of Statistics Sweden, was created in 1749.[15]

14 My summary is largely based on overviews by Sundin and Willner, *Social Change* and Karin Johannisson, "The People's Health: Public Health Policies in Sweden," in *The History of Public Health and the Modern State*, ed. D. Porter (Amsterdam & Atlanta: Editions Rodopi, 1994).

15 Identical developments occurred in Finland, which was still part of Sweden in the 18th century, and similar developments occurred in Denmark, Norway and Iceland; see Halvor

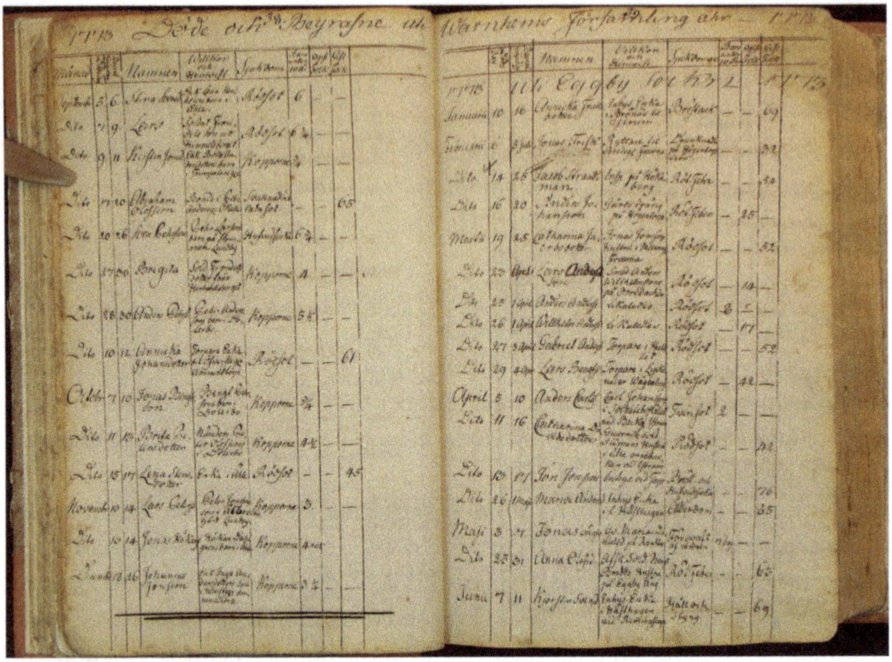

PLATE 17 *Sjukdomarna* [Diseases] registered by a parish priest in Varnhem, Sweden, 1773
Starting in the mid-18th century, Swedish parish priests had to register the causes of death of their deceased parishioners, and to report these regularly to "Tabellverket." For classification they could use a pre-printed list of diseases. This plate reproduces two pages from the "kirkebok" [church book] of Varnhem, a small municipality in the South of Sweden. "Rödsot" [dysentery] was the most frequent cause of death in the months covered by these pages.

The data were carefully studied by statisticians and medical scientists, and results were discussed in Swedish parliament where they gave rise to enlightened health policies, such as the creation of a system of provincial doctors who not only served the poor but also acted as officers of health. The scope of

Gille, "The Demographic History of the Northern European Countries in the Eighteenth Century," *Population Studies* 3, no. 1 (1949): 3–65. That the 18th century was a flowering period in Swedish science, is also clear from the European renown of Carl von Linné (1707–1778), who is famous as a founder of biological nomenclature, and also developed one of the earliest systematic disease classifications; see Johan P. Mackenbach, "Carl Von Linné, Thomas Mckeown, and the Inadequacy of Disease Classifications," *European Journal of Public Health* 14, no. 3 (2004): 225.

Sweden's public health policies was gradually expanded over time, to include measures like a national program for smallpox vaccination and provisions for the training of midwives in the 19th century, and early introduction of social security benefits, occupational health protection, and controls on the sales and consumption of alcohol in the first half of the 20th century.

All these measures contributed to early and strong improvements in population health, but so they did elsewhere in Europe. One additional reason why Sweden gained an advantage on other countries during the 19th century is that Sweden had a somewhat deviant pattern of industrialization. Unlike Great Britain and other industrializing countries in Western Europe, Sweden remained rural during most of the 19th century, even during the first phases of its industrialization, and this protected it from some of the high urban mortality of the early industrializers.[16]

Sweden subsequently managed to keep its population health advantage when, during the 20th century, infectious diseases and infant mortality were replaced by 'diseases of affluence' and middle- and old-age mortality. It was far from obvious that this would happen: several other countries, such as the Netherlands and Denmark, lost their pre-war advantage in the 1960s and 1970s because they were less successful in coping with the smoking epidemic than they had been in coping with puerperal fever and other pre-war health problems.[17]

Sweden's continued advantage cannot be simply due to an effective public health infrastructure that was already in place. In the second half of the 20th century, all countries including Sweden had to innovate their public health infrastructure to cope with cardiovascular disease, motor vehicle injuries and other 'diseases of affluence'. They had to develop new forms of expertise, new forms of organization, and new rationales for government intervention. It also was not simply a matter of prosperity: although Sweden is among the richest European countries, it has throughout the 20th century performed better than predicted by its national income.[18]

16 This has been analysed in Sandberg and Steckel, "Was Industrialization Hazardous."

17 On the Netherlands, see section below. On Denmark, see Knud Juel, Peter Bjerregaard, and Mette Madsen, "Mortality and Life Expectancy in Denmark and in Other European Countries," *European Journal of Public Health* 10, no. 2 (2000): 93–100. There were other European countries in which a strong state apparatus developed relatively early, such as England and France, but in which population health trends were not as favourable as Sweden's, so this cannot be the only explanation.

18 The difference between Sweden's observed life expectancy and its expected life expectancy, estimated from the association between GDP and life expectancy across all European countries, was in the order of 5 years in the first half of the 20th century. It continued

To understand Sweden's consistent advantage we therefore need to identify the conditions which helped Swedish society to cope effectively with a range of different health problems over more than two centuries. At first sight, political factors seem to be a good candidate. In the 16th and 17th centuries, Sweden had a large empire in Central-eastern and Eastern Europe, based on military might, and this left a relatively strong state apparatus with a competent bureaucracy. Somehow, in contrast to the Danes and the Dutch, the Swedes also accepted the state to be present in their lives, which must be based on the experience of a consistently benign state that can be expected to act for the benefit of all.[19]

During the 20th century, the remarkable success of Sweden's Social-Democratic Party, which has governed for decades in a row, may also have played a role. Many of Sweden's successes in the fight against (diseases of) poverty as well as 'diseases of affluence' have been enacted by Social-Democratic governments. Comparative analyses show that across Europe there is a positive association between left-wing government and indicators of population health, as well as with health policies in the areas of tobacco and alcohol control. But if left-wing politics would be the explanation of the Swedish success, the next question should be: why do the Swedes vote for left-wing parties?[20]

At second sight, therefore, it seems likely that cultural factors also play an important role in Sweden's remarkable health achievements. One aspect to this may be Lutheranism: historically, almost all Swedes were Lutherans, and although Sweden now is one of the most secularized countries in Europe, the Lutheran church is still very present. As explained in Chapter 3, over the last centuries Protestantism in Europe has been associated with several factors

---

to be positive, but smaller, after World War II, gradually diminishing to become less than 1 year in the early 2010s.

19 Despite their proximity, there are important differences between Sweden and Denmark in health policy. Whereas Danish health policies focus on behaviours and individual choice, and are averse to paternalism, Swedish health policies emphasize social determinants and collective responsibility; see Signild Vallgårda, "Addressing Individual Behaviours and Living Conditions: Four Nordic Public Health Policies," *Scandinavian Journal of Public Health* 39, no. 6 (Suppl) (2011): 6–10.

20 The association between left-party government and population health is actually not very strong. A negative correlation between social-democratic government and infant mortality was found in Vicente Navarro et al., "Politics and Health Outcomes," *Lancet* 368, no. 9540 (2006): 1033–037, but it is unclear whether this is a causal effect; see Enrique Regidor et al., "The Role of Political and Welfare State Characteristics in Infant Mortality," *International Journal of Epidemiology* 40, no. 5 (2011): 1187–195. For a more elaborate analysis, see Johan P. Mackenbach and Martin McKee, "Social-Democratic Government and Health Policy in Europe," *International Journal of Health Services* 43, no. 3 (2013): 389–413.

conducive to health: higher levels of literacy, early take-off of modern economic growth, early fertility decline, lower levels of cardiovascular risk factors ...[21]

This is an explanation shared by many observers of the Swedish health advantage, but Sweden has been more successful than other Protestant or Lutheran countries, so this can – again – not be the entire explanation. And why have the Swedes become Lutherans in the first place? At a certain point in history, i.e., the foundation of the Swedish (Lutheran) Church in the last decades of the 16th century, this was a choice that could have been made differently.[22]

Present-day studies of cultural values, such as Inglehart's two-value system of 'secular-rationalism' and 'self-expression', show Sweden to occupy an extremely advanced pole of the European cultural spectrum. This suggests that deeper cultural differences than those captured by religious affiliation are involved as well. My best guess is that the secret of Sweden's health advantage lies in the combination of a specific political legacy with a very 'enlightened' culture.[23]

On a final and more pragmatic note, it is important to acknowledge that more shallow explanations also go some way in explaining Sweden's success. On at least two occasions, Sweden has been simply lucky. The first was when Sweden could remain neutral in two World Wars, partly because of its geographical position aside from the main European conflict zones between the great continental powers. This saved it from destruction and was even highly profitable, because Sweden could export massive amounts of iron ore for use in the German weapons industry. Tactful foreign policy also played a role in

21 The health advantage of Estonians as compared to Latvians and Lithuanians is sometimes attributed to the fact that Estonians have become Lutherans under Swedish occupation. The Swedes also instituted a school system in Estonia, which has endowed it with higher levels of literacy than its neighbours; see Mackenbach, "Cultural Values"; Andres Kasekamp, *A History of the Baltic States* (London: Palgrave Macmillan 2017).

22 That the likelihood of choosing for Protestantism was greater in Northern than in Southern Europe has been attributed to a combination of greater distance from Rome and a Germanic cultural heritage (which was averse to hierarchy, perhaps because agriculture in the North did not permit the build-up of large surpluses and the creation of a hierarchical society); see Geert Hofstede, *Culture's Consequences* (Thousand Oaks etc.: Sage, 2001); Michael Minkov, *Cultural Differences in a Globalizing World* (Bingley: Emerald Group Publishing, 2011).

23 For the role of cultural values in explaining between-country differences in population health, health-related behaviour, and health policies, see Mackenbach and McKee, *Successes*; Mackenbach, "Cultural Values." See also Chapter 3.

maintaining its neutrality, but Sweden's geographical position was of course simply a matter of good luck.[24]

The second piece of good luck is that Sweden has 'snus', a form of smokeless snuff tobacco that, when inserted under the upper lip, releases nicotine but carries far fewer health risks than smoking cigarettes or using other forms of smoked tobacco. Snus was invented in the early 1800s and became very popular in Sweden, probably because it could easily be used during manual labour. It was the most popular form of tobacco use until the 1940s when it was overtaken by the cigarette, but when the harmful effects of smoking became known in the 1960s, use of snus rose again, partly as an aid to quit smoking.

As a result, lung cancer mortality in Sweden has peaked at a considerably lower level than in many other European countries, which has contributed importantly to Sweden's continued health advantage in the latter parts of the 20th century. Although the state has not been entirely absent in this story, and has regulated the contents of snus thereby ensuring its harmlessness, this is again difficult to explain otherwise than as a piece of good luck.[25]

Dutch Comfort: We Were the Champions

Most Continental-European countries did less well than the Nordic countries during most of the 19th and 20th centuries, with two exceptions: the Netherlands and Switzerland. In terms of life expectancy, the Netherlands did extremely well during the first half of the 20th century, and actually was the record holding country in some single calendar-years up to the early 1960s. However, it later fell back to second rank, due to stronger stagnation of life expectancy than that observed in other European countries. (The other exception, Switzerland, also came from second rank in the 19th century, but its life expectancy rose almost uninterruptedly during the 20th century, and ultimately surpassed that of Sweden at the end of the century.) What explains the remarkable performance of the Netherlands in the first half of the 20th century, and its falling behind in the second half?[26]

---

24 On Sweden's role in World War II, see Christian Leitz, *Nazi Germany and Neutral Europe During the Second World War* (Manchester: Manchester University Press, 2000), Chapter 3.

25 For the history of snus, see Lars E. Rutqvist et al., "Swedish Snus and the Gothiatek® Standard," *Harm Reduction Journal* 8, no. 1 (2011): 11. For the effect of snus on smoking in Sweden, see Jonathan Foulds et al., "Effect of Smokeless Tobacco (Snus) on Smoking and Public Health in Sweden," *Tobacco Control* 12, no. 4 (2003): 349–59. For a different view, see Maria R. Galanti et al., "Use of Snus and Lung Cancer Mortality: Unwarranted Claim of Causal Association," *Scandinavian Journal of Public Health* 38 (2010): 332–33.

26 Oeppen and Vaupel, "Broken Limits" analysed the evolution of world record life expectancy.

In the 19th century, the Netherlands had unfavourable indicators of population health. The West of the Netherlands had very high mortality, which was already well-known in the 18th century. According to British demographer Thomas Malthus (1766–1834), Holland was "Germany's grave" because so many German immigrants found their untimely death in this country. This dismal situation contrasted sharply with the country's glorious past: in the 17th century, the Dutch Republic had been the most prosperous, enlightened and powerful country in North-western Europe. Religiously inspired schooling campaigns during and after the Dutch Revolt (1568–1648) had also raised literacy levels to record heights (Figure 8). However, in the early 18th century the Dutch Republic lost its dominant position in world trade to Britain, and the resulting decline of its economy was further aggravated by the damage done by the Napoleonic Wars in the early 19th century.[27]

In more specific terms, the high level of mortality in the Netherlands during the 19th century was probably due to a combination of high population density and lack of good drinking water, which both increased the risk of infection. Public health measures were also slow to develop in the Netherlands. This situation changed around 1870, when infant mortality started to decline, probably more as a result of cultural change (e.g., the spread of modern concepts of hygiene and infant care) than as a result of economic growth. High levels of literacy – a remnant of the country's glorious past – may have facilitated these rapid improvements.[28]

In the first half of the 20th century, trends in life expectancy were still strongly determined by trends in infant mortality. Due to a remarkable decline of infant mortality to record-low levels in the 1930s, Dutch life expectancy jumped up. This favourable situation continued until the early 1960s, and as this did not go unnoticed in the rest of the world, public health experts from the Netherlands were asked by the US government to explain this remarkable success. They concluded that

---

27 The history of the rise, greatness and fall of the Dutch Republic has been analysed in Jonathan I. Israel, *The Dutch Republic: Its Rise, Greatness, and Fall, 1477–1806* (Oxford etc.: Clarendon Press Oxford, 1995). 'Dutch Republic' is the name usually given to what was officially named 'United Provinces of the Netherlands' (1581–1795). After the Napoleonic Wars, the Kingdom of the Netherlands was formed. This originally included Belgium, but the latter separated itself in 1830.

28 The demographic history of the Netherlands has been analysed in Hofstee, *Demografische Ontwikkeling*; Evert W. Hofstee, *Korte Demografische Geschiedenis van Nederland van 1800 tot Heden* (Haarlem: Fibula-Van Dishoeck, 1981). For the 19th century history of public health in the Netherlands, see Houwaart, *Hygiënisten*.

> the favourable situation in the Netherlands reflects a long tradition of basic infant care in the family, aided by district nurses and welfare centres and supported by social security measures and a rising standard of living.

Although not explicitly mentioned in this report, we have seen in Chapter 5 that the Netherlands also was an early adopter of a national system of well-trained midwives.[29]

Accepting these factors as at least a partial explanation, we may then want to ask how the Netherlands – still behind the more advanced European countries in the third quarter of the 19th century – managed to join the Scandinavian countries at the top of the European rank-list. Part of the explanation is that, as suggested in the quotation given above, the Dutch economy indeed grew very rapidly, both before, during and immediately after World War I. This was due to a combination of factors, including the fact that it benefited from rapid economic growth in its immediate hinterland and main trading partner, Germany.[30]

However, rapid economic development is certainly not the only explanation, because levels of infant mortality and life expectancy in the Netherlands during the 1920s were far more favourable than can be accounted for by its level of prosperity. Like in Sweden, cultural factors played a role as well, but the state was less central to population health improvements in the Netherlands in the first half of the 20th century. Since the 1880s, the 'pillarization' (*verzuiling*) of Dutch society, i.e., the organization of social life in separate Protestant, Roman-Catholic, Socialist and Liberal 'pillars', stimulated a successful 'civilization offensive' within each 'pillar', covering all aspects of life including infant care. 'Private initiative' also created separate public health and health care organizations within each 'pillar'. At the same time, consensus seeking between

29 Quoted from Haas-Posthuma and Haas, *Infant Loss*, p. 27. This report identified as main contributors to the Dutch success the quality of midwifery, the high proportion of pregnant women receiving antenatal care, the availability of maternity home help, and the performance of infant welfare centres. On the role of well-trained midwives in achieving low levels of maternal mortality in the Netherlands, see Loudon, *Death in Childbirth*, Chapter 24–26.

30 The Netherlands also remained neutral in World War I, so that it not only escaped the war's damages, but actually benefitted through increased exports of agricultural and industrial products; see Jan Luiten van Zanden, *The Economic History of the Netherlands 1914–1995* (London and New York: Routledge, 1998). There is a parallel with the remarkable performance of Sweden and Switzerland which remained neutral not only in World War I, but also in World War II.

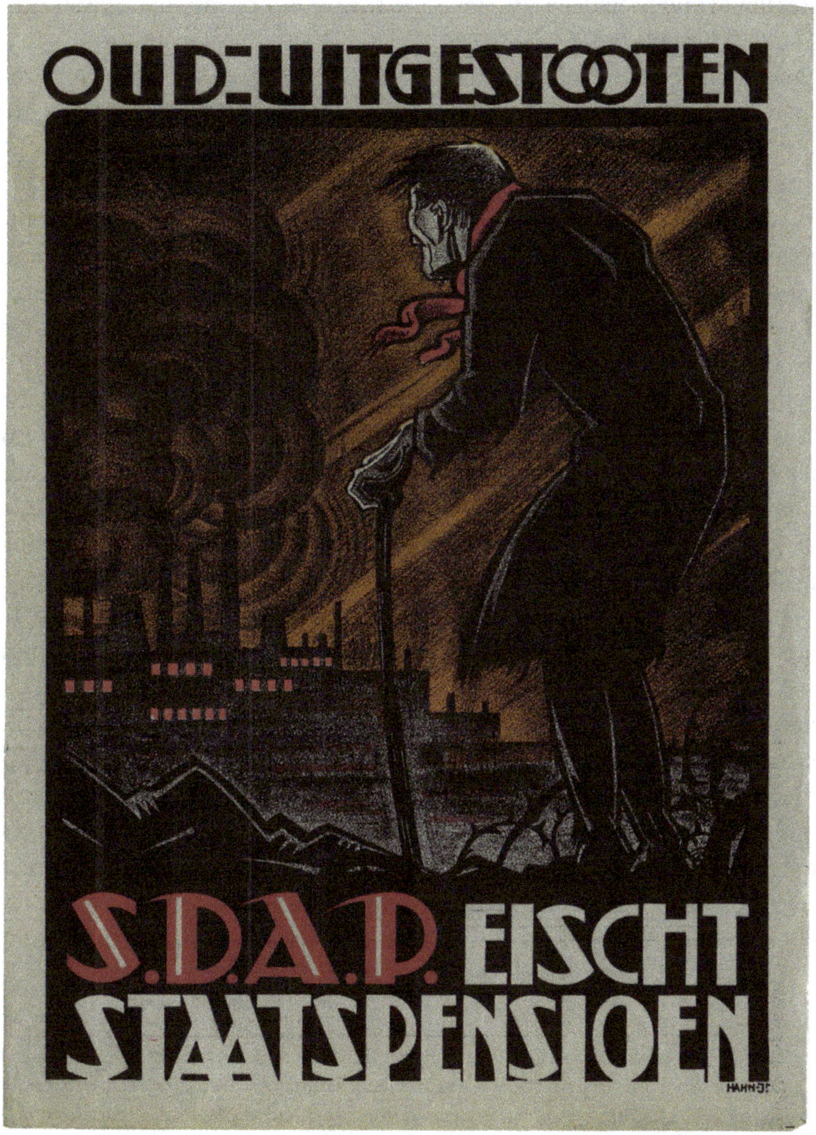

PLATE 18 "Social-democratic party demands state pension." Dutch election poster, 1929
*Like social-democratic parties in other European countries, the Dutch Labour party advocated state intervention to create a system of social security for workers, including a system of state-funded old-age pensions. A state pension was finally introduced in 1947 by Willem Drees (1886–1988), the first Labour prime minister in the Netherlands. The translation of the Dutch text at the top is: "Old. Expelled," and that at the bottom: "*SDAP *[Social-Democratic Labour Party] demands state pension."*

POSTER CREATED BY ALBERT HAHN JR. COLLECTION INTERNATIONAL INSTITUTE OF SOCIAL HISTORY (AMSTERDAM). REPRODUCED WITH PERMISSION

confessional and socialist politicians laid the basis for a rapidly expanding welfare state (Plate 18).[31]

Unfortunately, the Netherlands lost its advantage in the 1980s and 1990s, when a complete stagnation of mortality decline occurred in some age-groups in the Netherlands, while other high-income countries continued their rapid mortality declines. This happened both among the very young (perinatal mortality) and among the very old (80+). Although the over-all performance of the Netherlands remained well above the European average, this was cool comfort to those who believed the Netherlands to be capable of something better.

The obstetric professions at first attributed the high levels of perinatal mortality to more complete registration in the Netherlands than elsewhere, but this position became untenable with the publication of carefully harmonized figures which confirmed that the Netherlands compared unfavourably with other European countries. More detailed studies then found that stagnation of perinatal mortality decline resulted from lack of progress in perinatal care. This was due to the fact that a system that relied on midwives was less capable of absorbing new high-tech diagnostics and interventions. This suggests that the competitive advantage that the Netherlands had enjoyed in an earlier phase of mortality decline, had turned into a disadvantage in a later phase. When the government was finally convinced that something needed to be done, a government commission was installed that recommended better integration of extramural and intramural obstetric care.[32]

Stagnation of mortality decline among the elderly resulted partly from lack of progress in reducing smoking, which had reached extremely high levels among the cohorts dying in the 1980s and 1990s, partly from budgetary restrictions in the health care system. Interestingly, a similar stagnation of mortality decline among the elderly occurred around the same time in a small number

---

31 The affinity between the Netherlands and Scandinavia in social policy is illustrated by the fact that Danish sociologist Gøsta Esping-Andersen classified the Netherlands with the Scandinavian countries in a group of 'social-democratic' welfare systems. In reality, the Netherlands has always mixed a 'social-democratic' and a 'Christian-democratic' welfare system, but achieved a degree of poverty reduction similar to that in the Nordic countries; see Gøsta Esping-Andersen, *The Three Worlds of Welfare Capitalism* (Cambridge: Polity Press, 1990).

32 Mika Gissler et al., "Perinatal Health Monitoring in Europe: Results from the Euro-Peristat Project," *Informatics for Health and Social Care* 35, no. 2 (2010): 64–79; Judith H. Wolleswinkel-van Den Bosch et al., "Substandard Factors in Perinatal Care in the Netherlands," *Acta Obstetricia et Gynecologica Scandinavica* 81, no. 1 (2002): 17–24. Recent comparative studies suggest that perinatal mortality has declined somewhat more in the Netherlands than in other countries, but levels are still higher than in the Nordic countries; see EURO-Peristat Project, *European Perinatal Health Report.*

of other countries, particularly the US and Denmark. However, progress resumed in Denmark around 1995, after a government committee recommended improvements in cardiovascular disease prevention and treatment, and in the Netherlands around 2002, after the government decided to lift the budgetary restraints, and health care utilization (and health care costs) started to rise rapidly again.[33]

One common factor between the Netherlands and Denmark is the high prevalence of smoking. The Netherlands and Denmark share a history of small trading nations in which a tradition of libertarianism developed in conjunction with the requirements of free trade. In the Netherlands, the idea that everyone should be free to smoke was also strongly stimulated by the national tobacco industry, which used to be one of the largest in Europe. This libertarian trait has helped the Netherlands to develop rational policies in controversial areas like heroin treatment, AIDS prevention and euthanasia, but clearly also has its disadvantages.[34]

Southern Miracles: from Rear-guard to Forefront

One of the most remarkable features of the history of population health in Europe is that Southern European countries have moved from the rear-guard, having very low life expectancies in the late 19th and early 20th centuries, to the forefront, having very high life expectancies in the last decades of the 20th century. With a life expectancy at birth of around 40 years at the beginning of the 20th century, Spain, Portugal, Italy and Greece lagged far behind countries in Northern and Western Europe, but in a spectacular catch-up movement reached similar life expectancy levels as North-western European countries in the 1960s, and then surpassed many of them in the 1980s.

A somewhat similar trend can be seen for national income and other indicators of socioeconomic development. Southern European countries were late industrializers, and had a relatively low national income at the beginning of

33 For a comparative analysis, see Meslé and Vallin, "Diverging Trends." For a more in-depth analysis of the Netherlands, see Johan P. Mackenbach et al., "Sharp Upturn of Life Expectancy in the Netherlands," *European Journal of Epidemiology* 26, no. 12 (2011): 903–14; Fanny Janssen, Johan P. Mackenbach, and Anton E. Kunst, "Trends in Old-Age Mortality in Seven European Countries, 1950–1999," *Journal of Clinical Epidemiology* 57, no. 2 (2004): 203–16. For an analysis of Denmark, see Juel et al., "Mortality."

34 Should this be regarded as a form of 'antagonistic pleiotropy' which, like certain genetic traits, reduces some health risks at the expense of increasing others (see Chapter 3, note 19)? On Dutch tobacco control policies, and the cultural, political and commercial background to the reluctance of the Dutch government to implement stricter tobacco control measures, see Marc C. Willemsen, *Tobacco Control Policy in the Netherlands*, Palgrave Studies in Public Health Policy Research, (n.p.: Palgrave Macmillan, 2018).

the 20th century. Although they never caught up entirely with Northern and Western Europe, their national incomes grew impressively, particularly after World War II (see Suppl. Figure 6). While this indicates that Southern European countries' economic development may partly explain their life expectancy trajectories during the 20th century, life expectancy catch-up actually preceded economic catch-up.[35]

That rising living standards were not the only factor in the rapid rise in life expectancy in Southern Europe is also clear when we plot European countries' life expectancies against their national incomes in a series of successive Preston-curves. Southern European countries were 'under-performers', as compared to what could be expected on the basis of their level of economic development, in the beginning of the 20th century. However, they became 'over-performers', doing substantially better than expected, at the end of the century. What explains this puzzling phenomenon?

As we have seen in the disease-specific chapters above, in the first decades of the 20th century Southern European countries clearly lagged behind Northern and Western European countries in the decline of infectious diseases as well as in infant mortality. Mortality rates from smallpox, typhus, malaria, tuberculosis, syphilis, diphtheria, pneumonia – to name but a few – which had already declined in the North and West, were still high in Spain, Portugal, Italy and Greece. The decline of infant mortality also started later. This suggests that these countries were late in taking countermeasures against these health conditions.[36]

Unfortunately, a comparative history of public health covering all European regions has never been written. However, national histories of public health in, for example, Spain and Portugal show very clearly that large-scale measures to control the infectious diseases just mentioned only started after the turn of the century, i.e., with a considerable delay as compared to Northern and Western

35 This was shown in a recently published analysis of long-term trends in mortality in Spain; see Moreda et al., *Conquista*. In addition to pointing at the discrepancy in timing between the rise in national income and the rise in life expectancy, the authors also show that in the first half of the 20th century improvements in nutrition in Spain were quite modest, and left large sections of the Spanish population in a state of malnutrition (pp. 302–25).

36 National data-series for Southern European countries start in the last decades of the 19th century. However, regional data stretch back further in time. Infant and childhood mortality in Central-Spain can be followed since the late 18th century, suggesting that Spain's mortality rates were already comparatively high at this early point in time; see Diego Ramiro Fariñas and Alberto G. Sanz, "Childhood Mortality in Central Spain, 1790–1960," *Continuity and Change* 15, no. 2 (2000): 235–67.

Europe. There, important advances in vaccination, sanitation, malaria eradication etc. had already been made in the 19th century.

For example, a history of public health in Spain suggests that the birth of public health took place in the first two decades of the 20th century – indicating its late arrival. It is only in this period that the first large-scale sanitation measures were taken and that the first large campaigns against smallpox, tuberculosis and syphilis were held. In the 1930s and 1940s these campaigns were continued and broadened to include ancylostomiasis (hookworm disease) and malaria, with important assistance from the Rockefeller Foundation.[37]

In Portugal, public health similarly started in the first years of the 20th century, when after a small outbreak of bubonic plague in and around the harbour city of Oporto, the 'father of Portuguese public health', Ricardo Jorge (1858–1939), was appointed *Inspector-Geral de Saúde* in Lisbon. Acutely aware of the backwardness of his country in the fight against infectious diseases, he led campaigns against influenza, smallpox, typhus and diphtheria in the 1920s.[38]

The reasons for the delays in public health, as well as in economic development, of Southern Europe must be sought in previous centuries. Throughout the 19th century, and into the 20th century, these countries were low in human resources: levels of literacy were much lower than in Northern and Western Europe (Figure 8 and Plate 19). Even in 1975 20% of the Portuguese population

37 For histories of public health in Spain, see Esteban Rodríguez Ocaña and Ferran Martinez Navarro, *La Salud Pública en España. De la Edad Media al Siglo XX*, vol. 68 (Granada: Escuela Andaluza de Salud Publica, n.d.); Esteban Rodríguez Ocaña, *Salud Pública en España: Ciencia, Profesión y Política, Siglos XVIII–XX* (Granada: Unversidad de Granada, 2005). An envoy to Spain from the Rockefeller Foundation described the situation in the 1920s as "catastrophic"; see Esteban Rodriguez Ocaña, "El Informe sobre la Sanidad Española (1926) de Charles A. Bailey," *Cronos* 4, no. 1–2 (2001): 63–79. The role of the Rockefeller Foundation, and the sanitary policies of the Republican and Franco governments in the interbellum period are detailed in Josep Lluís Barona and Josep Bernabeu-Mestre, *La Salud y el Estado* (Valencia: Universitat de València, 2011), Chapter VI. For the Spanish anti-malaria campaign of the 1920s and 1930s, see Esteban Rodriguez Ocaña, "International Health Goals and Social Reform," in *Facing Illness in Troubled Times*, ed. Iris Borowy and Wolf Gruner (Frankfurt am Main: Peter Lang, 2005).

38 A history of public health in Portugal can be found in F.A. Gonçalves Ferreira, *História da Saúde e dos Serviços de Saúde em Portugal* (Lisbon: Edição da Fundação Calouste Gulbenkian, 1990). Specific periods or aspects are detailed in Jorge Fernandes Alves and Marinha Carneiro, "Saude Publica e Politica do «Codigo Sanitario» ao Regulamento Geral de 1901," *Cultura, Espaço & Memória* 5 (2018): 27–43; Rita Garnel, "Disease and Public Health (Portugal)," in *International Encyclopedia of the First World War*, ed. Ute Daniel et al. (Berlin: Freie Universitat Berlin, 2014). The life and works of Ricardo Jorge have been described in Jorge Fernandes Alves, "Ricardo Jorge e a Saúde Pública em Portugal," *Arquivos de Medicina* 22, no. 2–3 (2008): 85–90; Luis Graça, "História e Memória da Saúde Pública," *Revista Portuguesa de Saúde Pública* 33, no. 2 (2015): 125–27.

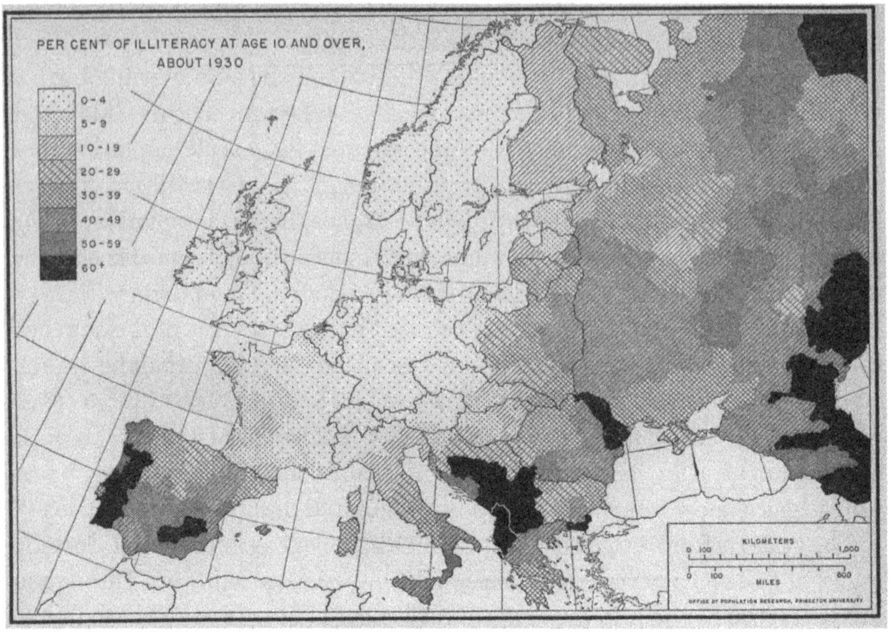

PLATE 19 Map of illiteracy levels in Europe, 1930

This map, from a book on Europe's population in the Interbellum produced for the League of Nations, shows the very high levels of illiteracy in Southern, South-eastern and Eastern Europe persisting into the early 1930s. For most European countries, the data on illiteracy, defined as the inability to both read and write, were taken from a population census

DUDLEY KIRK, "EUROPE'S POPULATION IN THE INTERWAR YEARS" (PRINCETON: OFFICE FOR POPULATION RESEARCH, 1946). REPRODUCED WITH PERMISSION

was illiterate. This reflected serious delays in the uptake of schooling, which had never been promoted as vigorously as in Protestant countries.[39]

Southern European countries were also held back in their development by long histories of autocratic government. These had installed extractive institutions that did little to promote economic growth, and were supported by a conservative Roman-catholic church which did little to promote social change. Nevertheless, around the turn of the 20th century Spain, Portugal and other

39 Houston, *Literacy*. See also Chapter 3.

Mediterranean countries started to modernize, probably as a result of the diffusion of ideas, knowledge and technology from North-western Europe.[40]

A recently published analysis of long-term trends in mortality in Spain concludes that the "conquest of health" in this country during the first half of the 20th century was due in large part to the modernization of public and private hygiene. This involved modernization of the sanitary infrastructure (but only in the cities – rural areas had to wait till the second half of the century), dedicated campaigns to get rid of epidemic diseases (e.g., obligatory smallpox vaccination, drainage of marshes, pasteurization of milk), and campaigns to improve infant care (e.g., education to promote breast-feeding, creation of a system of health visitors).[41]

One of the remarkable aspects of the 20th century history of population health in Southern Europe is, that some of the most dramatic improvements were achieved under autocratic or even fascist governments. For extended periods, autocratic governments replaced democratic governments in Spain, Portugal, Italy and Greece. In Spain, a bloody Civil War (1936–1939) replaced the Second Republic by an authoritarian nationalist government under General Francisco Franco, who stayed in power until 1975. The Civil War left deep traces in the health of the Spanish population, both in the form of hundreds of thousands of direct casualties, and of a resurgence of infectious diseases and nutrient deficiencies. Together, these caused a deep dent in Spain's rising life expectancy curve (Figure 1).[42]

Despite this catastrophe, however, population health improvement resumed in the 1940s, at an even more rapid speed than before the Civil War. As some observers have noted,

> undoubtedly, this is one of the most shocking and most 'remarkable' findings [of our analysis], because it relates above all to the mortality effects of the population policy of the Franco dictatorship.

Although this and other dictatorships in Southern Europe had a stifling effect on many other developments, they did often engage in large-scale health

40 For the role of extractive institutions, not only on the Iberian peninsula but also as exported to Latin America, see Daron Acemoğlu and James A. Robinson, *Why Nations Fail* (London: Profile Books, 2012). See also Chapter 3.

41 Moreda et al., *Conquista*, Chapter 4 and 7, presents a detailed cause-by-cause analysis of declines in infant, childhood, and adult mortality, relating the timing of decline to the introduction of various health-related policies in Spain.

42 For the effects of the Spanish Civil War on population health in Spain, see Barona and Bernabeu-Mestre, *Salud*, Chapter IX.

improvement campaigns, usually with pro-natalist or population-strengthening aims and with an authoritarian and socially-conservative character. Like Franco's government in Spain was effective in lowering infant mortality, Mussolini's government succeeded in mounting an effective anti-malaria campaign.[43]

Miraculously, after having finally pushed back mortality from infectious diseases, Southern European countries experienced much less of a rise in 'diseases of affluence', particularly ischaemic heart disease, than Northern and Western European countries. This is the immediate explanation for the puzzling fact that life expectancy in Southern Europe did not only catch up with, but even surpassed life expectancy in the North and West in the last third of the 20th century.[44]

As we have seen in Figure 22, mortality from ischaemic heart disease peaked early and at an extremely low level in Southern Europe. This is, however, likely due to a lucky coincidence, and not to superior health policies. Late economic and social 'modernization' of these countries also implied a delay of the 'modernization' of dietary and other consumption habits. One important factor is the Mediterranean diet. Mediterranean diets are rich in components which are cardioprotective: monounsaturated fats (in olive oil, nuts), omega-3 polyunsaturated fatty acids (in fat fish, vegetables, nuts, plant oils), and a variety of antioxidants (in fruits, vegetables, wine, olive oil), etc. This nutritional pattern could still commonly be found in Spain, the South of France, Italy, Dalmatia, and Greece in the 1950s and 1960s, but has more recently been eroded by the 'westernization' of life-styles which has accompanied economic progress and European integration.[45]

---

43 For the health policies of the Franco government, see Barona and Bernabeu-Mestre, *Salud*. The contribution of these policies to population health improvement have been analysed in Moreda et al., *Conquista*, from which the quote comes (p. 392). For infant mortality decline under European dictatorships, see Regidor et al., "Role of Political." For Mussolini's '*Bonifica*' program, a large-scale anti-malaria campaign carried out with the help of the Rockefeller Foundation, see Bruce-Chwatt and De Zulueta, *Malaria*; Darwin H. Stapleton, "Lessons of History?," *Public Health Reports* 119, no. 2 (2004): 206–15. For the remarkable performance of autocratically governed countries, see also Chapter 3.

44 This is not the only explanation: Spain (and other Southern European countries) also continued to have rapid declines in other causes of death, including causes amenable to medical intervention and liver cirrhosis, suggesting adoption of effective health policies in a range of areas. For the rapid introduction of HAART therapy in Spain, see Enrique Regidor et al., "Major Reduction in AIDS-Mortality Inequalities after HAART," *Social Science & Medicine* 68, no. 3 (2009): 419–26.

45 For the traditional Mediterranean diet and its cardioprotective effects, see Daan Kromhout, Alessandro Menotti, and Henry Blackburn, *Prevention of Coronary Heart Disease* (Dordrecht: Kluwer Academic Publishers, 2002); Ancel Keys, "Coronary Heart Disease in

The fact that these traditional diets could still be observed in the 1950s and 1960s can at least partly be explained from the economic 'backwardness' of these countries, as compared to most countries in Northern and Western Europe. The frugality of the Mediterranean diet probably was partly a necessity: bread, pasta and vegetables (instead of meat), fruits for dessert (instead of cakes and ice-creams), and green leaves picked in the wild were cheap solutions for the hardship that lasted into the 1950s and 1960's in many areas in the South of Europe.[46]

A second factor contributing to low ischaemic heart disease mortality in Southern Europe is a delay in the rise of smoking. As we have discussed above, the smoking epidemic started a few decades later in Southern Europe, mostly after World War II, instead of in the 1920s and 1930s as in Northern and Western Europe, with even further delays among women. This is not only reflected in a later peak in lung cancer mortality (among men – among women the rates are still rising), but also in a lower peak (Figure 27). This is probably because smoking prevalence has never had the chance to rise to the absurdly high levels in Western Europe, which were reached in a time when the health risks of smoking were still unknown to the public at large.

And while Southern European populations were still relatively protected against ischaemic heart disease by their Mediterranean diets and low smoking rates, medical interventions for the prevention and treatment of cardiovascular disease were developed in other parts of the world. These were available in Southern Europe to stop any rise caused by a change towards a 'Western' style diet, or by a rise in smoking.[47]

Seven Countries," *Circulation* 41, no. 1 (1970): 186–95; Kromhout et al., *Prevention of Coronary Heart Disease*. For a discussion of "why" a diet composed of products grown in the Mediterranean area is more cardioprotective than a diet composed from products grown in other parts of Europe, see Johan P. Mackenbach, "The Mediterranean Diet Story Illustrates That "Why" Questions Are as Important as "How" Questions," *Journal of Clinical Epidemiology* 60, no. 2 (2007): 105–09. For recent changes, see Walter C. Willett et al., "Mediterranean Diet Pyramid: A Cultural Model for Healthy Eating," *American Journal of Clinical Nutrition* 61, no. 6 (1995): 1402S-06S, Laurenzi Martino et al., "Is Italy Losing the 'Mediterranean Advantage'?," *Preventive Medicine* 18, no. 1 (1989): 35–44.

46 Fernand Braudel, *Les Structures du Quotidien: Le Possible et l'Impossible* (Paris: Armand Colin, 1979); Angus Maddison, *The World Economy* (Paris: Organization for Economic Cooperation and Development (OECD), 2001).

47 This argument has been further elaborated in Ivana Kulhanova et al., "Why Does Spain Have Smaller Inequalities in Mortality?," *European Journal of Public Health* 24, no. 3 (2014): 370–77, which also discusses another remarkable feature of population health in Southern Europe: socioeconomic inequalities in mortality are smaller than elsewhere in Europe.

As these favourable conditions developed in the 1970s and later, they were facilitated by the important political and economic changes happening in this period. Spain, Portugal and Greece shook off their autocratic governments in the 1970s. They then went through a period of rapid changes, both in their external relationships (an end to international isolation, membership of the European Union) and in their internal conditions (creation of a national health service and a more generous system of social security, institutional reforms).[48]

Balkan Troubles: the Weight of the Past

Most of South-eastern Europe has long been part of the Ottoman Empire, and these countries therefore have rather different economic, political and socio-cultural histories. The geographical position of the Balkans between the great European powers (Ottoman Empire, Habsburg Empire, expanding Russia) has also made it a contested area, frequently visited by war and ethnic conflict.[49]

In the early 19th century, the Ottoman Empire still nominally included current Bosnia, Serbia, North Macedonia, Montenegro, Albania, Romania, Bulgaria and Greece, as well as current Moldova and Southern Russia. Only Slovenia and Croatia belonged to the Habsburg Empire. However, during the 19th century growing feelings of nationalism led to uprisings and to forms of self-government or real independence for several of these countries: first Greece, then Serbia, then Romania, then Bulgaria. After World War I, both the Habsburg and Ottoman Empires collapsed which led to the independence of the 'Kingdom of Serbs, Croats and Slovenes' (later renamed Yugoslavia) and Albania.

The Ottoman Empire of the 18th and 19th centuries has often been characterized as 'backward', and for good reasons, if we take the industrializing countries of North-western Europe or the Habsburg Empire as our benchmark. The underdevelopment of the Ottoman Empire made itself felt in many areas of life, and some of the problems of South-eastern European countries can, long after independence, still be traced back to the economic, political and socio-cultural conditions prevailing under Ottoman occupation.

The Ottoman Empire kept itself shielded from Western influences. Although it repeatedly tried to reform itself (e.g., in the modernizing '*Tanzimat*' period of the mid-19th century), these reforms were imposed from above, and met with resistance from the Islamic clergy and the upper classes which benefited from

48 See Mackenbach et al., "Democratization" and Chapter 3.

49 See Misha Glenny, *The Balkans, 1804–1999* (New York etc.: Viking Penguin, 2000) for a comprehensive political history of the Balkans, and an analysis of how this history still shapes the present. A compact but insightful history is Mark Mazower, *The Balkans: From the End of Byzantium to the Present Day* (London: Weidenfeld & Nicolson, 2000).

the traditional organization of society. The Empire treated its subjects brutally, it made very little investments in education, and government was based on clientelism. This all contributed to economic stagnation while North-western and later Southern Europe were already booming.[50]

Slovenia and Croatia escaped these unfavourable conditions, partly because they belonged to the Habsburg Empire which followed a more 'enlightened' path in the 18th and 19th centuries, for example by promoting education. Both countries were also predominantly Roman-catholic which oriented them towards the West, whereas most of the other countries in South-eastern Europe were predominantly Eastern Orthodox, or Muslim as in the case of Albania. Slovenia and Croatia were even for some time occupied by Napoleon, and later by Italy, which had some extra modernizing influence.

Because of space we cannot review the population health history of the whole of South-eastern Europe, but must limit ourselves to the Western Balkans, i.e., former Yugoslavia plus Albania. Albania has for a few decades had a surprisingly good performance in life expectancy, and its neighbour Yugoslavia is interesting for comparison. Yugoslavia was also the arena for the last big war (so far) on the European subcontinent, after which the country split up and life expectancies between the former Yugoslav republics diverged.

Trends in life expectancy in Yugoslavia can be traced back to the early 1930s for the country as a whole, and to the 1950s for its constituent parts. Life expectancy in Yugoslavia was still very low in the 1930s – but comparable to that in Spain – and rose rapidly during the 1940s, 1950s and 1960s. Yet, in the 1980s life expectancy started to diverge within the country, and this divergence accelerated after the country split up, with relative stagnation in Serbia, a more favourable trend in Croatia, and rapid improvement in Slovenia (Figure 32).

As a result of this divergence, the differences are currently striking. In 2016, Slovenia had the highest life expectancy of the former Yugoslav republics, comparable to the best of North-western and Southern European countries: 78 years among men, 84 years among women. Serbia, Montenegro and North Macedonia had the lowest life expectancy: in the low 70s among men, and in the high 70s among women. Croatia was in-between, and semi-independent Kosovo had the lowest life expectancy of all: 69 years among men, and 74 years among women.

Trends in life expectancy in Albania can be traced back to 1950. At first, Albanian life expectancy was similar to, and rose in parallel with, that of

50 Şevket Pamuk, *Uneven Centuries: Economic Development of Turkey since 1820* (Princeton: Princeton University Press, 2018).

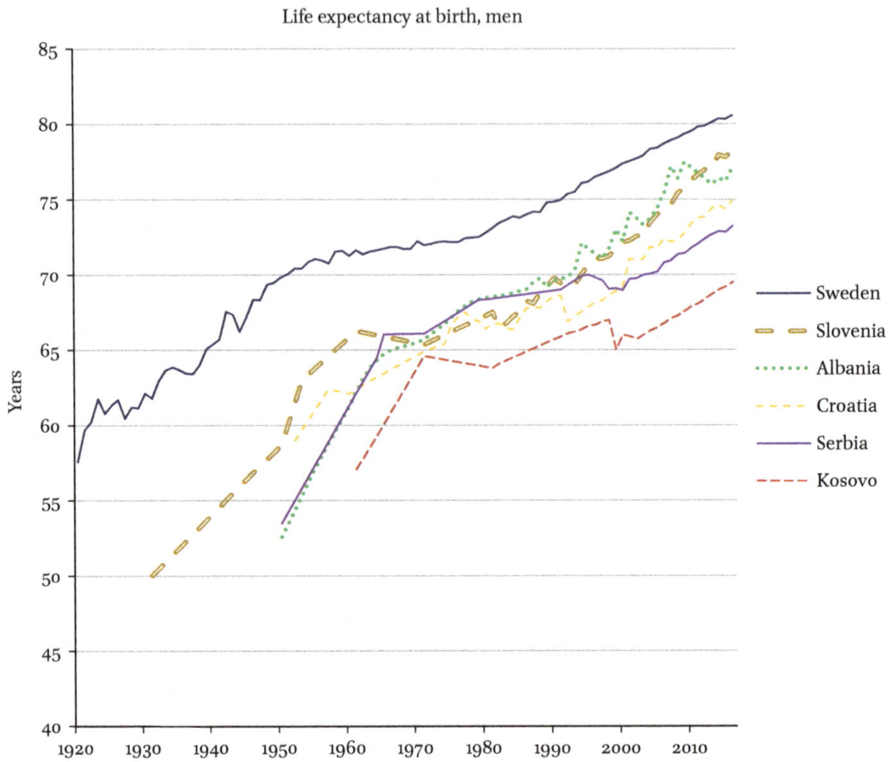

FIGURE 32 Trends in life expectancy in the Western Balkans, 1920–2015
SOURCE OF DATA: SEE SUPPL. TABLE 1

Yugoslavia. However, in the 1980s it moved away and started to follow a more favourable, but erratic, upward trajectory. This resulted in a remarkably high life expectancy in 2016: 76 years among men, and 80 years among women – much higher than expected on the basis of Albania's low national income.

Let's now try to understand these trends and variations. Taking it historically, so starting with the low levels of life expectancy in the 1930s which undoubtedly also applied to Albania, it is immediately clear that these mirrored the general underdevelopment of both countries. In North-western Europe, average national income in 1930 had already grown to around \$4300 per head per year, whereas in Yugoslavia it was still around \$1400 (much lower than in Spain!). In Albania national income was even lower, i.e., around \$900 per head per year. The differences in prevalence of illiteracy were even more striking: the percentage of people who could not read and write was between 0 and 5%

in almost all North-western European countries, whereas it was still around 45% in Yugoslavia and around 70% in Albania.[51]

We can also safely assume that the upward swing in life expectancy around World War II has a similar explanation as the catch-up movements in Southern Europe discussed in the previous section (and the catch-up movements in Eastern Europe that will be discussed in the next section). Although these trends have been less well researched for Yugoslavia and Albania, some of the same ingredients were in place, particularly massive public health campaigns: vector control against malaria, vaccinations against childhood diseases, elimination of endemic syphilis, ... These were supported by international organizations: the Rockefeller Foundation was even more enthusiastically at work in Yugoslavia than in many other Southern European countries. In addition, both countries created a primary health care system covering the whole of the country with basic facilities, which could administer the new miracle drugs: antibiotics.[52]

This rapid modernization of the health infrastructure was pushed through by political regimes which were autocratic but – certainly at first – inspired by high ideals. Advances in population health were supported by rapid modernization of the economy, and by reforms of the educational system and dedicated literacy campaigns. As a result, the prevalence of illiteracy fell rapidly (see Chapter 3). Both countries adopted a specific strand of communism

51 Estimates of Gross Domestic Product (in 1990 I$) are from Maddison, *World Economy*. Estimates of illiteracy (calculated from census data and counted among the population 10 years and older) are from Dudley Kirk, *Europe's Population in the Interwar Years* (Geneva: League of Nations, 1946), App. II. Within Yugoslavia, illiteracy varied between 7% in the Drav region (part of current Slovenia) and 71% and 73%, respectively, in the Vardar region (current North Macedonia) and the Vrba region (current Bosnia & Herzegovina).

52 The set-up of public health institutions in newly independent Yugoslavia, with the help of the Rockefeller Foundation, has been documented in Zeljko Dugac, "New Public Health for a New State," in *Facing Illness in Troubled Times*, ed. Iris Borowy and Wolf Gruner (Frankfurt am Main: Peter Lang, 2005). Croatian public health pioneer Andrija Stampar (1888–1958), who played an important role in the League of Nations Health Organization (LNHO), was instrumental in forging good links between the Rockefeller Foundation and the Yugoslav health authorities; see Zeljko Dugac, "Andrija Stampar (1888–1958): Resolute Fighter for Health and Social Justice," in *Of Medicine and Men*, ed. Iris Borowy and Anne Hardy (Frankfurt am Main etc.: Peter Lang, 2008). Stampar also led the movement for strengthening primary care, particularly in rural areas, both in Yugoslavia and internationally. For anti-malaria campaigns in Macedonia, a region contested between Yugoslavia and Bulgaria, and its role in strengthening the borders of the newly formed Yugoslavian Kingdom, see Patrick Zylberman, "Mosquitoes and the Komitadjis," in *Facing Illness in Troubled Times*, ed. Iris Borowy and Wolf Gruner (Frankfurt am Main: Peter Lang, 2005).

and – in contrast to the other communist countries in Europe – distanced themselves from the Soviet Union. Yugoslavia experimented with somewhat more liberal economic policies than other communist countries in Europe, but this did not prevent it from undergoing a similar economic stagnation as these other countries in the 1980s. Albania estranged itself politically from all other European countries, and strove for an extreme form of autarky with only Maoist China as its ally, which resulted in a very low standard of living.

After the death of long-time Yugoslav president Josip Tito (1892–1980), the cohesion within the federal republic of Yugoslavia rapidly grew less. Old ethnic and nationalistic antagonisms were stirred up, and the three Yugoslav Wars of the 1990s broke out: a war in Croatia (1991–1995), a war in Bosnia (1992–1995), and a war in Kosovo (1998–1999). Together, these three wars cost around 140,000 deaths (see Suppl. Table 5), and led to a massive reshuffling of populations due to 'ethnic cleansing' and emigration. As mentioned above, this was followed by a strong divergence of life expectancy between the newly independent republics, but this had already started in the 1980s.[53]

Albania, on the other hand, followed a rather different trajectory. In the 1980s, Albania's life expectancy grew to unexpected heights. This was not due to very low infant or childhood mortality rates (these actually remained relatively high), but due to very low adult mortality rates. These had remained low as a result of the absence of a notable epidemic of ischaemic heart disease, and can be regarded as a paradoxical effect of the policy of relentless self-sufficiency. This kept the population poor and shielded it from the factors driving the ischaemic heart disease epidemic in other countries.

A study investigating the extraordinary health situation in Albania around 1990 concluded that "Albanians benefit from eating a rather extreme version of the classic Mediterranean diet now widely recommended by nutritionists." They had low caloric intake, a lower intake of animal products than any other European country, and the lowest alcohol consumption of the whole of Europe. Furthermore,

> the lack of private vehicles necessitated everyone taking regular exercise simply to carry out daily activities. In short, the very poverty of their circumstances was, paradoxically, a significant factor in keeping Albanians healthy. This is clearly an ironic situation.[54]

53 See Kunitz, "Making and Breaking" for some further reflections on the consequences of the 'breaking up' of Yugoslavia for population health.

54 The "paradoxes of Albania's health transition" have been analysed in Arjan Gjonca, "Mortality Transition in Albania" (University of London, 1999). The quotes are from Arjan

After the death of Enver Hoxha (1908–1985), who had been president of Albania since 1944, Albania went through a political revolution which at first left many of the old communist apparatchiks in power. After the collapse of the government-supported Ponzi pyramid scheme in 1996, in which many Albanians lost a lot of money, violent riots broke out which led to a remarkable spike in homicide mortality (Figure 9). This can also be related to the fact that in Albania, like in other remote areas, the state monopoly on violence has only been introduced (and enforced) relatively recently. A UN peace keeping force had to be brought in to restore peace and order.[55]

Since the late 1990s, life expectancy trends in Albania have been somewhat erratic, but the high levels have by-and-large stayed. Although ischaemic heart disease mortality started to rise during the 1990s, this seems to have stopped in the 2000s, but more recent data than 2010 were not available at the time of writing (2019).

Russian Roulette: the Value of Life

If it were not so cruel, the history of Russia's population health would rank first in Europe in terms of its spectacle. No other European country, perhaps with the exception of Russia's immediate neighbours Ukraine and Moldova, has experienced such wide swings in life expectancy throughout the 20th century – even during peaceful periods in which other countries' life expectancy had already arrived in much calmer waters (Figure 1).

When we take a long-term perspective it is, however, obvious that Russia has always been special. The earliest year for which we have an estimate of life expectancy at birth is 1896/1897 – which is an important fact in itself, illustrating the late arrival of modern methods of public administration in Tsarist Russia. In that year its life expectancy was 29 years for men and 32 years for women – values that have correctly been characterized as 'medieval'.[56]

Gjonca, Chris Wilson, and Jane Falkingham, "Paradoxes of Health Transition in Europe's Poorest Country: Albania 1950–90," *Population and Development Review* 23, no. 3 (1997): 585–609, pp. 603 and 605.

55 On the delayed fall of homicide mortality in remote European regions, see Chesnais, *Histoire*, Chapter 2. In the Albanian 'pyramid crisis' protests against the government derailed into looting of weapon depots and violence between individuals and competing gangs in which between 2000 and 4000 Albanians were killed (https://en.wikipedia.org/wiki/Albanian_Civil_War, accessed 28/08/2019).

56 Shkolnikov et al., "Recent Trends." On mortality patterns in Tsarist Russia, see K. David Patterson, "Mortality in Late Tsarist Russia: A Reconnaissance," *Social History of Medicine* 8, no. 2 (1995): 179–210.

It is important to understand Russia's health trajectory, if only because Russia's population makes up such a large part of the total European population. In 1897, Russia's population numbered around 67 million, or around 16% of the European population as a whole. Despite the demographic disasters of the 20th century, Russia still is Europe's largest country, with around 146 million people who make up 20% of the total.[57]

It is not difficult to understand why Russia's life expectancy in the late 19th century was still so low. Lying on the periphery of Europe, in a vast space between the more densely inhabited and dynamic countries to its West, and the Asian steppes to its East from where invaders had repeatedly come to devastate the country, Russia was a relative newcomer on Europe's political stage. It grew out of the smaller Grand Duchy of Muscovy (1283–1547), and started to take its current form only in the 17th century after conquests of large swathes of land towards the North, West, South and East.

It was governed by a Tsar whose powers were absolute – which was perhaps inevitable in such a vast empire that needed to be held together – and to whom even the Eastern Orthodox Church was subordinate. In contrast to Western Europe, where authority was often shared between the Church and the State, and where religious pluralism emerged during the Reformation, Russia thus missed the creative stimulus of competition between different centres of power. Modernization had to come from above, as in the case of Peter the Great (1672–1725) and Catherine the Great (r. 1762–1796) whose attempts at reform only reached the upper echelons of society.

Russia also missed out on many of the modernizing changes that during the 19th century occurred in Western Europe. The 19th century wave of political reforms largely bypassed Russia, so that in 1870 it was the only European country, together with the Ottoman Empire, to still have absolute government without a constitution. Serfdom – peasants living in bondage to the nobility who owned the land they were forced to work – remained common until it was abolished in 1861. At the 1897 census, the average literacy level in European Russia was a low 30%.[58]

---

57 The population estimate for 1897 is for Russia within its present borders. The Russian empire, which also included Poland, Finland, the Baltic states etc., then had around 100 million inhabitants.

58 For a general history of Russia, see Roberts, *The Penguin History of Europe*, especially pp. 301–07. Long-term trends in literacy in Russia and the Soviet Union have been analysed by Boris N. Mironov, "The Development of Literacy in Russia and the USSR from the Tenth to the Twentieth Centuries," *History of Education Quarterly* 31, no. 2 (1991): 229–52. Please note, that the figure of 30% is based on a definition of literacy different from that used in Figure 8.

Industrialization also came late to Russia, like it did to Southern and South-eastern European countries. Although industrial production rose rapidly in the last decades of the 19th century, at the start of World War I Russia was still predominantly an agrarian country. In a sense, therefore, the Bolshevik revolution (1917) was – again – an attempt at reform-from-above, but one that would turn out to have tremendous impact.[59]

After a few years of bloody civil war, the new communist regime settled in and started to modernize the economy, and society as a whole, at break-neck pace. Rapid industrialization, together with forced collectivization of agriculture (Plate 20), moved large numbers of people into newly built cities. Living standards gradually improved, although interrupted by the dramatic famines described in Chapter 4, and contributed to a fall in mortality in 'normal' years, as well as a strong rise in body height.[60]

One of the priorities of the new regime was also to reform Russia's health system. In the early 1920s, a Commissariat of Public Health was created under the directorship of Nicolai Semashko (1874–1949), a progressive physician and long-term ally of Vladimir Lenin. The Bolsheviks involved physicians in public health affairs, and had a vision of a new type of physician, to be trained in a new medical curriculum with an emphasis on social hygiene, in which social factors were considered the prime determinants of health and disease.[61]

This fitted well with the official commitment to social change in the 1920s, but by the end of the decade official enthusiasm diminished due to a combination of budgetary problems and distrust of technocracy. In 1930 Semashko was removed from his post, and the role of the socially conscious physician was replaced by that of the sanitary scientist – who during the 1930s and 1940s

59 Earlier revolutions occurred in 1905 and in February 1917. The Russian revolution of October 1917 succeeded because the Bolshevik leaders remembered the failure of the 1848 revolution, and were determined to succeed at all costs.

60 Average body height of military recruits in the Soviet Union grew by more than 4 centimetres between those born in the early 1920s and early 1950s; see Stephen G. Wheatcroft, "The Great Leap Upwards: Anthropometric Data and Indicators of Crises and Secular Change in Soviet Welfare Levels, 1880–1960," *Slavic Review* 58, no. 1 (1999): 27–60. Whether this was an extraordinary achievement of the communist regime has been disputed, however; see Millward and Baten, "Population and Living Standards."

61 Early Soviet health policies were inspired by communist ideology, but also stood in a long tradition in which medical police, public hygiene and social hygiene had merged with the social orientation of 19th century Russian medicine; see David L. Hoffmann, *Cultivating the Masses* (New York: Cornell University Press, 2011). Illustrative is an article by Semashko in which he shows, how Karl Marx's analysis of the negative effects of capitalism on labourers' well-being foreshadowed social-hygienic insights; see Nikolai A. Semashko, "Karl Marx Und Die Sozialhygiene," in *Der Rote Oktober und der Sowjetische Gesundheitsschutz*, ed. Kurt Winter et al. (Jena: VEB Gustav Fischer Verlag, 1977 [1933]).

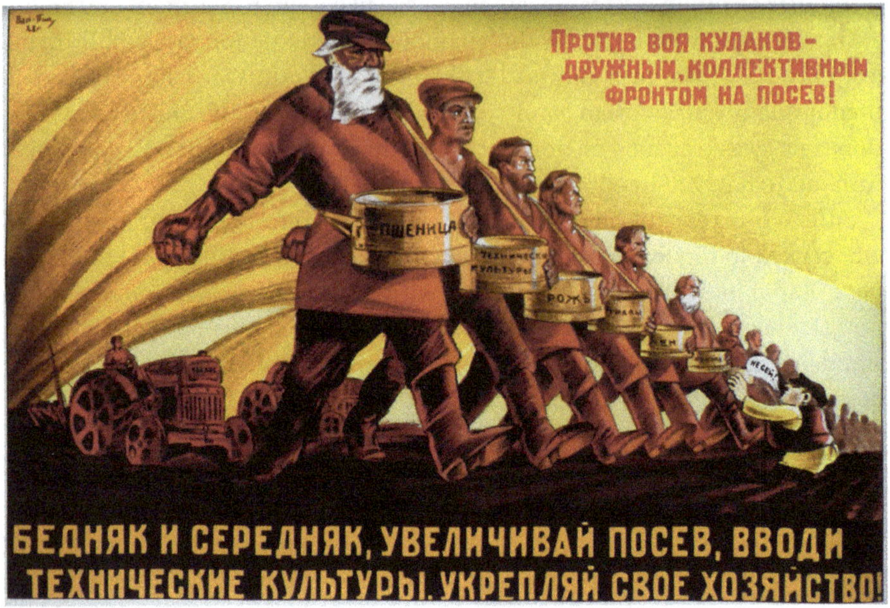
ПРОТИВ ВОЯ КУЛАКОВ –
ДРУЖНЫМ, КОЛЛЕКТИВНЫМ
ФРОНТОМ НА ПОСЕВ!
ПШЕНИЦА
РОЖЬ
БЕДНЯК И СЕРЕДНЯК, УВЕЛИЧИВАЙ ПОСЕВ, ВВОДИ
ТЕХНИЧЕСКИЕ КУЛЬТУРЫ. УКРЕПЛЯЙ СВОЕ ХОЗЯЙСТВО!

PLATE 20 "Against the kulak's howl." Soviet poster promoting collective farming, 1928
This Soviet propaganda poster was part of Stalin's campaign of forced collectivization of agriculture. It shows a large group of peasants marching against a 'kulak'. Kulaks were affluent peasants who were seen as enemies of communism. The translation of the text at the top is: "Against the kulak's howl – to sow by a concerted, collective front!." The translation of the text at the bottom is: "Poor and middle-class peasants, increase crop plantation, establish a technical culture, and strengthen your economy."
UNKNOWN ARTIST. SOURCE: SOVIET POSTERS (MIAMI, FL)

helped to create great successes in the battle against infectious diseases in the Soviet Union, some of which have been described in previous chapters.[62]

Between 1939, the last year before World War II, and 1964, the year in which it reached its highest level for decades to come, life expectancy in Russia

62 As far as I am aware, there is no biography of Semashko, although recent papers by Russian scholars have shed more light on his life and works (e.g., O.A. Trefilova and I.M. Sechenov, "Nikolai Semashko: Social Activist and Health Care Organizer," *History of Medicine* 1, no. 3 (2014): 65–72 and other papers in the same journal issue). See for the history of Russian and Soviet public health Susan Gross Solomon, "The Expert and the State in Russian Public Health," in *The History of Public Health and the Modern State*, ed. D. Porter (Amsterdam – Atlanta: Rodopi, 1994); Susan Gross Solomon and John F. Hutchinson, eds., *Health and Society in Revolutionary Russia* (Bloomington: Indiana University Press, 1990).

increased from 34 to 65 years among men, and from 42 to 75 years among women. It is difficult to overestimate the scale of this achievement, which was due to a huge reduction of mortality from a range of infectious diseases, and including infant mortality. Some improvement in living standards as well as rapid increases in literacy will have played a role, but large-scale public health campaigns were probably the most important factor. Interestingly, these campaigns did not so much focus on investments in sanitary infrastructure – for which the state did not have the money – but on measures, applied by massive detachments of health workers, to detect, isolate, decontaminate and treat anyone who might help spread an epidemic.[63]

These successes were highly admired in the West, particularly during the 1930s when many left-leaning intellectuals regarded the Soviet Union as a kind of 'Utopia come true'. There were also many admirers in the health professions, who saw their ideals of a truly 'social medicine', freely accessible to all and with an emphasis on prevention, put into practice. This is illustrated, for example, by Arthur Newsholme and John Kingsbury's *Red Medicine* (1933) and in Henry Sigerist's *Socialized Medicine in the Soviet Union* (1937). Both books were based on study tours through the Soviet Union in the 1930s, and both were written in a spirit of deep admiration for what the Soviet Union had achieved. The first book, but not the second, also contains a chapter with a critical evaluation of the autocratic character of the Soviet system. In neither of the two is there any awareness of the death toll of the man-made famines and political oppression in the Stalinist years. Sigerist even defended Stalin's show trials as a necessary defence against attempts to undermine the Soviet system.[64]

---

63 These improvements of life expectancy at birth should be balanced against the fact that of all men alive during the 1939 census, only 53% were still alive during the 1960 census; see Anatoly Vishnevsky, "Demographic Consequences of the Great Patriotic War," *Demographic Review (English Selection)* 3, no. 2 (2016): 6–42. Vaccines and antibiotics, which did not have to be imported but were produced in the Soviet Union, also helped to rapidly reduce mortality from infectious diseases. See Donald Filtzer, *The Hazards of Urban Life in Late Stalinist Russia* (Cambridge etc.: Cambridge University Press, 2010) for an analysis of public health in the Soviet Union during the late 1940s and early 1950s.

64 The first book arose from a study tour commissioned by the Milbank Memorial Fund (Arthur Newsholme and John Adams Kingsbury, *Red Medicine* (London: Heinemann, 1934)). Its patron Albert Milbank considered it left-wing "propaganda"; see Susan Gross Solomon, "A Matter of 'Reach'. Fact Finding in the Wake of World War I," in *Shifting Boundaries of Public Health*, ed. S. Gross Salomon, L. Murard, and P. Zylberman (Rochester: University of Rochester Press, 2008). Sir Arthur Newsholme (1857–1943) was one of England's greatest authorities in public health in the first decades of the 20th century; see John M. Eyler, *Sir Arthur Newsholme and State Medicine, 1885–1935* (Cambridge etc.: Cambridge University Press, 2002). The second book first appeared in 1933 and was republished in a slightly modified form shortly after World War II (Henry E. Sigerist, *Medicine and Health*

How, indeed, should these achievements be valued? The enormous leap forward in population health coincided with one of the most brutal periods in Russian history. After millions of people had lost their lives in the Civil War (1917–1922) and in famines (1927–1933), another 700,000 people were executed during Stalin's purges (1937–1938). While the ultimate gains in population health can of course not justify the brutality of the communist regime, it is important to understand that the intensive state involvement with improving population health on the one hand, and the massive state violence on the other hand, served the same purpose: a rapid social transformation to a new society in which social causes of ill-health would have been eliminated.[65]

After the mid-1960s life expectancy in Russia (and the Soviet Union) stalled among women and even declined among men. It increased again temporarily during Gorbachev's anti-alcohol campaign (1985–1987), and then declined even more strongly (among men) after the collapse of the Soviet Union. Russia's mortality experience since the mid-1960s has been extensively studied, and the main conclusion has been that stagnation and decline of life expectancy since the 1960s were due to lack of progress in the prevention and treatment of cardiovascular diseases, combined with high and fluctuating levels of alcohol consumption.

In its turn, the lack of progress in the prevention and treatment of cardiovascular diseases was partly the result of the Soviet Union's political situation. Under Leonid Brezhnev (general secretary of the Central Committee of the Communist Party between 1964 and 1982), the Soviet Union was engaged in an arms race with the West that absorbed resources that would otherwise have been available for health care expansion and innovation. Also, the Iron Curtain was a barrier for the diffusion of new knowledge on cardiovascular risk factors and their management. Furthermore, dogmatic Marxism did not go well together

in the Soviet Union (Binghamton: Citadel Press, 1947)). In the preface to this second edition, Sigerist writes "My book was given a very favorable reception when it appeared in Great Britain. At that time, the Left Book Clubs were flourishing […]. In the United States, the reception was decidedly cool. The country was under a heavy barrage of anti-Soviet propaganda. Girding to meet attack, and knowing by what methods the Nazis were striving to build up fifth columns in other countries, the Soviet Union got rid of its traitors in time. In the United States, however, few persons attempted to understand the meaning and significance of the Moscow trials." In these sentences, Sigerist, a Swiss-German medical historian who emigrated to the United States in the early 1930s and who has been highly admired, defends Stalin's show trials. For a short introduction to Sigerist's life and work, see Elizabeth Fee, "Henry E. Sigerist," *Milbank Quarterly* 67, no. Suppl. 1 (1989): 127–50.

65 Hoffmann, *Cultivating the Masses.*

with the application of modern epidemiological methods, such as Randomized Controlled Trials.

Partly because of the earlier successes in infectious disease control, the Soviet Union stuck to a public health system almost exclusively focused on sanitation, thereby turning an advantage in a previous stage of epidemiological development into a disadvantage in a later stage. After the collapse of the Soviet Union, life expectancy in Russia and other former republics of the Soviet Union fell even more dramatically, as a result of the disruptive economic and political changes of the 1990s, with large-scale unemployment, declining incomes, reduced access to health care, and high levels of psychosocial stress.[66]

Fortunately, Russian life expectancy has started to rise again in 2004, due to a reversal of the trend in mortality from cardiovascular diseases and injuries. In contrast to earlier mortality declines (in the mid-1980s and late-1990s) this recent mortality decline has now continued for more than 10 years. It has been attributed to a combination of factors, including decreases in alcohol consumption (partly in response to some tightening of alcohol control policies) and improvements in the prevention and treatment of cardiovascular disease (hypertension control, greater supply of advanced treatment).

Russian president Vladimir Putin, who for good reasons does not have a very good press in the West, may have contributed to this reversal by officially decreeing increases in life expectancy to be an important policy goal, and by

66 The literature on recent trends in life expectancy in Russia is very extensive. A good description up to the early 2000s is Vladimir M. Shkolnikov et al., "Mortality Reversal in Russia: The Story So Far," *Hygiea Internationalis* 4, no. 1 (2004): 29–80. An interpretation in terms of a "second epidemiological [transition] that never was" is offered in Anatoly Vishnevsky, "Mortality in Russia: The Second Epidemiological Revolution That Never Was," *Demographic Review (English Selection)* 1 (2014): 5–40. Medical scientists in the Soviet Union missed out on the developments in cardiovascular disease epidemiology in the West, partly because the uncertainty inherent in the idea of risk factors and multiple causes was incompatible with Marxism-Leninism (Vasiliy V. Vlassov, "Russian Medicine: Trying to Catch up on Scientific Evidence and Human Values," *Lancet* 390, no. 10102 (2017): 1619–620), and because Randomized Controlled Trials were similarly unpalatable (McKee, "Cochrane on Communism"). An early paper showing the role of fluctuations in excessive alcohol consumption is by David A. Leon et al., "Huge Variation in Russian Mortality Rates 1984–94: Artefact, Alcohol, or What?," *Lancet* 350, no. 9075 (1997): 383–88. The role of economic disruption during the transition from a communist to a capitalist economy was analysed in David Stuckler, Lawrence King, and Martin McKee, "Mass Privatisation and the Post-Communist Mortality Crisis," *Lancet* 373, no. 9661 (2009): 399–407. When Russia's life expectancy is plotted in a Preston-curve, it is clear that it is far below the expected value, showing that low living standards are not the main factor; see Vladimir M. Shkolnikov et al., "Patterns in the Relationship between Life Expectancy and Gross Domestic Product in Russia in 2005–15," *Lancet Public Health* 4, no. 4 (2019): e181–e88.

channelling government funds from increased oil revenues into health care programs.[67]

Over the 20th century, trends in Russia have to some extent been mirrored by trends in neighbouring countries, resp. other republics of the Soviet Union. The life expectancy trajectory of Ukraine has been similar to that of Russia, both before and after the collapse of the Soviet Union, but the decline of male life expectancy during the 1990s has been less severe, and the upturn of male life expectancy came earlier in Ukraine than in Russia. Interestingly, within Ukraine there is a clear East-West gradient, with Western regions having lower mortality than Eastern regions, suggesting that the Ukrainian health situation is partly determined by its position on a cultural fault-line between West and East.[68]

The Baltic countries also offer interesting trends for comparison with Russia's. As was already briefly mentioned in Chapter 3, the Baltic republics (still independent at that time) had relatively high life expectancies during the 1920s and 1930s, moving in parallel with Finland's and slowly converging towards Sweden's life expectancy. However, the Baltic republics lost their independence in World War II, when they were incorporated in the Soviet Union, and after 1960 their life expectancy trends began to follow the unfavourable trends in Russia. It was only after the breaking-up of the Soviet Union that life expectancy trends in the Baltic countries started to diverge again from Russia's.[69]

What then are the deeper causes of Russia's bad record in population health? Which factor, within the intertwined constellation of geographical, economic, political and sociocultural factors, is the ultimate driver of Russia's low life expectancy?

67 For an analysis of these recent trends, see Vladimir M. Shkolnikov et al., "Components and Possible Determinants of the Decrease in Russian Mortality in 2004–2010," *Demographic Research* 28 (2013): 917–50 Pavel Grigoriev et al., "The Recent Mortality Decline in Russia: Beginning of the Cardiovascular Revolution?," *Population and Development Review* 40, no. 1 (2014): 107–29. The recent expansion of myocardial infarction facilities has been analysed in Sergey Timonin et al., "Reducing Geographic Inequalities in Access Times for Acute Treatment of Myocardial Infarction," *International Journal of Epidemiology* 47, no. 5 (2018): 1594–602.

68 Johan P. Mackenbach, Adrianna Murphy, and Martin McKee, "Ukraine: Not Only a Matter of Geopolitics," *Lancet* 383, no. 9920 (2014): 848–50.

69 Within the Baltic countries, Russians now have lower life expectancies than ethnic Lithuanians, Latvians and Estonians. For life expectancy trends in the Baltic countries, see Mackenbach, "Political Conditions and Life Expectancy"; Jacques Vallin, Domantas Jasilionis, and France Meslé, "Does a Turbulent History Lead to Turbulent Life Expectancy Trends?," *Historical Methods* 50, no. 4 (2017): 191–209.

Excessive alcohol consumption, including the use of toxic surrogate alcohols, is certainly one of the more immediate causes, and the evidence for its role in creating the recent 'saw-tooth' pattern in mortality is rather overwhelming. Already in the 19th century consumption of spirits was very high in Russia, perhaps as a result of the start of industrial production of alcoholic drinks. Russian drinking culture, which permits drunkenness and stimulates intake of great amounts of alcohol on a single occasion, perhaps in response to the cold and darkness of long winters, also definitely plays a role. Furthermore, the state failed in its role as protector of the people's health, as it was dependent on income from alcohol taxes even in the Soviet period, and reluctant to take away a narcotic that kept people quiet. After the fall of communism, the international alcohol industry rapidly took possession of the huge Russian market with aggressive marketing strategies.[70]

Ultimately, however, excessive alcohol consumption cannot be the final explanation, because not all health problems that are more frequent in Russia are linked to alcohol, and because Russia's alcohol culture must itself also be explained. The specific factors involved in the Russian health disadvantage – alcohol and other forms of risk-taking behaviour, plus a suboptimal health care system – ask for a more general explanation. As alluded to in the first paragraphs of this section, this should perhaps be sought in Russia's culture, which has been shaped by its location on the inhospitable fringes of the European subcontinent, in-between the rest of Europe and Asia. Russia's cultural history has been characterized as one long search for a specifically Russian identity between West and East. Has this also influenced the value of human life, which – according to a recent study – has never reached the supreme levels it has in the West?[71]

---

70 Andrew Stickley, Yury Razvodovsky, and Michael McKee, "Alcohol Mortality in Russia: A Historical Perspective," *Public Health* 123, no. 1 (2009): 20–6; Martin McKee, "Alcohol in Russia," *Alcohol and Alcoholism* 34, no. 6 (1999): 824–29. See Chapter 6, Ischaemic heart disease, for the "saw-tooth" pattern in Russian mortality.

71 For a characterization of Russia's cultural history as an eternal hesitation between West and East, see Orlando Figes, *Natasha's Dance* (London: Allen Lane, 2002). Economists have compared the monetary value of human life (as estimated from decisions on health investments, or from life insurance and other compensation schemes) between Russia and other countries, concluding that in Russia the value of human life is lower than in other European countries with a similar level of income, and more similar to that of Asian countries with a lower level of income; see T. Karabchuk et al., "Как Оценить Стоимость Человеческой Жизни? [How to Evaluate the Value of Human Life?]," *Economic Sociology* 15, no. 1 (2014): 89–106.

CHAPTER 8

Outlook

Population health has improved enormously over the last centuries, and substantial further gains are certainly possible. Some further increases in life expectancy are even likely, whether we want them or not, as a result of on-going advances in the treatment of currently fatal conditions like cancer. If we do our best, we can undoubtedly also make progress against non-fatal diseases which cause a lot of illness and disability, particularly among elderly people. In addition to diabetes mellitus, depression and dementia, dealt with in this book, this includes musculoskeletal diseases and sensory disorders for which we have unfortunately found no space. This short final chapter, however, will not focus on the possibilities of further progress, but on the more fundamental question whether what has been achieved so far is sustainable in the longer run. This will also force us to have a closer look at some of the darker sides of progress.

Feathers of Icarus

"Feathers of Icarus," the title of this section, refers to a small book I wrote many years ago, in which I compared the rise of Dutch life expectancy to the flight of Icarus, and then asked how sustainable this rise is. A Greek myth tells us the story of Daedalus, who used wax to attach feathers to his own body and that of his son Icarus, in order to escape from his enemies. He warned his son not to fly too high, because the sun would melt the wax, but Icarus did not pay heed. He flew too high, his wings fell off, and he crashed into the part of the Mediterranean Sea that would later be named after him. We, Europeans, are flying high with our average life expectancies, often exceeding 80 years. To what extent are the conditions which have allowed us to live so long, and to live in such good health, sustainable?[1]

In this book I have argued that human health depends on whether we have 'favourable exchanges with the natural environment', and that effective 'human agency' against disease and premature death is dependent on economic,

1 For a summary, see, e.g., www.britannica.com/topic/Daedalus-Greek-mythology. The book I refer to analysed the epidemiologic transition in the Netherlands: Johan P. Mackenbach, *De Veren van Icarus* (Utrecht: Bunge, 1992).

political and sociocultural conditions. This suggests that, in the future, at least three factors may threaten the sustainability of today's high levels of population health: geopolitical instability, increasing inequality, and global environmental change. Closer scrutiny of these factors reveals that – without knowing it – Europe may have passed a tipping-point ushering in a new era with less rosy prospects for population health.[2]

Geopolitical Instability

Europe's early rise, both in terms of prosperity and population health, was partly based on its favourable geography. We may now, in the age of the internet, no longer be as strongly hindered by distance as our ancestors, but geography may well become important again in a different way. Europe is no longer the centre of the world, which is now dominated by two superpowers, the United States and China, and a few mighty competitors including Russia. With military, financial and technological support from the US, the Western part of the subcontinent built its post-World War II miracle. A prosperous peace provided the background to high and increasing levels of human welfare. The Eastern part of the subcontinent at first benefitted from the support of the Soviet Union but then fell back, and has only recently joined the world of liberal democracy, capitalism and modern health care, struggling in the transition.

The geopolitical situation in which Europe finds itself today does no longer look particularly stable. Even war is not completely unthinkable anymore. As the memories of World War II have begun to fade, the threshold to war may become lower again, and recent small-scale conventional wars between Russia and its neighbours (e.g., with Ukraine and Georgia) indeed illustrate that war is a real possibility. The inner core of the European Union probably has become too well integrated for war between its members ever to break out again, but the short period of intra-European *détente* after the collapse of the Soviet Union has reversed into renewed hostility which may over time develop into something more serious. If this happens it will hamper further progress in

2 The idea of such a "tipping-point" has been developed in Bayly, *Remaking the Modern World*, Chapter 9. It refers to a combination of economic, political and sociocultural changes occurring between the late 1970s and early 1990s, radically altering the relative stability after World War II which provided the background to the rapid improvement of living conditions (and population health). Slowing down of life expectancy increases since 2010 in some European countries (e.g., the United Kingdom) suggests that stability of the economic and social forces that facilitated these increases is not a given; see David A. Leon, Dmitry A. Jdanov, and Vladimir M. Shkolnikov, "Trends in Life Expectancy and Age-Specific Mortality in England and Wales, 1970–2016," *Lancet Public Health* 4, no. 11 (2019): e575–e82.

population health, or even cause outright deterioration, for example in the vulnerable Baltic states.

Another and more immediately important aspect of Europe's geographical position is, that its nearest neighbours to the South and South-east are the politically and economically unstable countries in North Africa and the Middle East. The involvement of European countries in the US-led war in Iraq has brought Islamic terrorism to Madrid, Paris, London and other European cities. The devastating war in Syria has sent millions of refugees into neighbouring countries and, through Turkey and North Africa, into a not-too-welcoming European Union. Lack of employment opportunities in countries with high fertility has created large migration streams from Africa and Asia into Europe, which has much lower fertility and – as a result – shrinking population numbers. All this has contributed to the rise of nationalist-populist political parties in many European countries, which reject many of the premises on which post-World War II national and international politics were built.

Finally, what to think of the rise of China? China is extending its influence around the world, not only to find markets for its increasingly sophisticated products, but also to get access to the mineral and agricultural resources that it needs for its economic growth and for the nutritional demands of its immense population. While China's moves have been peaceful so far, and may continue to be based on wielding 'soft power', in the long run there could well be negative effects on Europe's welfare. In a future world of 11 billion people, competition for minerals, food and other resources will be fierce. The uncertainty inherent in the rise of a new world power, together with the other two geopolitical uncertainties, warn against the assumption that – in a few decades from now – we will still live in a world in which we can quietly devote ourselves to improving population health.[3]

Increasing Inequality

High levels of average population health can only be attained, if health inequalities within populations are kept small. People with a higher income or level of education always manage to have good health, even if the conditions in their country are not conducive to health. They do so, e.g., by copying the behaviour of their likes in better-off countries, or by buying private health care if the publicly funded system does not offer what they want. As a consequence,

---

3 On geopolitical risks in Europe's future, see, e.g., Bruno Maçães, *The Dawn of Eurasia* (London: Allen Lane, 2018).

differences between countries in average population health are mainly determined by what happens to people with a lower income or level of education.[4]

Historically, the rise of the European welfare state has therefore been crucial for improvements in population health. The welfare state has created collective arrangements for financing public health and health care services, often subsidised or directly paid from taxes, which have ensured reasonably equal access regardless of individual financial means. The welfare state has also redistributed money from the rich to the poor, by social security arrangements and progressive taxation, which has helped to keep the prevalence of poverty low so that people at the bottom of the social hierarchy could at least partly share in the post-World War II improvements in living conditions.[5]

Since the 1970s, however, the welfare state has come under attack, initially because of the perceived necessity of reducing public expenditure and improving economic competitiveness, and later also because of the rise of neoliberalism with its preference for *laissez-faire* economics and free markets. Since the 1980s, many North-western European countries have reduced the scope of their welfare arrangements, sometimes substantially.

Also, income inequality has been rising again, partly as a result of globalization, partly as a result of the neoliberal distaste for income redistribution. The tendency for economic inequality to rise is inherent in market economies – a system of economic production that has been hugely successful in raising over-all living standards – and is another example of the flipside of progress. Inequalities in wealth are now startlingly high again all over Europe – as high as in the years immediately preceding World War I.

Even hard-core economists who believe in the societal benefits of some degree of economic inequality, regard this recent widening as dangerous. Too large inequalities may have major negative side-effects, such as reduced social mobility, higher rates of crime, and political instability, and may ultimately threaten the functioning of democracy. They may also and more directly threaten population health, when the increased social distance between groups in society erodes the solidarity underpinning the welfare state. More simply, when new medical treatments become increasingly unaffordable for publicly financed health care systems, we may reach a point at which only the rich can pay for them.[6]

4 See Mackenbach et al., "Socioeconomic Inequalities" for an empirical illustration.

5 Huber and Stephens, *Development and Crisis*; Kees van Kersbergen and Barbara Vis, *Comparative Welfare State Politics* (Cambridge etc.: Cambridge University Press, 2014).

6 On the rise of economic inequality, see Thomas Piketty, *Capital in the Twenty-First Century* (Cambridge (Mass): Harvard University Press, 2014); Branko Milanovic, *Global Inequality*

Global Environmental Change

Advances in population health have, unfortunately, gone hand-in-hand with degradation of the natural environment. As the Lancet Commission on Planetary Health wrote a few years ago,

> Far-reaching changes to the structure and function of the Earth's natural systems represent a growing threat to human health. And yet, global health has mainly improved as these changes have gathered pace. What is the explanation? As a Commission, we are deeply concerned that the explanation is straightforward and sobering: we have been mortgaging the health of future generations to realise economic and development gains in the present. By unsustainably exploiting nature's resources, human civilisation has flourished but now risks substantial health effects from the degradation of nature's life support.[7]

One example may suffice: the agricultural and industrial revolutions which unleashed modern economic growth, would have been impossible without the use of fossil fuels. Burning fossil fuels, in steam-machines and all the other technologies that followed, was necessary for tilling the fields, transporting food around the world, producing goods, building and warming houses, conducting public health programs, exchanging scientific information, and everything else that was necessary for population health improvement. The release into the atmosphere of massive amounts of carbon dioxide and other greenhouse gases is now creating world-wide climate change that threatens population health in geographical zones sensitive to, for example, flooding, drought or vector-borne diseases.

Climate change is just one of the environmental changes that are going on globally, and that risk to undermine human population health. Other dangerous changes include ocean acidification (due to absorption of atmospheric carbon dioxide, threatening marine life), freshwater depletion (due to extraction of groundwater, leading to shortages of water for human consumption and agriculture), land degradation (due to erosion and overexploitation, threatening food security), and biodiversity loss (due to habitat destruction, climate change and other factors, threatening ecosystem services such as pollination and climate control). Recent reports by international agencies and

(Cambridge & London: Belknap Press, 2016). On the dangers of rising economic inequality, see Joseph E. Stiglitz, *The Price of Inequality* (New York etc.: W.W. Norton & Co., 2012).

7 Sarah Whitmee et al., "Safeguarding Human Health in the Anthropocene Epoch," *Lancet* 386, no. 10007 (2015): 1973–2028. The quote is from p. 1973.

commissions have made alarming (and depressing) lists of all that is going wrong.[8]

One way to look at this, from an historical point of view, is to see this as an 'environmental risk transition'. This concept complements the 'demographic transition' and the 'epidemiologic transition', and focuses on the underlying transition in disease risks. According to this framework, over time a shift has occurred from risks at the household level (e.g., poor water, sanitation, indoor air pollution, food quality) to risks at the community level (e.g., outdoor air pollution, occupational hazards, traffic injury risks), and then from risks at the community level to risks at the global scale (e.g., climate change, freshwater depletion, ...). It is as if humans have put their environmental risks farther and farther away – but without losing their fundamental dependence on the natural environment.[9]

Pessimists have pointed out that this man-made degradation of the global environment may be inherent to the philosophy underlying our progress. In their reasoning, it is not just an unfortunate side-effect of our use of the Earth's resources, but reflects a deeper problem in the way we think. The Enlightenment and the scientific, economic and social advances that followed, may not only have given us the instruments to take better care of ourselves, but may also have reinforced our tendency to make human welfare our primary focus – if necessary, at the expense of everything else.[10]

The Way Ahead

The Public Health Paradigm

Needless, to say, public health is in a much better position to help humanity cope with the challenges of the future than medical care. Medical care may be able to treat the 'symptoms', but public health can deal with the 'causes'. Medical care offers solutions for when we are sick, and may be able to offer increasingly effective solutions for treating disease in the future, but what we really

8 In addition to Whitmee et al., "Safeguarding Human Health" this includes reports of the Intergovernmental Panel on Climate Change (IPCC) (Alistair Woodward et al., "Climate Change and Health: On the Latest IPCC Report," *Lancet* 383, no. 9924 (2014): 1185–189), and the World Health Organization (www.who.int/globalchange/environment/en/). On biodiversity loss, see also Stuart H.M. Butchart et al., "Global Biodiversity: Indicators of Recent Declines," *Science* 328, no. 5982 (2010): 1164–168.

9 See Kirk R. Smith and Majid Ezzati, "How Environmental Health Risks Change with Development," *Annual Review Environmental Resources* 30 (2005): 291–333.

10 For this and related 'dialectics', see Chapter 3, note 55.

need is not falling sick in the first place. In the past, public health has developed a powerful arsenal to bring prevention to the people, but how can it continue to be effective in the future?

Public health is a fuzzy area, with boundaries that are much less clear than those of medical care. It emerged in the form of public hygiene in the 19th century, morphed into social hygiene in the first half of the 20th century, and then took on the cloak of 'new public health' in the second half of the 20th century. To a large extent, these were adaptations to the most pressing health problems of their historical periods – suggesting that some degree of 'fuzziness' can be an advantage.

Today, like in the past, public health exists in the form of dedicated institutions delivering interventions (e.g., local and national institutes of public health), dedicated professions providing the manpower (e.g., 'public health specialists', health scientists), and a knowledge base from which institutions and professions draw their expertise (and which can be found in the expanding textbooks of the field). What keeps the field together, however, is something that could be called the 'public health paradigm'.[11]

This was shaped in the era of 'public hygiene', and can be characterized as follows: (a) The causes of disease are primarily sought in environmental factors. (b) These causes of disease are addressed proactively, preferably through measures protecting the entire population. (c) Taking these measures is seen as a collective responsibility, which requires intervention by local and national governments. It is this set of core ideas that lies at the basis of successes like compulsory smallpox vaccination, municipal sanitation, outreaching facilities for the prevention and treatment of tuberculosis and syphilis, alcohol and tobacco control strategies, breast cancer screening programs, and much more.[12]

It is not difficult to see that – although institutions, professions and knowledge base may need to be adapted – this paradigm will continue to be useful.

11 I am using this term, loosely, in the sense of Thomas S. Kuhn, *The Structure of Scientific Revolutions* (Chicago: University of Chicago Press, 1962). It refers to an all-encompassing collection of beliefs and assumptions that result in the organization of scientific worldviews and practices. Michel Foucault coined a somewhat similar concept, '*epistèmè*', for the "a priori which grounds knowledge"; see Michel Foucault, "Les Mots et les Choses," (Paris: Gallimard, 1966).

12 These ideas are still very much alive within the discipline of public health, as is clear from the popularity of Geoffrey Rose's (1926–1993) *The strategy of preventive medicine* which provides a modern incarnation of this paradigm. In this book, Rose argued that a 'population approach' to prevention had not only worked best against infectious diseases in the past, but would also be most effective in the struggle with cardiovascular diseases now (Geoffrey Rose, *The Strategy of Preventive Medicine* (Oxford etc.: Oxford University Press, 1992)).

'Endogenous' causes of disease may slowly gain more importance in the future, but there continues to be enormous scope for preventing disease by addressing 'exogenous' causes. High-risk approaches should be considered if population approaches are less effective, but health protection measures continue to be the fundamentally correct way of preventing disease.[13]

It is on the third point, collective responsibility, that the public health paradigm is suffering from a certain loss of credibility – or perhaps better: acceptability. There can be no doubt that the health challenges of today and the future can only be addressed collectively, because individual behaviour change or uptake of preventive interventions can only go a short way in keeping disease away. This applies to personal hygiene, smoking and obesity, and even more strongly to global environmental change. However, the acceptability of government intervention has been eroded by neoliberalism, and the rationale for collective intervention therefore needs to be re-articulated. Also, we need supra-national intervention to complement intervention by national and local governments, but we are currently lacking the international institutions that can deliver this.[14]

An Expanding Circle of Concern

In his book *The Expanding Circle*, Australian-American bioethicist Peter Singer describes how altruism began as a drive to protect one's kin and community members, but has since developed into a consciously chosen ethic with a gradually widening circle of moral concern. In the distant past, we were only concerned with the well-being of our family and fellow villagers, but in more recent times this developed into a concern for all our countrymen, and then from a concern with white people only, into a concern including people of colour. It is not so long ago that black Africans were not even considered human beings. Singer argues that there is no rational argument for limiting our altruistic concerns to the human species, and that we should also be concerned with the well-being of other living beings, particularly sentient species.[15]

If we accept this argument, we have a very big problem. The demographic transition, including the increase in human life expectancy, has been an important factor in the population explosion of the last centuries. Rising human

13 It has been estimated that approximately three quarters of the health gains due to prevention since 1970 were achieved by a population approach and approximately a quarter by a high-risk approach; see Johan P. Mackenbach et al., "The Population and High-Risk Approaches to Prevention," *European Journal of Public Health* 23, no. 6 (2012): 909–15.

14 Robert Beaglehole and Ruth Bonita, *Global Public Health: A New Era* (Oxford etc.: Oxford University Press, 2009).

15 Peter Singer, *The Expanding Circle* (Princeton: Princeton University Press, 1981).

population numbers, and the increase in resource use per human, have in their turn played an important role in the loss of biodiversity on Earth. While human life expectancy rose, whole species of other living beings have become extinct. The extinction rate of other living species is now 100 times higher than before humans rose to prominence on this planet, and many remaining species are rapidly decreasing in number.[16]

Is further lengthening of human life, and more generally, further improvement in human health, a priority now that we see other species being completely erased? I think that we should re-consider our goals if analyses show that human health goals are in conflict with the goal of preserving biodiversity. Some analysts have suggested that we can stop biodiversity loss and conserve at least 80% of preindustrial species richness, by protecting the remaining 50% of the Earth as intact ecosystems. A recently published analysis shows that it will still be possible to feed the future world population in such a "Half-Earth" strategy, but that a "Great Food Transformation" will be needed, in which all of us switch to a largely plant-based diet.[17]

Much more than switching to a vegan diet will be necessary to keep the other half of the Earth intact, and even then this will only save 80% of living species ... Whether such large transitions can and will be made on a voluntary basis remains to be seen. Democracy may have been an effective way of sharing population health improvements among humans, but can we realistically expect it to be effective in creating more equality between species?[18]

Re-thinking Utopia

We started this book by referring to Thomas More's 16th century Utopia, and its 19th century sequel written by Étienne Cabet. These utopian visions have served as a source of inspiration for all those who believed that a better world

16 Stuart L. Pimm et al., "The Biodiversity of Species and Their Rates of Extinction, Distribution, and Protection," *Science* 344, no. 6187 (2014): 1246752-1-10.

17 The "Half-Earth" strategy was proposed by American biologist Edward O. Wilson; see Edward O. Wilson, *Half-Earth: Our Planet's Fight for Life* (New York & London: W.W. Norton & Co., 2016). The implications for humanity's feeding patterns were outlined in Walter C. Willett et al., "Food in the Anthropocene," *Lancet* 393, no. 10170 (2019): 447–92.

18 For further reflection, readers are referred to the growing literature on the challenges to democracy of climate change. Even leaving non-human interests aside, it is unclear whether liberal democracies can effectively create the collective action necessary to mitigate climate change; see Marcello Di Paola and Dale Jamieson, "Climate Change and the Challenges to Democracy," *University of Miami Law Review* 72 (2017): 369–424. However, autocracies will not necessarily perform better, as argued in Daniel J. Fiorino, *Can Democracy Handle Climate Change* (Cambridge: Polity, 2018).

could be created, in which human welfare would be infinitely better than in the 16th or 19th centuries. Today, at the beginning of the 21st century, we do live in such a world, with longer lives spent in much better material conditions and in considerably better health. In North-western Europe, this has even been achieved without the restrictions on personal freedom that More believed to be necessary for realising Utopia. Nevertheless, when we allow ourselves to look at the price that other living species have paid for our development, it is difficult to suppress a feeling of guilt.

Did the Utopias that inspired our actions, perhaps guide us in the wrong direction? Well, actually, Utopias have come in all sorts, and while some Utopias described an ideal state of abundance, in which advances in technology would provide humans with incredible levels of luxury, other Utopias described an ideal state in which maximum satisfaction would be reached by moderation and self-restraint. As a matter of fact, Thomas More's Utopia is an example of the latter. It has no private property, and its inhabitants achieve happiness and spiritual fulfilment though harmony with nature.[19]

One wonders whether it is possible to imagine a modern version of Utopia, in which reasonable levels of human welfare, including high levels of health and personal freedom, are combined with a sufficient level of ecological sustainability. Writing Utopias has gone out of fashion, perhaps because utopian visions have become associated with lack of realism, or because attempts to realize utopian visions have often ended in authoritarianism. Yet, utopian visions may still be able to guide us, as illustrated by the popularity of Ernest Callenbach's book *Ecotopia* when it was published in 1975. This describes a small country on the West Coast of North America whose people live an egalitarian life close to nature. Ecological sustainability is achieved through local production and endless recycling, and marijuana is used on a large scale to achieve the higher states of consciousness required for complete ecological 'attunement'.[20]

While this solution may not sound 100% convincing, there is an urgent need for re-thinking our goals, and for developing a concrete vision of what an ecologically responsible 'Utopia' would look like. In any case, continuing in a 'business-as-usual' mode seems unwise, even if human health is all we care for.

19 Marius de Geus, *Ecological Utopias* (Utrecht: International Books, 1999).

20 For an analysis of the end of utopia-writing, see Krishan Kumar, "The Ends of Utopia," *New Literary History* 41, no. 3 (2010): 549–69. Full reference for *Ecotopia*: Ernest Callenbach, *Ecotopia* (Indore: Banyan Tree Books, 1975).

By Way of Conclusion

Through the Telescope of History

The history of population health sketched in this book spans more than three centuries: it starts in the early 1700s, when the first quantitative data begin to flow, and it ends just before today, several decades after other histories of population health have closed their pages. What have we seen through this very long 'telescope of history', that we would not have seen in a more myopic time-frame?

The most important thing we have seen – perhaps already over-emphasized in the preceding pages – is that most diseases have followed a trajectory of 'rise-and-fall'. When we go back far enough in time, we see smallpox, malaria, tuberculosis, the infectious diseases of childhood and many other 'diseases of pre-industrial and industrializing societies' rise to their 17th, 18th or 19th century highs, before they started their better-documented declines.

Similarly, when we study the health conditions that replaced these diseases, and dominated population health in the second half of the 20th century, we see almost all of them starting to fall, sometimes as recently as the 1990s. This does not only apply to the well-known examples of ischaemic heart disease and road traffic injury, but also to cancers of the breast, lung and other organs, liver cirrhosis, suicide and many other 'diseases of affluence' (for want of a better name).

These 'rises-and-falls' were experienced by Europeans whose structural and functional 'design' has not changed: the genes that determined the build-up and workings of their ancestors' bodies and minds are almost 100% the same as theirs. The only reasonable explanation for these striking changes in disease patterns is that something has changed in the interaction with their environment.

These changes have not happened once, but many times. Dozens of times there were negative trends first, but positive outcomes in the end. The implications of this regularity in our historical experience are many, and some of these have already been highlighted earlier. Here we will try to dig a bit deeper still, highlighting some of the profounder implications.

A theoretical implication of the fact that diseases had to 'rise' from low levels to become frequent at a later point in time, is that most diseases are, in a sense, 'man-made'. In the course of history, humans have actively produced their own diseases, or, in the case of diseases that already afflicted their distant ancestors, they have themselves raised the frequency with which they occurred. Most diseases do not originate in the inner workings of our cells, but in how we interact with the outside world. This also implies that medicine should – to repeat the famous words of Rudolf Virchow – be a social science as much as it is a branch of biology.[21]

A closely related implication is that most diseases are avoidable. The historical experience proves this empirically for the diseases of the 19th and 20th centuries which have since declined, or even disappeared. It must also be true for the diseases whose incidence has risen more recently but not yet declined, or not yet declined much. Even at the start of the 21st century, the theoretical scope for prevention is enormous. Most of today's cardiovascular disease, cancer, injury and other health problems would simply not occur, if we had eliminated their well-known behavioural or environmental determinants.

However, we do not sufficiently exploit this avoidability of disease. This starts when new health problems arise: is it really necessary for new diseases to reach epidemic proportions, before we start to tackle them? It is perhaps inevitable that we do not immediately recognize new health risks when we embark on new activities, and that we need a bit of time to develop an effective counter-strategy. Nevertheless, it usually takes far longer than strictly necessary before a 'rise' is reversed into a 'fall'. AIDS is the exception (at least in North-western Europe) that confirms the rule.

Powerful counterforces, in the form of commercial interests, cultural barriers, political inertia or simple silliness, often cause substantial delays. It was not necessary for cholera to still cause so many European deaths during the fifth pandemic (1881–96), or for lung cancer to rise until the 1980s, 1990s or even later in so many European countries.

Furthermore – and this should temper our enthusiasm about recent advances in population health – it has become much easier to control the health outcomes of our interactions with the environment, than to change these interactions themselves. The recent 'falls' of cardiovascular disease and cancer were to a large extent due to medical interventions, such as antihypertensive and cholesterol-lowering drugs and advanced cancer treatments. While the declines in mortality from these conditions are more than welcome, it would have been preferable if these had mainly been achieved by controlling the well-known behavioural and environmental risk factors of these diseases.

Finally, the 'telescope of history' also makes us see the 'epidemiologic transition' in a different perspective. The last decades of the 19th century and the first half of the 20th century were certainly special, in the sense that many important causes of mortality declined rapidly and simultaneously. Yet, the absence of natural dividing-lines with earlier and later periods, and the virtually continuous succession of diseases starting to fall in the 17th, 18th, 19th and

21 See Chapter 3 for the full quote, and what made Virchow say this.

20th centuries, suggest that the concept of one or even a few 'epidemiologic transitions' has limited usefulness.

The European Experience

It has been difficult to find a satisfactory explanation for the spectacular increase in life expectancy, and the somewhat less spectacular but still substantial improvements in other aspects of population health. Many authors, including this one, have found it easier to criticize McKeown's conclusion that improvements in living standards did the trick, than to come up with an explanation that better fits the facts, but can still be summarized in a few sentences.

Although recent scholarship has been able to demonstrate a neat causal relationship here, and another one there, the many interlinkages between the factors underlying population health improvement have made it impossible to empirically identify which factor was the most important. Logically, however, when one sees so many diseases 'fall', one after the other, it is impossible to escape the conclusion that some form of goal-directed 'human agency' played a crucial role. What this exactly was has been better documented for the more recent 'falls', but the consistency in the time-pattern clearly suggests that the same factor – human intervention in one form or another – was at work throughout.

This can be in the form of public health and medical care, but also in the form of less intentional changes in individual or collective behaviour that are – often implicitly – guided by concerns for human welfare. Everything in the European experience confirms this, and it is by studying variations between European countries' health trajectories that we can sometimes put a finger on what the necessary ingredients of this 'human agency' were.

One important conclusion is that – even if we include the most recent health improvements – the contribution of public health has been greater than that of medical care. The contribution of public health measures has also been greater than suggested by studies done in North-western Europe. In the first decades of the 20th century, mortality from the 'diseases of industrializing societies' was still high in Southern, Central-eastern, South-eastern and Eastern Europe. Introduction of public health measures therefore had a much larger impact on mortality decline there than it had in North-western Europe.

Another important conclusion is that the contribution of medical care has increased over time, and has become far greater than suggested by studies done up to the 1970s. It may be true that much of the mortality decline (in North-western Europe) until the 1970s antedated the introduction of effective medical treatments. However, this is not true for the mortality decline during and after the 1970s. Over the last decades, improvements in medical care have become a major driver of improvements in population health.

The European experience also shows that changes in economic conditions were undoubtedly important as a background factor, but also that these were not the direct or even the ultimate cause of population health improvements. There are just too many exceptions to the rule that economic development should have positive health consequences, and that health improvements should follow economic growth. Many advances in health have also preceded or coincided with countries' economic development.

The European experience suggests that changes in sociocultural conditions have been at least as important. For example, differences between countries in the penetration of the 'Enlightenment' made them front-runners or laggards in population health improvement. Sociocultural change is also the more plausible 'prime mover' of population health improvement. The development of a more rational way of thinking was the result of an autonomous process that some European countries had been following for centuries, and that probably set in motion all the other changes.

Through the rise of science and technology, it led to a better understanding of health and disease and the development of effective public health and medical interventions. Through the agricultural and industrial revolutions, it led to a rise in living standards. And through gradual political reforms and abrupt revolutions it led to the rise of the modern state, more democratic government, and the adoption of 'enlightened' social and health policies.

The Role of Politics

It has also been striking to see how closely population health followed European countries' political trajectories, and how effective some countries' political determination has been to get rid of infectious and other diseases. From malaria to tobacco, and from syphilis to air pollution, creating conditions for health improvement was a profoundly political enterprise. Usually, the state played a crucial role by providing the necessary infrastructure, legislation or funding. Decisions for and against were often hotly debated in parliaments, municipal councils, politburos and other political arenas. At first sight, therefore, the European experience also confirms the other part of Rudolf Virchow's famous one-liner: "politics is nothing else than medicine at a larger scale."

In terms of importance for population health, political conditions do not trump economic and sociocultural conditions, but politics has always had the special attention of public health professionals. It is not for nothing that Virchow's one-liner is one of the most widely quoted statements in public health. It summarises public health's biggest idea: human health and disease are the embodiment of the successes and failures of society as a whole, and the only way to radically improve health and reduce disease is by changing society, which – if it does not happen spontaneously – can only be achieved by political action. In milder form, modern textbooks of public health have come to see influencing government policy as a standard ingredient of public health practice.

However, throughout European history politics has not only been a benevolent but also a malicious force. Politics has not only been medicine at a larger scale, but also violence, exploitation and injustice at a larger scale. The apparatus of the modern state can be used for good and for bad things, and pursuing health improvement sometimes went hand-in-hand with brutal oppression. Stalin's ruthless reforms of Russian society ultimately saved the lives of millions of people, but cost the lives of millions of other people. *In extremis,* this is where Virchow's idea can lead to, if there are no moral restraints on the means that can be used to attain otherwise legitimate ends.

Another qualification of Virchow's idea – often ignored by public health professionals – is that it is not 'left' vs. 'right' that makes the difference. Throughout the 19th and 20th centuries, the most important cleavage in European politics was that between the 'left' (mainly represented by social-democratic and communist parties) and the 'right' (represented by conservative and fascist parties), with Christian-democratic parties and their predecessors often occupying the 'centre'. Which of these parties dominated government certainly did have an impact, for example on income distribution and social security, but on the whole was not decisive for population health.

What does make a difference is the relative importance given to health improvement as compared to other political objectives, steadfast resistance to commercial and other interests which detract from prioritizing health, and the use of effective policies to achieve good health outcomes. Although the track record of left-wing parties is somewhat better than that of right-wing parties, health policies and health outcomes have over time gradually converged, probably because 'health' has become an almost universally accepted touchstone of government policy. Nevertheless, engaging with politics was, is, and will remain necessary for attaining high levels of population health.

The Future

When non-historians write history, they often have a 'hidden agenda'. McKeown wanted to demonstrate that the more important role of medicine was to care, not to cure. When I started writing this book, I hoped that it would demonstrate that "we can": just like we create our own diseases, we have the power to get rid of them. Yet, while such a positive vision is certainly defensible in light of the European experience, a more pessimistic vision is also possible.

This book is a story of tremendous progress, but we can no longer close our eyes to the darker sides of this history. First of all, and continuing in the mode of human self-interest, it is uncertain whether our current levels of population health can be sustained. To a large extent, they have been mortgaged on the health of future generations, by ruthlessly exploiting and – if we do not stop this very soon – destroying our habitat. We have to a large extent controlled the health threats in our immediate environment, but have created new health threats at the planetary level that may turn out to be fatal flaws in our survival strategy.

While this alone already makes it difficult to end this book on a 100% positive note, there is more bad news. We can also no longer look away when other species disappear from the earth as a result of human expansion. It is a bitter irony that proving McKeown wrong proves him right at another level. McKeown argued that we should not think too highly of medicine's capacity to save lives, and that we should place our trust in low-tech solutions, like a full stomach and good nursing care. We now believe that we can trust public health and medical technologies to really save lives, but we are no longer fully convinced that we have done well to – in this way – help multiply humanity's ecological footprint.

We must therefore re-think the role of public health and medical care, making sure that whatever we do to further improve population health in the future, fits within ecologically sustainable boundaries. Most of all, in order to save the large majority of other living species on this planet, we may need to scale down our activities and consumption substantially. Less humans, or less health per human, may be the price to pay for preserving biodiversity. Achieving this is a tall order, but – in a final leap of the imagination – I am inclined to believe that the historical experience shows that "we can."

Appendix

Suppl. Part I, Chapters 1–3

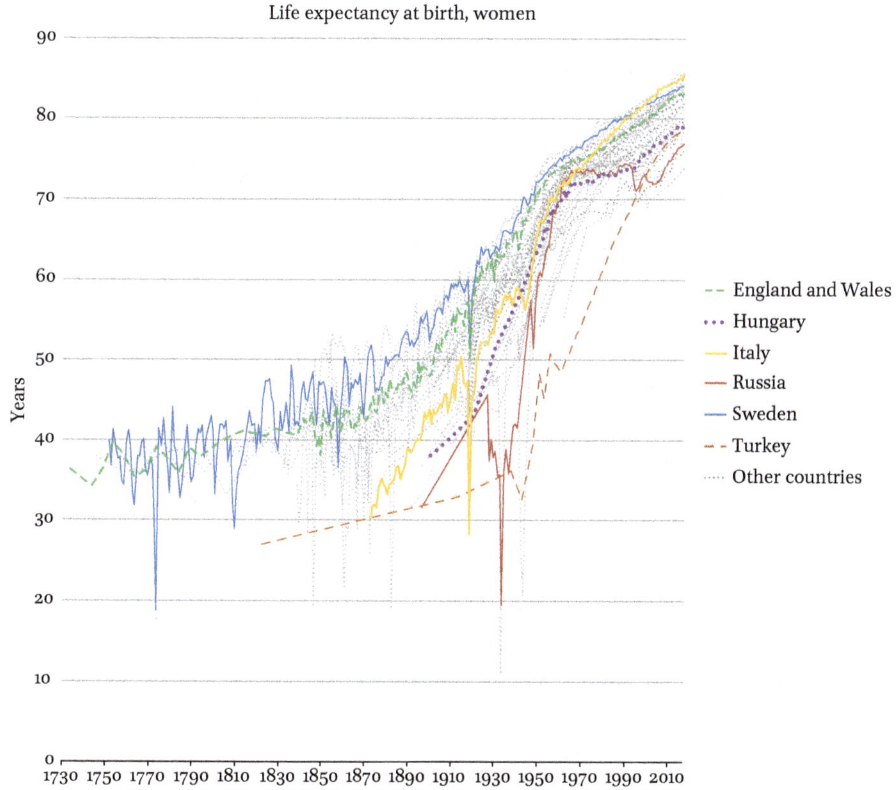

SUPPL. FIGURE 1 Trends in life expectancy in Europe, 1730–2015, women
SOURCE OF DATA: SEE SUPPL. TABLE 1

SUPPL. TABLE 1 Sources of mortality data

Indicator	Data sources
Life expectancy	Human Mortality Database (mortality.org; accessed 23/11/2018) Human Lifetable Database (lifetable.de; accessed 23/11/2018) WHO Health for All Databases (gateway.euro.who.int/en/datasets/european-health-for-all-database; accessed 22/11/2018) Eurostat (ec.europa.eu/eurostat/data/database; accessed 22/11/2018) World Bank (data.worldbank.org; accessed 23/11/2018) Country-specific data sources
Crude mortality rates	Mitchell: International Historical Statistics 1750–2010 (Volume 3: Europe; published 2013) Chesnais: The demographic transition (Table A3; published 1992) WHO Health for All Databases (gateway.euro.who.int/en/datasets/european-health-for-all-database; accessed 09/07/2018) Eurostat (ec.europa.eu/eurostat/data/database; accessed 20/12/2018) Gille: Demographic history of the Northern European countries (appendix III; published 1949) Country-specific data sources
Infant mortality rates	Mitchell: International Historical Statistics 1750–2010 (Volume 3: Europe; published 2013) WHO Health for All Databases (gateway.euro.who.int/en/datasets/european-health-for-all-database; accessed 09/07/2018) Eurostat (ec.europa.eu/eurostat/data/database; accessed 30/11/2018) Country-specific data sources
Age-specific mortality rates	Human Mortality Database (mortality.org; accessed 23/11/2018) Human Lifetable Database (lifetable.de; accessed 23/11/2018)

SUPPL. TABLE 1 Sources of mortality data (*cont.*)

Indicator	Data sources
Cause-specific mortality	Alderson: International Mortality Statistics (published 1981) WHO International Mortality Database (who.int/healthinfo/mortality_data; accessed 14/02/2019) Cause-specific data sources
Maternal mortality	Alderson: International Mortality Statistics (published 1981) WHO International Mortality Database (who.int/healthinfo/mortality_data; accessed 14/02/2019) Loudon: Death in childbirth (appendix 6; published 1992) Country-specific data sources
Still-births	Mitchell: International Historical Statistics 1750–2010 (Volume 3: Europe; published 2013) Masuy-Stroobant: Infant health and infant mortality in Europe (table 1A.2; published 1997) Country-specific data sources
Other	Data sources listed below tables and graphs

SUPPL. TABLE 2 ICD-codes for causes of death

	ICD-1	ICD-5	ICD-8	ICD-10
	ca. 1901-	**1938-**	**ca. 1965-**	**ca. 1990-**
Cholera	12	4	0	A00
Typhoid, paratyphoid	1,164	1,2,177	001–003	A01
Bacillary dysentery	14	27	4	A03
Resp. tuberculosis	26,27	13	010–012	A15–A16
Syphilis	36,62,67	30	090–097	A50–A52
Scarlet fever	7	8	34	A38
Measles	6	35	55	B05
Whooping cough	8	9	33	A37
Diphtheria	9	10	32	A36
HIV/AIDS	N/A	N/A	N/A	B20–B24
All infectious diseases	1–9,11,12, 14–24, 26–38,61, 62,67,72, 107,111	1–32,34–43, 44,177	000–136	A00–B99
Pneumonia	92,93	107–109	480–486	J12–J18
Influenza	10	33	470–474	J10–J11
All respiratory diseases	10,87,88, 90–96,98,99	33,104–111, 113–115	460–519	J00–J98
Ischaemic heart disease	N/A	92ac,93cd,94	410–414	I20–I25
Cerebrovascular disease	64–66,82a	83	430–438	I60–I69
All cardiovascular diseases	64–66,82a, 77–86,142	83,90b, 91–103,111a	393–458	I00–I99
Stomach cancer	40	46b	151	C16
Colorectal cancer	41	46cd	152–154	C18–C21
Lung cancer (incl. trachea and bronchus)	N/A	47b	162	C33–C34
Breast cancer	43	50	174	C50
Prostate cancer	N/A	51b	185	C61

SUPPL. TABLE 2 ICD-codes for causes of death (*cont.*)

	ICD-1	ICD-5	ICD-8	ICD-10
	ca. 1901-	**1938-**	**ca. 1965-**	**ca. 1990-**
All neoplasms	39–46,53, 74,129,131	44b,45–55,74	140–239	C00–D48
Diabetes mellitus	50	61	250	E10–E14
Peptic ulcer	103	117	531–533	K25–K27
Appendicitis	118	121	540–543	K35–K37
Liver cirrhosis	112	124	571	K70, K74
Dementias	N/A	N/A	N/A	F01–03,G30
Maternal mortality	134–141	140–150	630–678	O00–O99
Motor vehicle injuries	N/A	170	E810–E823	V02–V04, V09, V12–V14, V20–V79, V82–V87, V89
Suicide	155–163	163–164	E950–E959	X60–X84
Homicide	182–184	165–168,198	E960–E978	X85–Y09
All non-natural causes	57,59,153, 155–172, 174–176	78,79,40–43, 163–176, 178–198	E800–E999	V01–Y89

Notes: Selection of years only. Some countries (e.g., Portugal, countries of former Soviet Union) used different codes in certain periods

SUPPL. TABLE 3 Correlations between determinants and life expectancy, 1870–2010s

A.	Cross-sectional correlation (level of determinant vs. level					
	Men	**Women**	**Men**	**Women**	**Men**	**Women**
	1870	**1870**	**1900**	**1900**	**1930**	**1930**
National income	−0.10	−0.12	0.38	0.43	**0.73**	**0.77**
Level of democracy	−0.07	−0.10	0.23	0.30	**0.71**	**0.81**
Protestant legacy	**0.69**	**0.80**	**0.57**	**0.65**	**0.63**	**0.63**
Average education	**0.77**	**0.79**	**0.69**	**0.71**	**0.73**	**0.74**

B.	Cross-sectional correlation (level of determinant vs. level					
	Men	**Women**	**Men**	**Women**	**Men**	**Women**
	1870	**1870**	**1900**	**1900**	**1930**	**1930**
National income	−0.51	**−0.53**	−0.10	−0.07	0.25	0.32
Level of democracy	0.55	**0.53**	−0.12	−0.04	−0.01	0.14
Protestant legacy	**0.65**	**0.64**	**0.53**	**0.54**	**0.44**	**0.38**
Average education	**0.51**	**0.54**	0.54	0.51	0.40	0.27

C.	Longitudinal correlation (level of determinant vs.			
	Men	**Women**	**Men**	**Women**
	1870–1900	**1870–1900**	**1900–1930**	**1900–1930**
National income	−0.13	0.10	**0.47**	0.38
Level of democracy	−0.24	−0.04	0.15	0.24
Protestant legacy	−0.50	−0.66	0.30	0.00
Average education	−0.66	−0.60	0.37	0.14

of life expectancy; univariate)

Men	**Women**	**Men**	**Women**	**Men**	**Women**
1960	**1960**	**1990**	**1990**	**2010**	**2010**
0.74	**0.78**	**0.62**	**0.79**	**0.70**	**0.80**
0.66	**0.67**	**0.72**	**0.75**	**0.60**	**0.50**
0.54	**0.50**	**0.37**	**0.45**	**0.35**	**0.34**
0.41	**0.38**	0.24	0.32	0.34	0.30

of life expectancy; multivariate)

Men	**Women**	**Men**	**Women**	**Men**	**Women**
1960	**1960**	**1990**	**1990**	**2010**	**2010**
0.03	0.40	0.55	**0.83**	**0.81**	**0.95**
0.35	0.21	0.43	0.31	**0.49**	**0.39**
0.26	0.16	−0.05	−0.10	**−0.26**	**−0.31**
0.25	0.15	−0.11	−0.22	−0.03	−0.14

change in life expectancy; univariate)

Men	**Women**	**Men**	**Women**	**Men**	**Women**
1930–1960	**1930–1960**	**1960–1990**	**1960–1990**	**1990–2010**	**1990–2010**
−0.72	**−0.71**	−0.31	**−0.45**	**0.46**	0.02
−0.72	**−0.74**	0.10	−0.07	**0.51**	0.29
−0.51	−0.55	−0.19	−0.20	0.19	−0.11
−0.72	−0.68	0.09	0.03	0.20	−0.18

SUPPL. TABLE 3 Correlations between determinants and life expectancy, 1870–2010s (*cont.*)

D.	**Longitudinal correlation (change in**			
	Men	**Women**	**Men**	**Women**
	1870–1900	**1870–1900**	**1900–1930**	**1900–1930**
National income	−0.41	−0.29	0.41	0.13
Level of democracy	−0.40	−0.53	0.17	−0.10
Protestant legacy	N/A	N/A	N/A	N/A
Average education	0.40	0.35	−0.07	0.14

Notes: This table shows correlation coefficients for the association between countries' level of determinants and their life expectancy. Correlation coefficients can take values between -1 and +1, with positive values indicating that a higher level of the determinant goes together with higher life expectancy. Table A: simple correlations between level of determinant and level of life expectancy at same point in time. Table B: multiple correlations between level of determinant and level of life expectancy at same point in time, controlling for the correlation with other determinants. Table C: simple correlations between level of determinant at begin of period and change in life expectancy during that period. Table D: simple correlations between change in determinant during a period and change in life expectancy during the same period. National income = Gross Domestic Product in 1990 I$ (source: www.clio-infra.eu); average education = average number of years of education (source: www.clio-infra.eu); protestant legacy = percent of population protestant ca. 1950 (source: www.qog.gu.se); level of democracy = polity_2 score (source: www.qog.gu.se). For Protestantism, no data on changes over time were available, and this variable is therefore missing in table D. In bold: statistically significant (p<.05)

determinant vs. change in life expectancy; univariate)

Men	Women	Men	Women	Men	Women
1930–1960	1930–1960	1960–1990	1960–1990	1990–2010	1990–2010
−0.59	**−0.54**	−0.08	−0.20	**0.51**	0.18
−0.35	−0.28	0.22	0.31	−0.25	−0.06
N/A	N/A	N/A	N/A	N/A	N/A
0.52	**0.54**	**−0.53**	**−0.54**	0.03	0.28

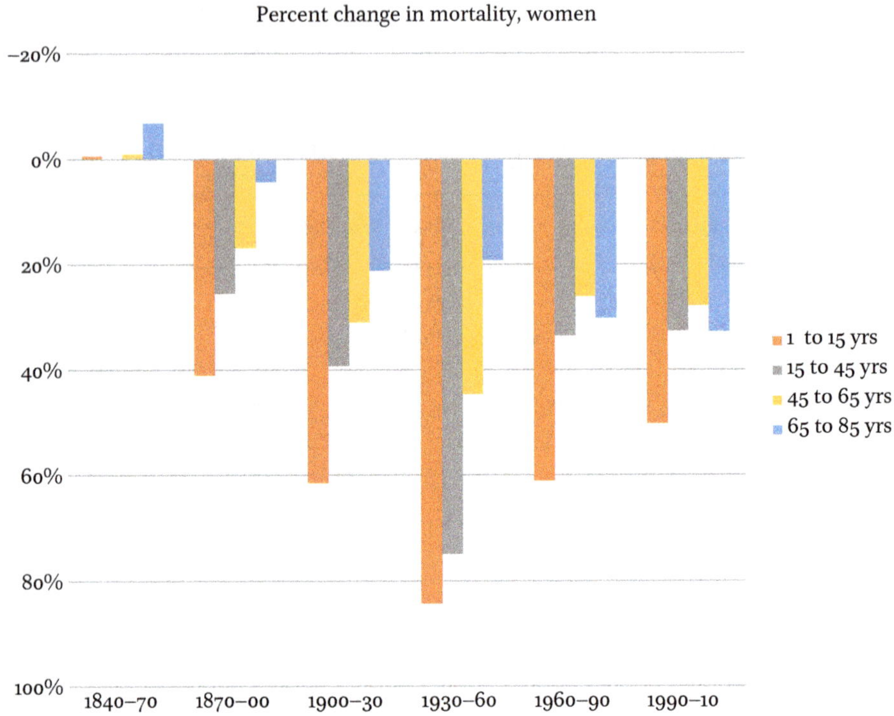

SUPPL. FIGURE 2 Mortality decline in Europe, by age and sex, 1870–2010
Notes: Calculated from arithmetic average of age-adjusted mortality rates (in each of the age-groups mentioned) for all countries with available data in 1840, 1870, 1900, 1930, 1960, 1990 and 2010
SOURCE OF DATA: SEE SUPPL. TABLE 1

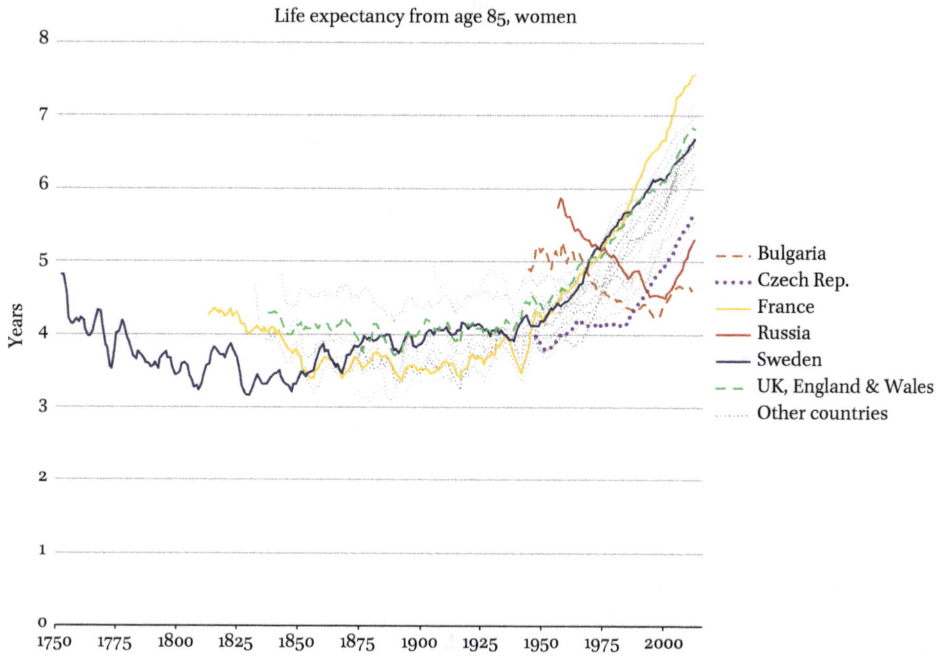

SUPPL. FIGURE 3 Life expectancy from age 85 in Europe, 1750–2015
Notes: Five-year moving averages. Women only; men similar
SOURCE OF DATA: SEE SUPPL. TABLE 1

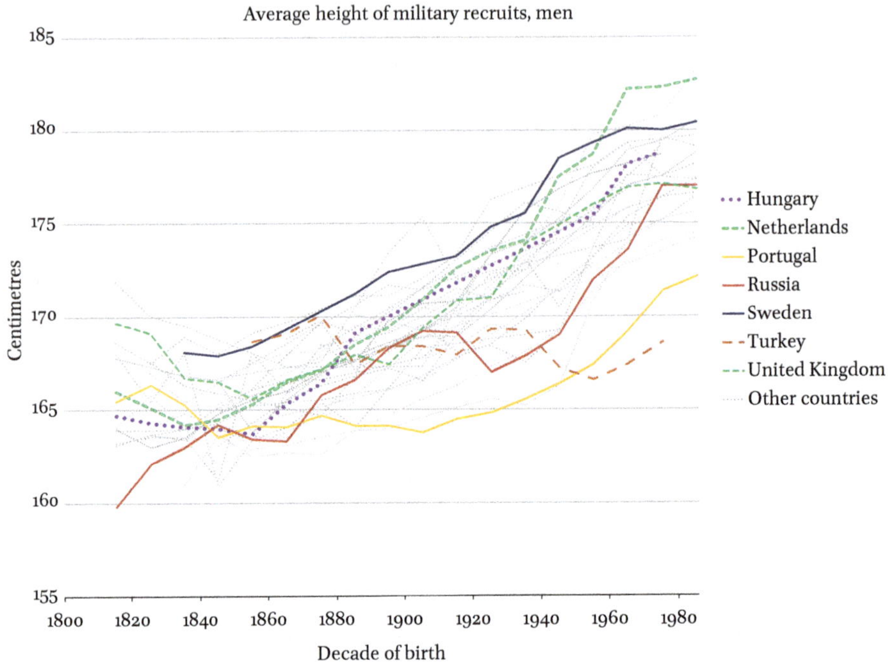

SUPPL. FIGURE 4 Trends in height of military recruits in Europe, 1800–1985
SOURCE OF DATA: WWW.CLIO-INFRA.EU (ACCESSED 07/12/2018)

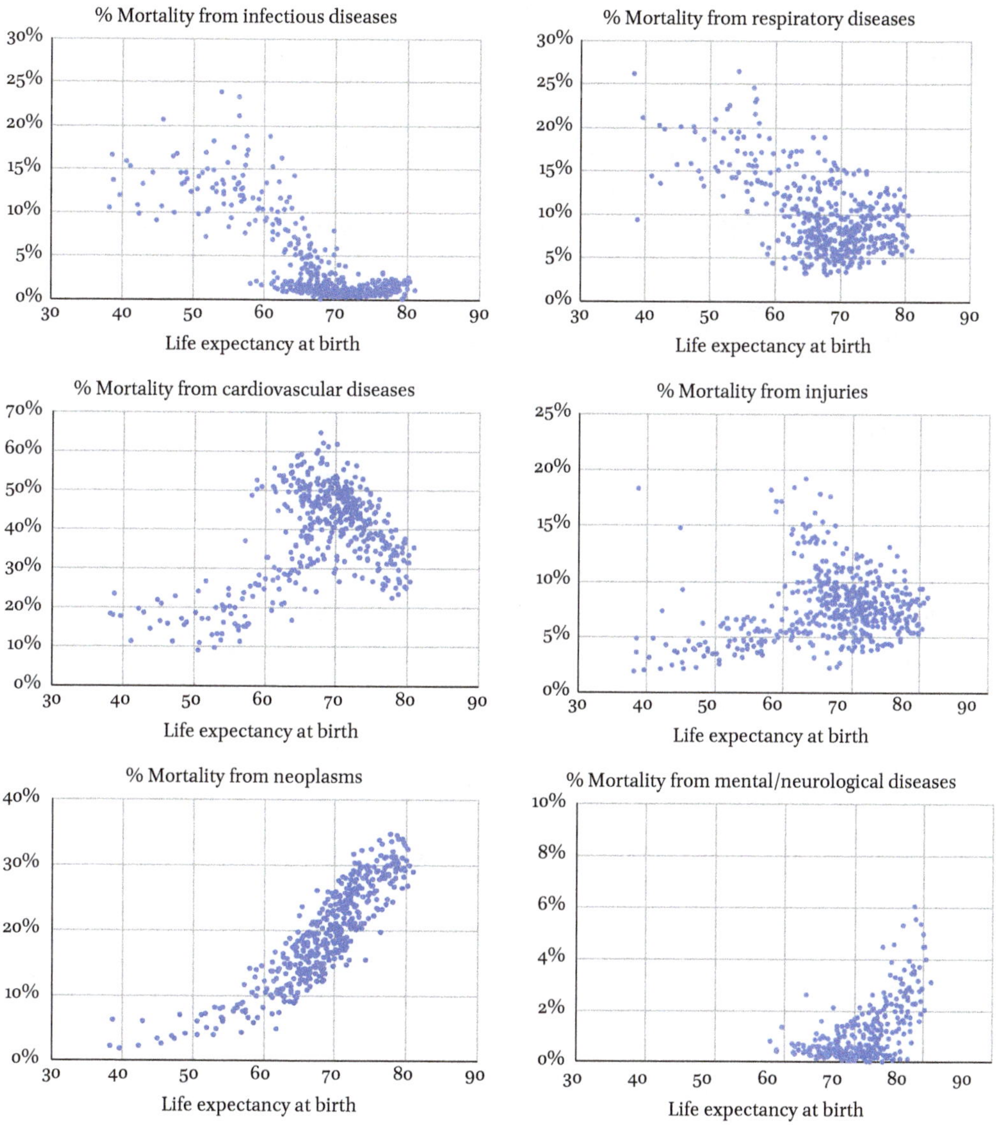

SUPPL. FIGURE 5 Shifts in cause-of-death patterns in Europe, ca. 1900–2015
Notes: Percent mortality calculated from age-standardized mortality rates. Each dot represents one country/decade combination
SOURCE OF DATA: SEE SUPPL. TABLE 1

SUPPL. TABLE 4 Differences in population health trends between European countries

		Variation in annual mortality rates, 1880–1900[a]	Year in which female life expectancy surpassed 50 years	Year in which infant mortality declined below 10%	Year in which female life expectancy surpassed 65 years	Year in which % male CVD deaths declined below 40%	Year in which female life expectancy surpassed 80 years
North	Finland	10%	1920	1925	1948	2005	1994
	Sweden	5%	1882	1902	1933	2005	1989
	Norway	6%	1883	1900	1930	2000	1991
	Denmark	7%	1894	1917	1937	1995	2005
West	England and Wales	5%	1902	1916	1942	2000	2000
	Ireland	4%	[<1911]	1905	1948	2005	2002
	Netherlands	9%	1901	1912	1930	1990	1994
	Belgium	7%	1901	1931	1947	1985	1994
	Germany	8%	1909	1927	*N/A*	2005	1997
	Austria	7%	1920	1933	1948	2005	1996
	Switzerland	7%	1901	1912	1936	1995	1984
South	France	4%	1907	1930	1947	*N/A*	1987
	Spain	7%	1927	1943	1952	1990	1987
	Portugal	6%	1941	1950	1958	1990	2000
	Italy	8%	1922	1946	1949	1990	1989
	Greece	*N/A*	1932	1940	[<1950]	2010	1993
Centre-east	Czech Republic	*N/A*	1921	1939	1947	n/y	2007
	Hungary	9%	1928	1948	1952	n/y	2010
	Poland	*N/A*	1922	1952	1953	n/y	n/y

SUPPL. TABLE 4 Differences in population health trends between European countries (*cont.*)

		Variation in annual mortality rates, 1880–1900[a]	Year in which female life expectancy surpassed 50 years	Year in which infant mortality declined below 10%	Year in which female life expectancy surpassed 65 years	Year in which % male CVD deaths declined below 40%	Year in which female life expectancy surpassed 80 years
South-east	Slovenia	*N/A*	[<1931]	*N/A*	1951	1995	2001
	Croatia	8%	*N/A*	*N/A*	1955	n/y	2011
	Serbia	11%	*N/A*	1969	[<1964]	n/y	n/y
	Yugoslavia (former)	*N/A*	[<1932]	1958	1961	n/y	n/y
	Albania	*N/A*	[<1950]	1956	1962	*N/A*	n/y
	Romania	10%	*N/A*	1953	1956	n/y	n/y
	Bulgaria	19%	1933	1952	1953	n/y	n/y
East	Lithuania	*N/A*	*N/A*	*N/A*	[<1952]	n/y	n/y
	Latvia	*N/A*	*N/A*	*N/A*	[<1952]	n/y	n/y
	Estonia	*N/A*	*N/A*	*N/A*	[<1952]	n/y	2009
	Russia	10%	1947	1953	1955	n/y	n/y
	"Early"	<8%	<1900	<1920	<1940	<2000	<2000
	"Mid"	8–10%	1900–1920	1920–1945	1940–1955	2000–2015	2000–2015
	"Late"	>10%	>1920	>1945	>1955	n/y	n/y

n/y not yet in 2015
[...] not directly observed, but inferred from other points in the time-series
N/A no data available
a coefficient of variation

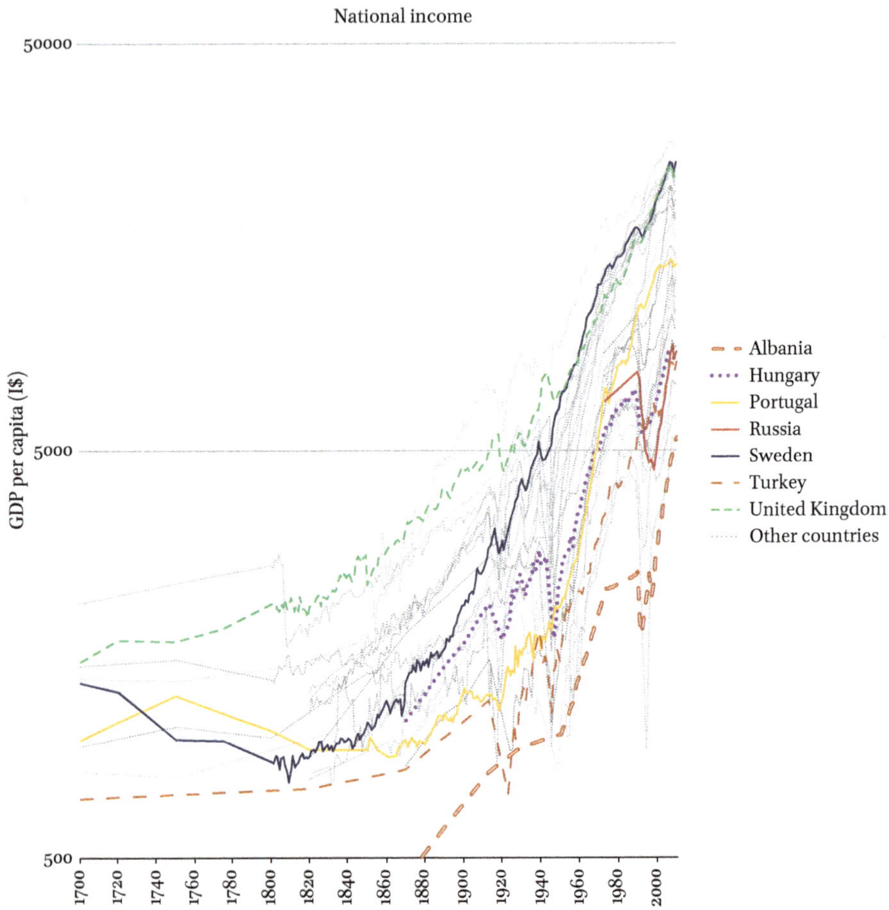

SUPPL. FIGURE 6 Trends in national income in Europe, 1700–2015
Notes: Sparse data before 1800
SOURCE OF DATA: OECD 'HOW WAS LIFE' PROJECT (WWW.CLIO-INFRA.EU), ACCESSED 28/08/2018

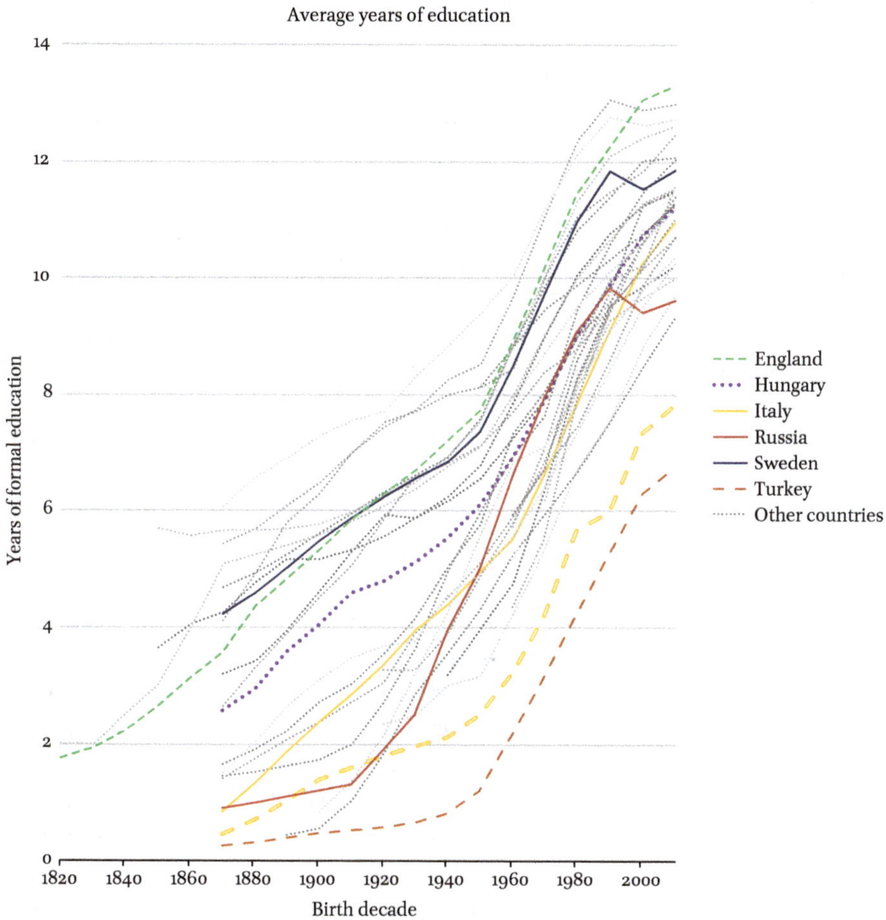

SUPPL. FIGURE 7 Trends in education levels in Europe, 1820–2010
Notes: Average number of years of formal education in the population aged 15 years and older
SOURCE OF DATA: WWW.CLIO-INFRA.EU (ACCESSED 28/08/2018)

Suppl. Part II, Chapters 4–6

SUPPL. TABLE 5 European war deaths, 1700–2010

Century	War	Deaths
Eighteenth century	Spanish succession (1701–1713)	1,000,000
	Great Northern War (1700–1721)	400,000
	Austrian succession (1740–1748)	500,000
	Seven Years War (1755–1763)	1,300,000
Nineteenth century	French/Napoleonic wars (1792–1815)	2,000,000
	Russo-Turkish war (1806–1812)	225,000
	Russo-Turkish war (1828–1829)	190,000
	First Carlist war (1832–1840)	100,000
	Crimean war (1854–1856)	300,000
	Franco-Prussian war (1870–1871)	200,000
	Russo-Turkish war (1877–1878)	250,000
Twentieth century	Balkan Wars (1912–1913)	140,000
	First World War (1914–1918)	10,000,000
	Russo-Polish War (1918–1920)	1,00,000
	Russian civil War (1917–1922)	2,000,000
	Greco-Turkish War (1919–1922)	400,000
	Spanish Civil War (1936–1939)	365,000
	Russo-Finnish War (1939–1940)	150,000
	Second World War (1939–1945)	41,000,000
	Greek Civil War (1943–1949)	158,000
	Yugoslav Wars (1991–2001)	140,000

Notes: Direct military and civilian deaths from war-related violence, and only if total number >100,000. Please note that most of these estimates are disputed, and have wide margins of uncertainty

SOURCE OF DATA: MEDIANS OF ESTIMATES PRESENTED ON (WWW.NECROMETRICS.COM ACCESSED 28/04/2019), EXCEPT THE NUMBERS FOR WORLD WARS I AND II WHICH ARE BASED ON NORMAN DAVIES. *EUROPE: A HISTORY*. LONDON: PIMLICO, 1997, PP. 1328–9

SUPPL. TABLE 6 A selection of major European famines, 1700–2010

Period	Name	Countries	Cause
1740–43	'Great Frost'	Northern Europe, Ireland	Extremely cold weather leading to crop failures and destruction of livestock
1816–17	'Year without a Summer'	Western and Continental Europe	Cold and wet weather due to eruption of Mount Tambora; economic and political upheaval after Napoleonic wars
1845–50	'Potato Famine'	Western and continental Europe	Potato Blight causing several crop failures in a row
1866–68	'The Great Hunger Years'	Northern and Eastern Europe	Cold and wet weather causing a succession of crop failures
1927–33	'Holodomor'	Ukraine, Russia, Kazakhstan	Drought causing a succession of crop failures; forced collectivization of agriculture
1946–47	-	Moldova, Ukraine	Drought causing crop failure; economic destruction after World War II

SOURCE OF DATA: GUIDO ALFANI AND CORMAC Ó GRÁDA. "FAMINES IN EUROPE: AN OVERVIEW." IN *FAMINE IN EUROPEAN HISTORY*, EDITED BY GUIDO ALFANI AND CORMAC Ó GRÁDA, 1–24. CAMBRIDGE ETC.: CAMBRIDGE UNIVERSITY PRESS, 2017, VARIOUS TABLES

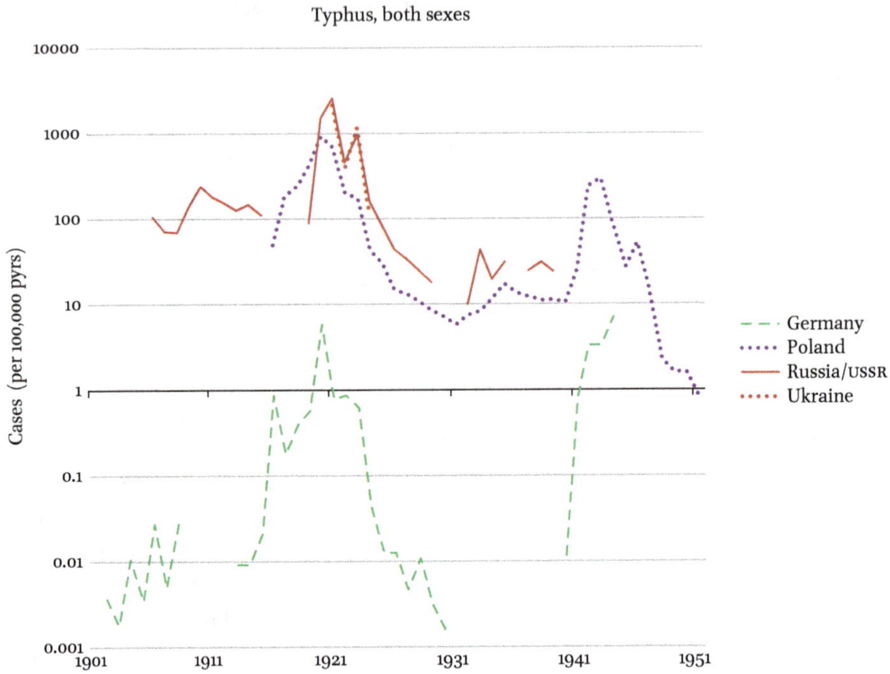

SUPPL. FIGURE 8 Trends in typhus incidence in selected European countries, 1901–1951
Notes: Logarithmic scale. Please note that country borders changed over time. For Poland 1915–1918, Rajchman's higher numbers have been selected for presentation; for Russia/Soviet Union, the officially published lower numbers have been selected for presentation
SOURCE OF DATA: ABSOLUTE NUMBER OF CASES FROM PAUL WEINDLING, *EPIDEMICS AND GENOCIDE IN EASTERN EUROPE, 1890–1945*. OXFORD ETC.: OXFORD UNIVERSITY PRESS, 2000, APP. 1.

SUPPL. TABLE 7 Deaths from cholera in selected European countries, 1831–1923

	Pandemic				
	Second (1831–32)	Third (1846–60)	Fourth (1863–75)	Fifth (1881–96)	Sixth (1899–23)
England & Wales	55,201	54,398	24,516	135	ca. 0
Netherlands	9543	22,078	21,286	276	ca. 0
Germany	N/A	N/A	ca. 120,000	10,361	ca. 0
France	ca. 100,000	ca. 150,000	44,202	8550	ca. 0
Spain	ca. 300,000	ca. 236,000	ca. 35,000	ca. 120,000	93
Italy	N/A	N/A	ca. 113,000	14,299	7236
Russia	ca. 100,000	>1,000,000	ca. 90,000	267,890	>500,000

Notes: N/A Not available (Germany and Italy were not yet united, so no national figures were collected)

SOURCE OF DATA: VARIOUS (NATIONAL AND INTERNATIONAL) PUBLICATIONS

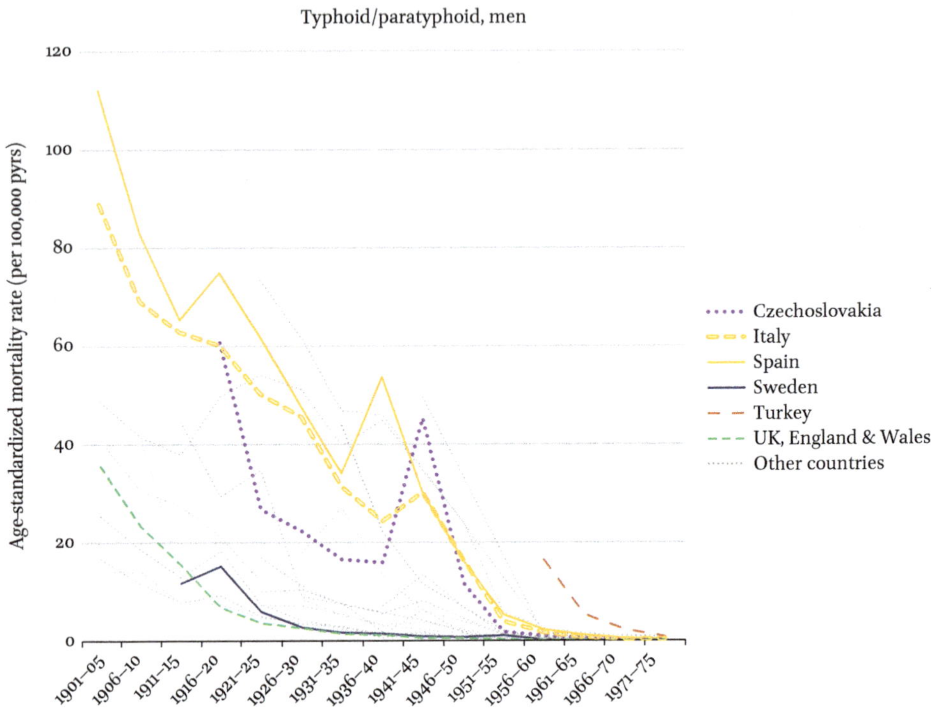

SUPPL. FIGURE 9 Trends in mortality from typhoid and paratyphoid fever in Europe, 1901–1975
Notes: Quinquennial data
SOURCE OF DATA: SEE SUPPL. TABLE 1

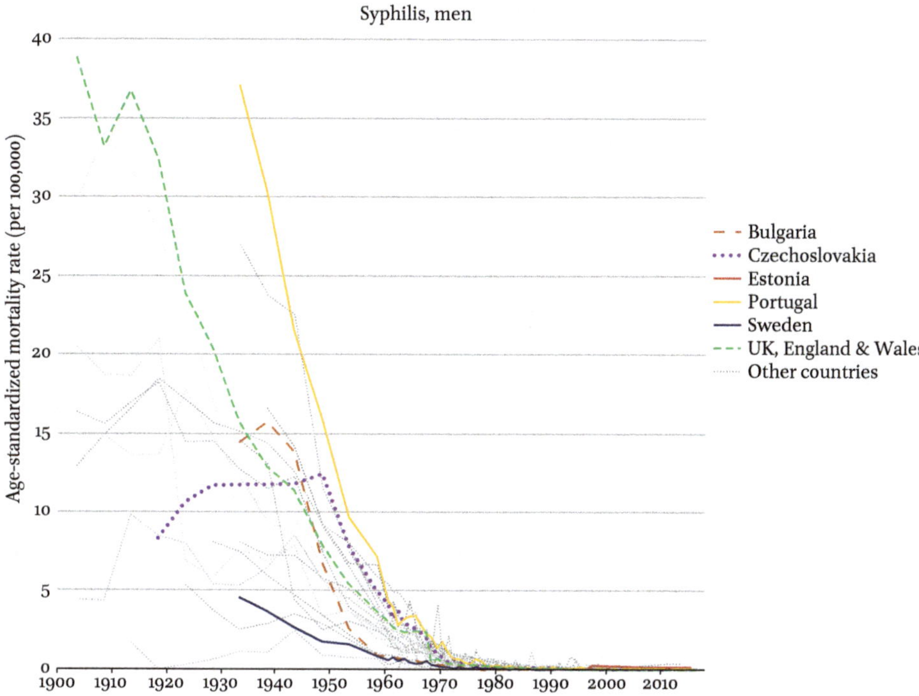

SUPPL. FIGURE 10 Trends in syphilis mortality in Europe, 1900–2015
Notes: Between 1900 and 1960: quinquennial data
SOURCE OF DATA: SEE SUPPL. TABLE 1

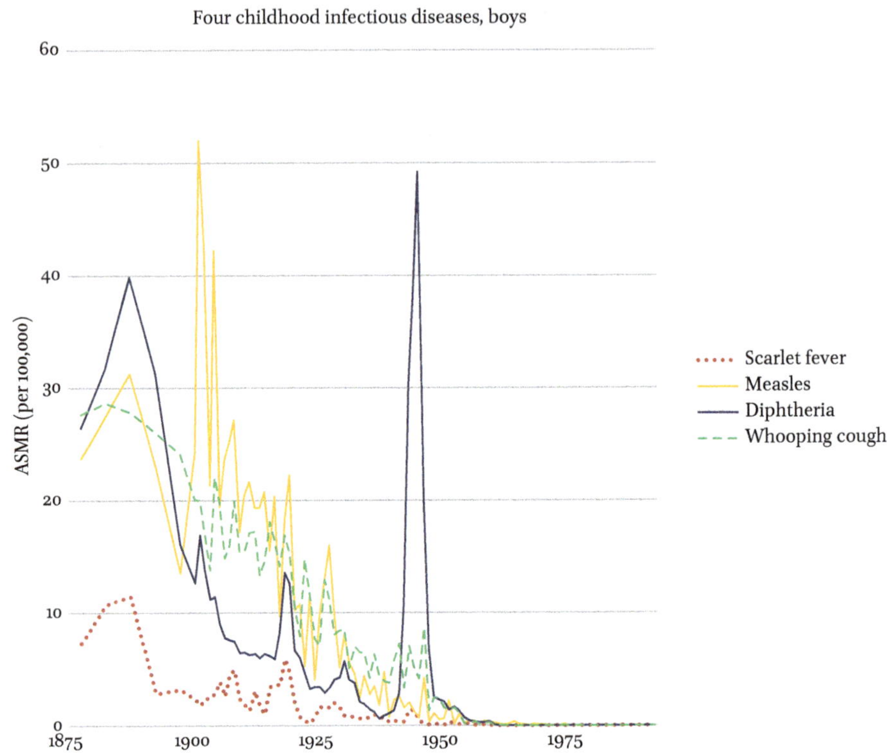

SUPPL. FIGURE 11 Trends in mortality from childhood infections in the Netherlands, 1875–1992

Notes: Before 1900: quinquennial data

SOURCE OF DATA: JUDITH H. WOLLESWINKEL-VAN DEN BOSCH. *THE EPIDEMIOLOGICAL TRANSITION IN THE NETHERLANDS*. ERASMUS UNIVERSITY, 1998

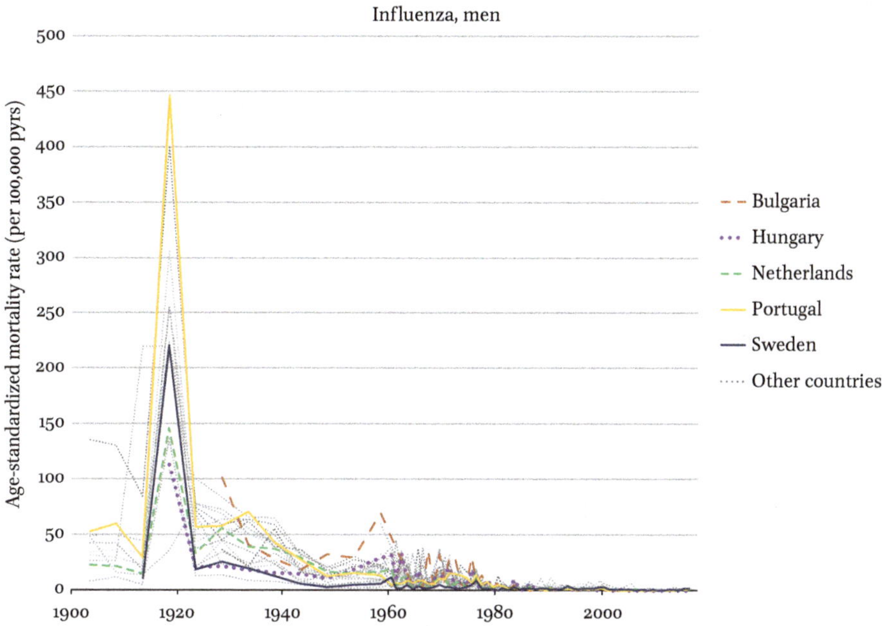

SUPPL. FIGURE 12 Trends in influenza mortality in Europe, 1900–2015
Notes: Between 1900 and 1960: quinquennial data
SOURCE OF DATA: SEE SUPPL. TABLE 1

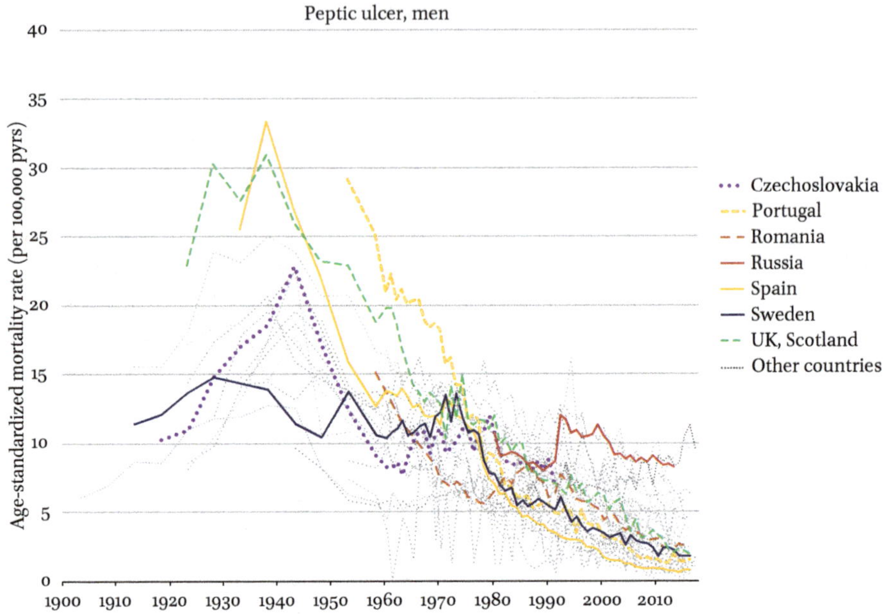

SUPPL. FIGURE 13 Trends in peptic ulcer mortality in Europe, 1900–2015
Notes: Quinquennial data before 1960
SOURCE OF DATA: SEE SUPPL. TABLE 1

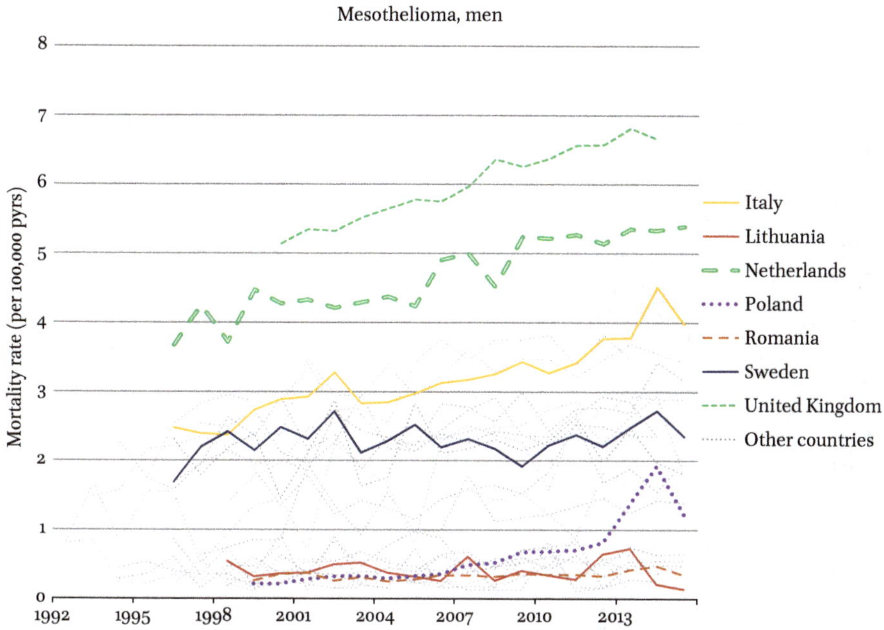

SUPPL. FIGURE 14 Trends in mesothelioma mortality in Europe, 1992–2015
SOURCE OF DATA: SEE SUPPL. TABLE 1

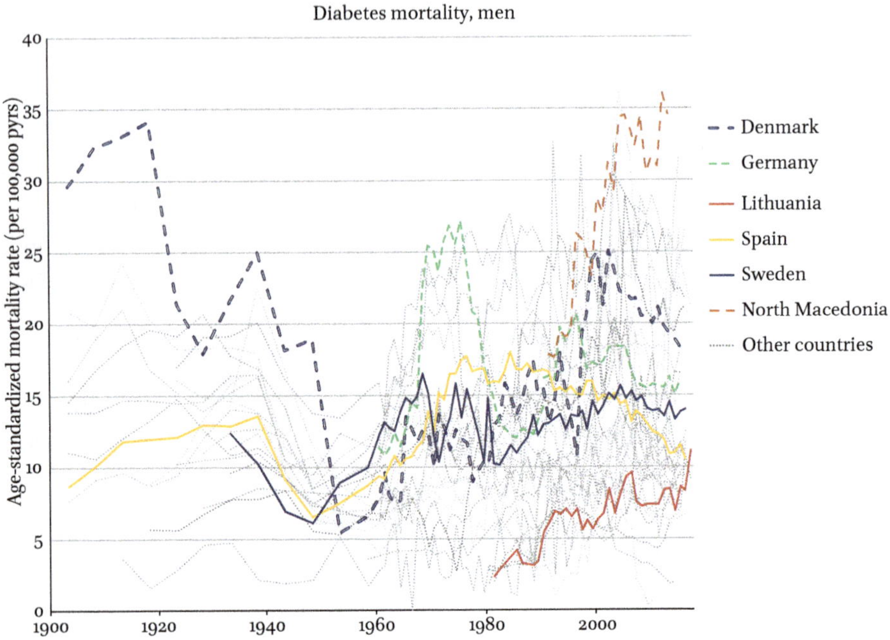

SUPPL. FIGURE 15 Trends in diabetes mortality in Europe, 1900–2015
Notes: Quinquennial data before 1960
SOURCE OF DATA: SEE SUPPL. TABLE 1

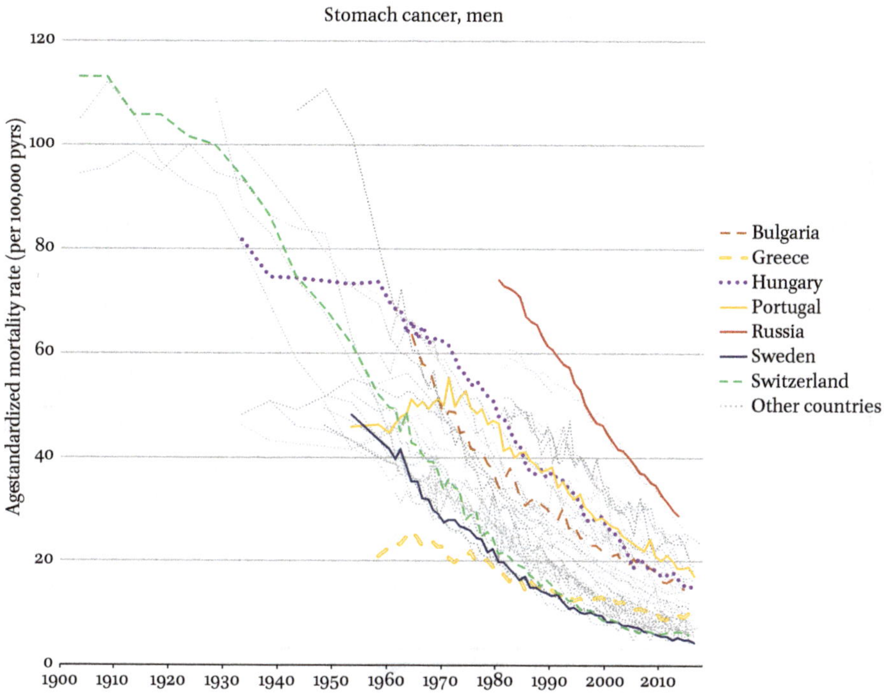

SUPPL. FIGURE 16 Trends in stomach cancer mortality in Europe, 1900–2015
Notes: Quinquennial data before 1960
SOURCE OF DATA: SEE SUPPL. TABLE 1

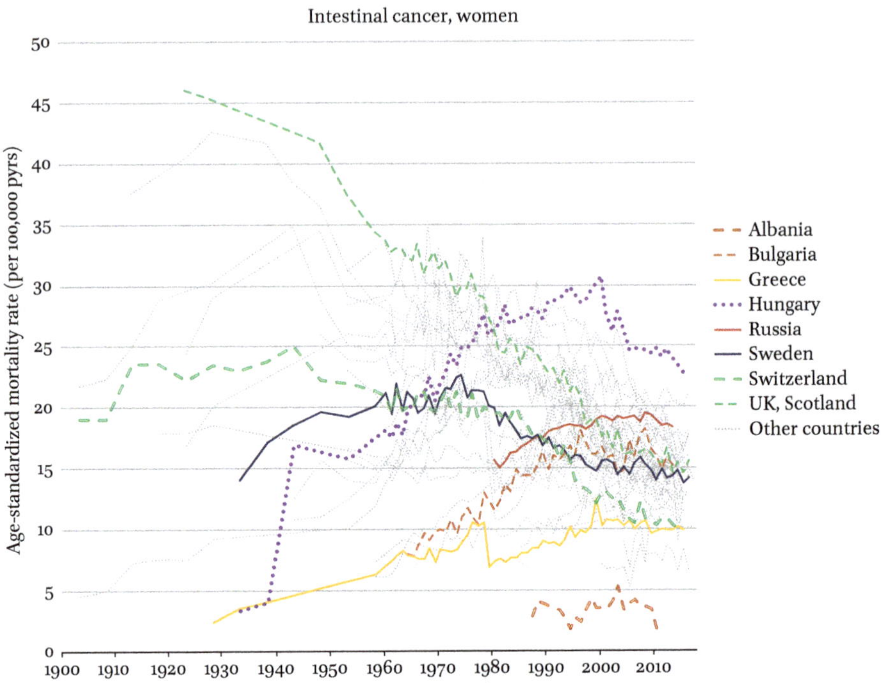

SUPPL. FIGURE 17 Trends in colorectal cancer mortality in Europe, 1900–2015
Notes: This is cancer in colorectum plus small intestine; likely to include other abdominal cancers as well before 1950. Quinquennial data before 1960
SOURCE OF DATA: SEE SUPPL. TABLE 1

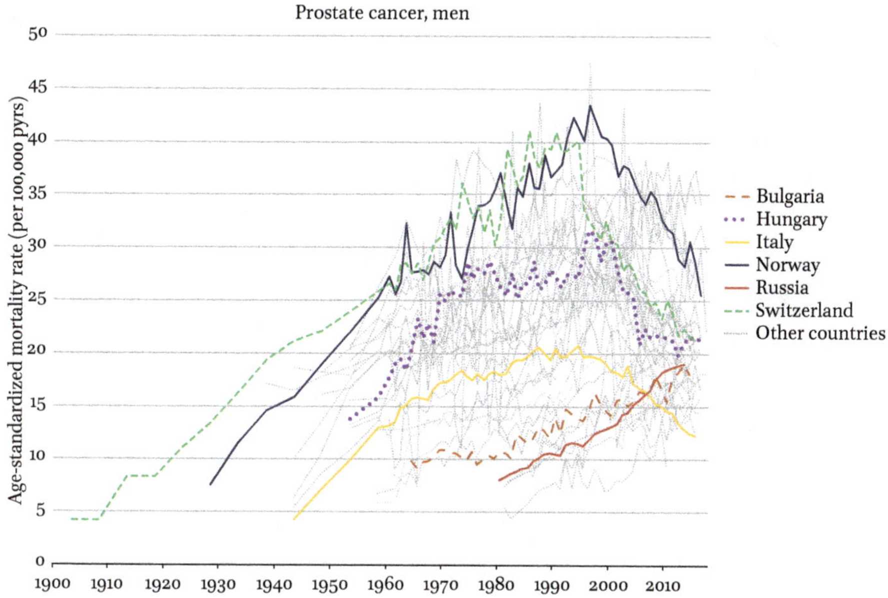

SUPPL. FIGURE 18 Trends in prostate cancer mortality in Europe, 1900–2015
SOURCE OF DATA: SEE SUPPL. TABLE 1

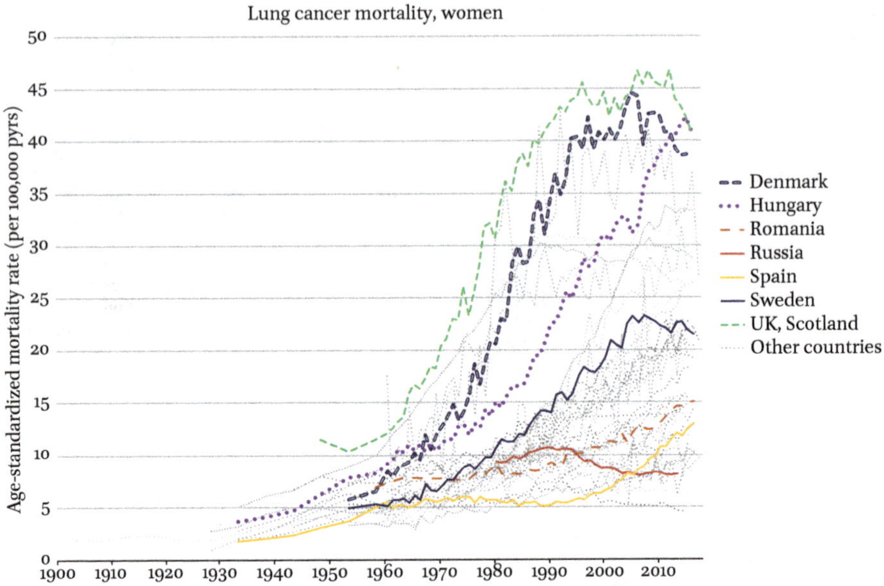

SUPPL. FIGURE 19 Trends in lung cancer mortality in Europe, women, 1900–2015
SOURCE OF DATA: SEE SUPPL. TABLE 1

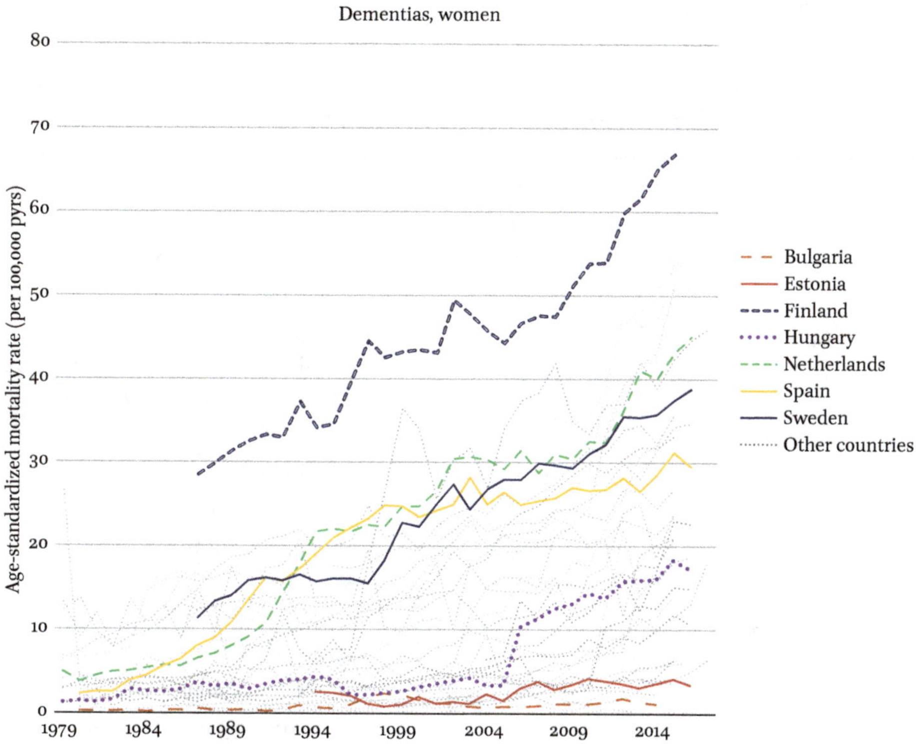

SUPPL. FIGURE 20 Trends in dementia mortality in Europe, 1979–2017
SOURCE OF DATA: SEE SUPPL. TABLE 1

Suppl. Part III, Chapters 7–8

SUPPL. TABLE 8 Contributions of specific diseases to mortality decline, ca. 1870–1950

		% Contribution to mortality decline (both sexes)	Remarks
Health problems of pre-industrial societies	War	[crisis]	Strong fluctuations; positive contribution, but magnitude inestimable
	Homicide	0.7%	European average (source: www.clio-infra.eu)
	Famine	[crisis]	Strong fluctuations; positive contribution, but magnitude inestimable
	Plague	.	Plague had been practically eliminated by 1870
	Smallpox	2.7%	Estimate for England & Wales (Logan 1950); probably higher elsewhere
	Typhus	[crisis]	Strong fluctuations; positive contribution, but magnitude inestimable
	Malaria	3.6%	Estimate for Italy (Bruce-Chwatt & De Zulueta 1980); lower elsewhere
Health problems of industrializing societies	Cholera, intestinal infections	21.0%	Estimate for England & Wales (Logan 1950); probably similar elsewhere
	Respiratory tuberculosis	28.0%	Estimate for England & Wales (Logan 1950); probably lower elsewhere
	Syphilis	0.4%	Estimate for England & Wales (Logan 1950); probably higher elsewhere
	Childhood infections	21.7%	Estimate for England & Wales (Logan 1950); probably similar elsewhere

SUPPL. TABLE 8 Contributions of specific diseases to mortality decline, ca. 1870–1950 (*cont.*)

		% Contribution to mortality decline (both sexes)	**Remarks**
Health problems of industrializing societies	Pneumonia	6.3%	Estimate for England & Wales (Logan 1950); probably similar elsewhere
	Influenza	[crisis]	Strong fluctuations; positive contribution, but magnitude inestimable
	Puerperal fever	0.5%	Estimate for England & Wales (Logan 1950); probably similar elsewhere
	Infant mortality [g]	[32.1%]	European average (sources: see Suppl. Table 1)
	Pellagra	15.5%	Estimate for Italy (source: Ginnaio 2011); much lower elsewhere
	Rickets	.	Rickets already had negligible mortality in 1870
	Goitre	.	Localized problem with low case fatality
	Peptic ulcer	–	Rise and fall within period (source: see Suppl. Figure 13); 1870 level unknown
	Appendicitis	0.3%	European average (source: see Figure 20); contribution 1900–1950
	Pneumoconiosis	–	No mortality data available
	Stomach cancer	1.6%	European average (source: see Suppl. Figure 16) ; contribution 1900–1950

Notes: For this period, data on trends in cause-specific mortality are limited, and usually cover only one or a few countries, from which an extrapolation needed to be made to Europe as a whole. The figures in this table were calculated by taking the difference between the cause-specific mortality rate at the beginning and the end of the study-period, and divide that by the difference between the all-cause mortality rate at the beginning and end of the study-period.

SUPPL. TABLE 9 Contributions of specific diseases to mortality decline, ca. 1970–2015

		Contribution to mortality decline (both sexes)	
		Average	**Standard deviation**
Health problems of industrializing societies	(Para)typhoid, dysentery	1.9%	4.5%
	Resp. tuberculosis	2.6%	2.3%
	Syphilis	0.2%	0.1%
	Diphtheria	0.0%	0.0%
	Measles	0.2%	0.6%
	Pneumonia	5.2%	5.6%
	Influenza	2.3%	2.4%
	Peptic ulcer	0.9%	1.0%
	Appendicitis	0.2%	0.1%
	Stomach cancer	5.3%	2.6%
Health problems of affluent societies	Ischaemic heart disease	29.1%	23.7%
	Cerebrovascular disease	19.9%	7.1%
	Colorectal cancer	-0.1%	2.0%
	Breast cancer	0.1%	1.9%
	Prostate cancer	-1.0%	2.0%
	Lung cancer	-0.8%	2.5%
	Liver cirrhosis	0.4%	2.1%
	Road traffic injuries	2.6%	1.6%
	Suicide	1.5%	2.0%

Notes: The figures in this table were calculated from data on 28 countries, representing all European regions. For each country, the starting point of the analysis was chosen by selecting, within the time-window 1960–1981, the year in which all-cause mortality peaked, and the end-point was chosen by selecting, within the time-window 2010–2017, the most recent year for which data were complete. For each country and each cause of death, the difference between the age-standardized mortality rate at the starting point and at the end-point was calculated, as well as the contribution of each cause of death to the decline of all-cause mortality in that country. The figures in the table represent the cross-country averages and standard deviations of these country-specific contributions. Please note the huge variation between countries, indicated by the large standard deviations. Negative values imply rising mortality (and thus a negative contribution to all-cause mortality decline)

SOURCE: WHO MORTALITY DATABASE (SEE SUPPL. TABLE 1)

Bibliography

A'Hearn, Brian, Jörg Baten, and Dorothee Crayen. "Quantifying Quantitative Literacy: Age Heaping and the History of Human Capital." *Journal of Economic History* 69, no. 3 (2009): 783–808.

Aaby, Peter, *et al.* "Severe Measles in Sunderland, 1885." *International Journal of Epidemiology* 15, no. 1 (1986): 101–07.

Acemoğlu, Daron, Simon Johnson, and James Robinson. "The Rise of Europe: Atlantic Trade, Institutional Change, and Economic Growth." *American Economic Review* 95, no. 3 (2005): 546–79.

Acemoğlu, Daron, and James A. Robinson. *Why Nations Fail.* London: Profile Books, 2012.

Ackerknecht, Erwin H. "Anticontagionism between 1821 and 1867." *Bulletin of the History of Medicine* 22 (1948): 562–93.

Ackerknecht, Erwin H. "Hygiene in France, 1815–1848." *Bulletin of the History of Medicine* 22 (1948): 117–55.

Ackerknecht, Erwin H. *History and Geography of the Most Important Diseases.* New York & London: Hafner, 1965.

Adminaite, Dovile, *et al. Ranking EU Progress on Road Safety.* Brussels: European Transport Safety Council, 2018.

Ahmed, Awad M. "History of Diabetes Mellitus." *Saudi Medical Journal* 23, no. 4 (2002): 373–78.

Alderson, Michael. *International Mortality Statistics.* New York: Facts on File, 1981.

Aleshina, Nadezhda, and Gerry Redmond. "How High Is Infant Mortality in Central and Eastern Europe and the Commonwealth of Independent States?." *Population Studies* 59, no. 1 (2005): 39–54.

Alfani, Guido, and Cormac Ó Gráda. "Famines in Europe: An Overview." In *Famine in European History*, edited by Guido Alfani and Cormac Ó Gráda, 1–24. Cambridge etc.: Cambridge University Press, 2017.

Alter, George, and James C. Riley. "Frailty, Sickness, and Death: Models of Morbidity and Mortality in Historical Populations." *Population Studies* 43, no. 1 (1989): 25–45.

Alvarez-Dardet, Carlos, and I Hernandez Aguado. "AIDS in Spain: Lessons Learned from a Public Health Disaster." *Journal of Epidemiology and Community Health* 48, no. 4 (1994): 331–32.

Alves, Jorge Fernandes. "Ricardo Jorge e a Saúde Pública em Portugal." *Arquivos de Medicina* 22, no. 2–3 (2008): 85–90.

Alves, Jorge Fernandes, and Marinha Carneiro. "Saúde Pública e Política do «Código Sanitário» ao Regulamento Geral de 1901." *Cultura, Espaço & Memória* 5 (2018): 27–43.

Anderson, Gaylord W. "Foreign and Domestic Trends in Diphtheria." *American Journal of Public Health and the Nations Health* 37, no. 1 (1947): 1–6.

Anderson, Peter. "Alcohol." In *Successes and Failures of Health Policy in Europe*, edited by Johan P. Mackenbach and Martin McKee, 41–57. Maidenhead: Open University Press, 2013.

Anderson, Roy M., Bryan T. Grenfell, and R.M. May. "Oscillatory Fluctuations in the Incidence of Infectious Disease and the Impact of Vaccination." *Epidemiology & Infection* 93, no. 3 (1984): 587–608.

Andersson, Tobias, U. Hogberg, and S. Bergstrom. "Community-Based Prevention of Perinatal Deaths: Lessons from Nineteenth-Century Sweden." *International Journal of Epidemiology* 29, no. 3 (2000): 542–48.

Andreev, Evgueni M., *et al.* "The Evolving Pattern of Avoidable Mortality in Russia." *International Journal of Epidemiology* 32, no. 3 (2003): 437–46.

Ansart, S., *et al.* "Mortality Burden of the 1918–1919 Influenza Pandemic in Europe." *Influenza Other Respiratory Viruses* 3, no. 3 (2009): 99–106.

Anttila, Ahti, and José M. Martin-Moreno. "Cancer Screening." In *Successes and Failures of Health Policy in Europe*, edited by Johan P. Mackenbach and Martin McKee, 179–92. Maidenhead: Open University Press, 2013.

Awofeso, Niyi. "What's New About the "New Public Health"?." *American Journal of Public Health* 94, no. 5 (2004): 705–09.

Bailar III, John C., and Elaine M. Smith. "Progress against Cancer?." *New England Journal of Medicine* 314, no. 19 (1986): 1226–32.

Bailar, John C., and Heather L. Gornik. "Cancer Undefeated." *New England Journal of Medicine* 336, no. 22 (1997): 1569–74.

Baili, Paolo, *et al.* "Age and Case Mix-Standardised Survival for All Cancer Patients in Europe 1999–2007." *European Journal of Cancer* 51, no. 15 (2015): 2120–29.

Baláz, V., *et al.* "Prevalence of Ischaemic Heart Disease Risk Factors in Warsaw and Bratislava. Part II: Hypertension." *Cor et Vasa* 22, no. 3 (1980): 140–46.

Baldwin, Peter. *Contagion and the State in Europe, 1830–1930.* Cambridge: Cambridge University Press, 1999.

Balińska, Marta A. *For the Good of Humanity.* Budapest: Central European University Press, 1998.

Barbagli, Marzio. *Farewell to the World.* Cambridge & Malden: Polity Press, 2015.

Barberis, I., *et al.* "History and Evolution of Influenza Control through Vaccination." *Journal Prevention Medical Hygiene* 57, no. 3 (2016): e115-e20.

Barker, David J. "Acute Appendicitis and Dietary Fibre: An Alternative Hypothesis." *British Medical Journal* 290, no. 6475 (1985): 1125–27.

Barker, David J. "Rise and Fall of Western Diseases." *Nature* 338, no. 6214 (1989): 371–27.

Barker, David J., and C. Osmond. "Diet and Coronary Heart Disease in England and Wales During and after the Second World War." *Journal of Epidemiology & Community Health* 40, no. 1 (1986): 37–44.

Barnes, David S. *The Great Stink of Paris and the Nineteenth-Century Struggle against Filth and Germs.* Baltimore: Johns Hopkins University Press, 2006.

Barona, Josep Lluís, and Josep Bernabeu-Mestre. *La Salud y el Estado.* Valencia: Universitat de València, 2011.

Barrett, Ronald, *et al.* "Emerging and Re-Emerging Infectious Diseases: The Third Epidemiologic Transition." *Annual Review of Anthropology* 27, no. 1 (1998): 247–71.

Barry, John M. *The Great Influenza.* Harmondsworth: Penguin, 2005.

Baten, Joerg, ed. *A History of the Global Economy.* Cambridge etc.: Cambridge University Press, 2016.

Baten, Joerg, and Matthias Blum. "Growing Tall but Unequal." *Economic History of Developing Regions* 27, no. Suppl. 1 (2012): S66-S85.

Baten, Joerg. "Why Are You Tall While Others Are Short?." *European Review of Economic History* 18, no. 2 (2014): 144–65.

Baum, Frances. *The New Public Health: An Australian Perspective.* Melbourne etc.: Oxford University Press, 1998.

Baxter, Peter J., *et al. Hunter's Diseases of Occupations* [*Tenth Edition*]. London: Arnold 2010.

Bayly, Christopher A. *Remaking the Modern World 1900–2015.* Chichester: John Wiley & Sons, 2018.

Beaglehole, Robert, and Ruth Bonita. *Global Public Health: A New Era.* Oxford etc.: Oxford University Press, 2009.

Beddington, John, *et al.* "The Mental Wealth of Nations." *Nature* 455, no. 7216 (2008): 1057–60.

Beeck, Eduard F. van, Gerard J.J. Borsboom, and Johan P. Mackenbach. "Economic Development and Traffic Accident Mortality in the Industrialized World, 1962–1990." *International Journal of Epidemiology* 29, no. 3 (2000): 503–09.

Beeck, Eduard F. van, Caspar W. Looman, and Johan P. Mackenbach. "Mortality Due to Unintentional Injuries in the Netherlands, 1950–1995." *Public Health Reports* 113, no. 5 (1998): 427–39.

Bell, Frances, and Robert Millward. "Public Health Expenditures and Mortality in England and Wales, 1870–1914." *Continuity and Change* 13, no. 2 (1998): 221–49.

Benatru, Isabelle, *et al.* "Stable Stroke Incidence Rates but Improved Case-Fatality in Dijon, France, from 1985 to 2004." *Stroke* 37, no. 7 (2006): 1674–79.

Bengtsson, Tommy, and Martin Dribe. "The Late Emergence of Socioeconomic Mortality Differentials." *Explorations in Economic History* 48, no. 3 (2011): 389–400.

Bengtsson, Tommy, and Frans van Poppel. "Socioeconomic Inequalities in Death from Past to Present: An Introduction." *Explorations in Economic History* 48, no. 3 (2011): 343–56.

Berghöfer, Anne, *et al.* "Obesity Prevalence from a European Perspective: A Systematic Review." *BMC Public Health* 8, no. 1 (2008): 200.

Berkman, Lisa F., *et al.* "From Social Integration to Health: Durkheim in the New Millennium." *Social Science & Medicine* 51, no. 6 (2000): 843–57.

Berridge, Virginia. "AIDS in the UK: The Making of Policy, 1981–1994." In *Sex, State and Society: Comparative Perspectives on the History of Sexuality*, edited by Lars-Göran Tedebrand, 15–23. Umeå: Nyheternas tryckeri, 1996.

Berridge, Virginia. *Marketing Health: Smoking and the Discourse of Public Health in Britain, 1945–2000.* Oxford etc.: Oxford University Press, 2007.

Berridge, Virginia. *Demons: Our Changing Attitudes to Alcohol, Tobacco, and Drugs.* Oxford etc.: Oxford University Press, 2013.

Berridge, Virginia. *Public Health: A Very Short Introduction.* Oxford etc.: Oxford University Press, 2016.

Berridge, Virginia, and Philip Strong, eds. *AIDS and Contemporary History.* Cambridge etc.: Cambridge University Press, 1993.

Besley, Timothy, and Masayuki Kudamatsu. "Health and Democracy." *Political Economy* 96, no. 2 (2006): 313–18.

Biraben, Jean Noël. *Les Hommes et la Peste en France et dans les Pays Européens et Méditerranéens.* Paris: Mouton, 1975.

Black, Douglas, *et al. Inequalities in Health (the Black Report).* London Department of Health and Social Services, 1980. Penguin Books, 1982.

Bland, Edward F. "Declining Severity of Rheumatic Fever: A Comparative Study of the Past Four Decades." *New England Journal of Medicine* 262, no. 12 (1960): 597–99.

Blanning, Timothy C.W. *The Pursuit of Glory: Europe, 1648–1815.* London: Allen Lane, 2007.

Blood Pressure Lowering Treatment Trialists' Collaboration. "Effects of Different Blood-Pressure-Lowering Regimens on Major Cardiovascular Events." *Lancet* 362, no. 9395 (2003): 1527–35.

Bloom, David E., and David Canning. "Commentary: The Preston Curve 30 Years On: Still Sparking Fires." *International Journal of Epidemiology* 36, no. 3 (2007): 498–99.

Bloom, David E. *Population Health and Economic Growth.* Health and Growth. Vol. 24, Washington, DC: World Bank (Commission on Growth and Development), 2009.

Bloom, David E., David Canning, and Jaypee Sevilla. *Economic Growth and the Demographic Transition.* NBER Working Papers. Cambridge, Mass: National Bureau of Economic Research, 2001.

Boffetta, Paolo. "Epidemiology of Environmental and Occupational Cancer." *Oncogene* 23, no. 38 (2004): 6392–403.

Bollet, Alfred J. "Politics and Pellagra: The Epidemic of Pellagra in the US in the Early Twentieth Century." *Yale Journal of Biology and Medicine* 65, no. 3 (1992): 211–21.

Boonstra, O.W.A. *De Waardij van eene Vroege Opleiding.* Wageningen: Wageningen University, 1993.

Borch-Johnsen, K., S. Kreiner, and T. Deckert. "Mortality of Type 1 (Insulin-Dependent) Diabetes Mellitus in Denmark." *Diabetologia* 29, no. 11 (1986): 767–72.

Borowy, Iris. "Road Traffic Injuries: Social Change and Development." *Medical History* 57, no. 1 (2013): 108–38.

Borowy, Iris, and Wolf Gruner, eds. *Facing Illness in Troubled Times.* Frankfurt am Main: Peter Lang, 2005.

Bos, Kirsten I., *et al.* "A Draft Genome of Yersinia Pestis from Victims of the Black Death." *Nature* 478, no. 7370 (2011): 506–10.

Bosetti, Cristina, *et al.* "Worldwide Mortality from Cirrhosis: An Update to 2002." *Journal of Hepatology* 46, no. 5 (2007): 827–39.

Bourdelais, P. *Les Épidémies Terrassées. Une Histoire de Pays Riches.* Paris: Éditions de la Martinière, 2003.

Boyle, Peter, Patrick Maisonneuve, and Stanley B. Kaye. "Therapy for Testicular Cancer in Central and Eastern Europe." *Lancet* 335, no. 8696 (1990): 1033.

Boys, Richard J., Donald P. Forster, and Peter Jozan. "Mortality from Causes Amenable and Non-Amenable to Medical Care: The Experience of Eastern Europe." *British Medical Journal* 303, no. 6807 (1991): 879–83.

Brandt, Allan M. *No Magic Bullet.* Oxford etc.: Oxford University Press, 1987.

Brandt, Allan M. *The Cigarette Century.* New York: Basic Books, 2007.

Braudel, Fernand. *Les Structures du Quotidien: Le Possible et l'Impossible.* Paris: Armand Colin, 1979.

Brennan, P., and Issy Bray. "Recent Trends and Future Directions for Lung Cancer Mortality in Europe." *British Journal of Cancer* 87, no. 1 (2002): 43–48.

Brinkhof, Martin W., *et al.* "Influenza-Attributable Mortality among the Elderly in Switzerland." *Swiss Medical Weekly* 136, no. 19–20 (2006): 302–09.

Brinton, Louise A., Mia M. Gaudet, and Gretchen L. Gierach. "Breast Cancer." In *Cancer Epidemiology and Prevention (Fourth Edition)*, edited by Michael Thun, Martha S. Linet, James R. Cerhan, Christopher A. Haiman and David Schottenfeld, 1–111. Oxford etc.: Oxford University Press, 2017.

Broadberry, Stephen, eds. *Cambridge Economic History of Modern Europe: Volume 1: 1700–1870.* Cambridge etc.: Cambridge University Press, 2010.

Broadberry, Stephen, and Kevin H. O'Rourke, eds. *Cambridge Economic History of Modern Europe. Volume 2: 1870 to the Present.* Cambridge etc.: Cambridge University Press, 2010.

Brown, George W., and Tirril Harris. *Social Origins of Depression.* London: Tavistock Publications, 1978.

Bruce-Chwatt, Leonard J., and Julian De Zulueta. *The Rise and Fall of Malaria in Europe.* Oxford etc.: Oxford University Press, 1980.

Brunekreef, Bert, and Stephen T. Holgate. "Air Pollution and Health." *Lancet* 360, no. 9341 (2002): 1233–42.

Bunker, John P. "The Role of Medical Care in Contributing to Health Improvements within Societies." *International Journal of Epidemiology* 30, no. 6 (2001): 1260–63.

Bunker, John P., Howard S. Frazier, and Frederick Mosteller. "Improving Health: Measuring Effects of Medical Care." *Milbank Quarterly* 72, no. 2 (1994): 225–58.

Burdorf, Alex, Bengt Järvholm, and Anders Englund. "Explaining Differences in Incidence Rates of Pleural Mesothelioma between Sweden and the Netherlands." *International Journal of Cancer* 113, no. 2 (2005): 298–301.

Burney, Peter G.J., *et al.* "Global and Regional Trends in Copd Mortality, 1990–2010." *European Respiratory Journal* 45, no. 5 (2015): 1239–47.

Butchart, Stuart H.M., *et al.* "Global Biodiversity: Indicators of Recent Declines." *Science* 328, no. 5982 (2010): 1164–68.

Cabet, Étienne. *Voyage et Aventures de Lord William Carisdall en Icarie.* Paris: H. Souverain, 1840.

Caldwell, John C. *Theory of Fertility Decline.* New York: Academic, 1982.

Caldwell, John C. "Routes to Low Mortality in Poor Countries." *Population and Development Review* 12, no. 2 (1986): 171–220.

Callenbach, Ernest. *Ecotopia.* Indore: Banyan Tree Books, 1975.

Campbell, Maurice. "Death Rate from Diseases of the Heart: 1876 to 1959." *British Medical Journal* 2, no. 5356 (1963): 528–35.

Campbell, Stephen, *et al.* "Quality of Primary Care in England with the Introduction of Pay for Performance." *New England Journal of Medicine* 357, no. 2 (2007): 181–90.

Cancer Registry of Norway. *Survival of Cancer Patients - Cases Diagnosed in Norway 1968–1975.* Oslo: Cancer Registry of Norway, 1980.

Canfora, Luciano. *Democracy in Europe.* Oxford: Blackwell, 2006.

Cantor, Norman F. *In the Wake of the Plague.* New York: Free Press, 2001.

Carmichael, Ann. "Diphtheria." In *Cambridge World History of Human Disease,* edited by K.F. Kiple, 680–83. Cambridge etc.: Cambridge University Press, 1993.

Carpenter, Thomas O., *et al.* "Rickets." *Nature Reviews Disease Primers* 3 (2017): 17101.

Caselli, Graziella. "Health Transition and Cause-Specific Mortality." In *The Decline of Mortality in Europe,* edited by Roger S. Schofield, David S. Reher and Alain Bideau, 68–96. Oxford: Clarendon Press, 1991.

Centers for Disease Control and Prevention. "Ten Great Public Health Achievements-- United States, 1900–1999." *MMWR. Morbidity and mortality weekly report* 48, no. 12 (1999): 241.

Centers for Disease Control and Prevention. "Ten Great Public Health Achievements-- United States, 2001–2010." *MMWR. Morbidity and mortality weekly report* 60, no. 19 (2011): 619.

Cervellati, Matteo, and Uwe Sunde. *Demographic Change and Long-Run Development.* Cambridge (Mass.) & London: MIT Press, 2017.

Chamberlain, Geoffrey. "ABC of Antenatal Care. Vital Statistics of Birth." *British Medical Journal* 303, no. 6795 (1991): 178–81.

Chang, Shu-Sen, *et al.* "Impact of 2008 Global Economic Crisis on Suicide: Time Trend Study in 54 Countries." *British Medical Journal* 347 (2013): f5239.

Charlton, John, and Mike Murphy. *The Health of Adult Britain 1841–1994. Decennial Supplement No. 12.* London: The Stationery Office, 1997.

Charlton, John, and Ramon Velez. "Some International Comparisons of Mortality Amenable to Medical Intervention." *British Medical Journal* 292, no. 6516 (1986): 295–301.

Chen, Lei, Dianna J. Magliano, and Paul Z. Zimmet. "The Worldwide Epidemiology of Type 2 Diabetes Mellitus—Present and Future Perspectives." *Nature Reviews Endocrinology* 8, no. 4 (2012): 228–36.

Chesnais, Jean-Claude. *Histoire de la Violence en Occident de 1800 à Nos Jours.* Paris: Robert Laffont, 1981.

Chesnais, Jean-Claude. *La Transition Démographique.* Paris: Presses Universitaires de France, 1986.

Chick, Harriette. "Study of Rickets in Vienna 1919–1922." *Medical History* 20, no. 1 (1976): 41–51.

Chirot, Daniel. "The Rise of the West." *American Sociological Review* 50, no. 2 (1985): 181–95.

Christie, A.B. "Smallpox." In *World Geography of Human Diseases*, edited by G. Melvyn Howe, 255–70. London etc.: Academic Press, 1977.

Cliff, Andrew D., Matthew R. Smallman-Raynor, and Peta M. Stevens. "Controlling the Geographical Spread of Infectious Disease: Plague in Italy, 1347–1851." *Acta Medico-Historica Adriatica* 7, no. 2 (2009): 197–236.

Coale, Ansley J., and Susan C. Watkins, eds. *The Decline of Fertility in Europe*. Princeton: Princeton University Press, 1986.

Cockburn, Thomas A. "The Origin of the Treponematoses." *Bulletin of the World Health Organization* 24, no. 2 (1961): 221–28.

Cohn, Samuel K. "Epidemiology of the Black Death and Successive Waves of Plague." *Medical History* 52, no. S27 (2008): 74–100.

Coleman, William. "Health and Hygiene in the Encyclopédie: A Medical Doctrine for the Bourgeoisie." *Journal of the History of Medicine and Allied Sciences* 29, no. 4 (1974): 399–421.

Commission on Social Determinants of Health. *Closing the Gap in a Generation.* Geneva: World Health Organization, 2008.

Cooper, Richard. "Smoking in the Soviet Union." *British Medical Journal* 285, no. 6341 (1982): 549–51.

Corbin, Alain. *Les Filles de Noce.* Paris: Flammarion, 1982.

Correia, Manuel, *et al.* "Prospective Community-Based Study of Stroke in Northern Portugal." *Stroke* 35, no. 9 (2004): 2048–53.

Crayen, Dorothee, and Joerg Baten. "Global Trends in Numeracy 1820–1949 and Its Implications for Long-Term Growth." *Explorations in Economic History* 47, no. 1 (2010): 82–99.

Crimmins, Eileen M., Yasuhiko Saito, and Dominique Ingegneri. "Changes in Life Expectancy and Disability-Free Life Expectancy in the United States." *Population and Development Review* 15, no. 2 (1989): 235–67.

Crosby, Alfred W. "The Early History of Syphilis: A Reappraisal." *American Anthropologist* 71, no. 2 (1969): 218–27.

Crosby, Alfred W. "Influenza." In *Cambridge World History of Human Disease*, edited by Kenneth F. Kiple, 807–11. Cambridge etc.: Cambridge University Press, 1993.

Cross-National Colaborative Group. "The Changing Rate of Major Depresion: Cross-National Comparisons." *Journal of the American Medical Association* 268 (1992): 3098–105.

Currie, Laura, and Anna B. Gilmore. "Tobacco." In *Successes and Failures of Health Policy in Europe*, edited by Johan P. Mackenbach and Martin McKee, 23–40. Maidenhead: Open University Press, 2013.

Cutler, David, and Grant Miller. "The Role of Public Health Improvements in Health Advances." *Demography* 42, no. 1 (2005): 1–22.

Cutler, Richard G., and Henry Rodriguez. *Critical Reviews of Oxidative Stress and Aging*. New York: World Scientific Publishing, 2003.

Da Costa, Bruno R., and Edgar Ramos Vieira. "Risk Factors for Work-Related Musculoskeletal Disorders." *American Journal of Industrial Medicine* 53, no. 3 (2010): 285–323.

Dahlgren, Göran, and Margaret Whitehead. *Policies and Strategies to Promote Social Equity in Health*. Stockholm: Institute for Future Studies, 1991.

Dale, Henry H. "Advances in Medicinal Therapeutics." *British Medical Journal*, no. 4644 (1950): 1–7.

Danaei, Goodarz, *et al.* "National, Regional, and Global Trends in Systolic Blood Pressure since 1980." *Lancet* 377, no. 9765 (2011): 568–77.

Davidson, Roger. *Dangerous Liaisons*. Amsterdam & Atlanta: Rodopi, 2000.

Davies, Norman. *Europe: A History*. London: Pimlico, 1997.

Dawood, Fatimah S., *et al.* "Estimated Global Mortality Associated with the First 12 Months of 2009 Pandemic Influenza a H1N1 Virus Circulation." *Lancet Infectious Diseases* 12, no. 9 (2012): 687–95.

De Brouwere, Vincent. "The Comparative Study of Maternal Mortality over Time." *Social History of Medicine* 20, no. 3 (2007): 541–62.

De Martel, Catherine, and Julie Parsonnet. "Stomach Cancer." In *Cancer Epidemiology and Prevention (Fourth Edition)*, edited by Michael Thun, Martha S. Linet, James R. Cerhan, Christopher A. Haiman and David Schottenfeld, 1–70. Oxford etc.: Oxford University Press, 2017.

Deaton, Angus. *The Great Escape*. Princeton: Princeton University Press, 2013.

Delpech, Valerie, and J. Lundgren. "Death from AIDS Is Preventable, So Why Are People Still Dying of AIDS in Europe?." *Eurosurveillance* 19, no. 47 (2014): 20973.

Department of Health. *Public Health in England* (*the Acheson Report*). London: Her Majesty's Stationery Office, 1988.

Désesquelles, Aline, *et al.* "After the Epidemiologic Transition." *International Journal of Public Health* 60, no. 8 (2015): 961–67.

Detels, Roger, *et al. Oxford Textbook of Global Public Health*. 5 ed. Oxford etc.: Oxford University Press, 2015.

Di Paola, Marcello, and Dale Jamieson. "Climate Change and the Challenges to Democracy." *University of Miami Law Review* 72 (2017): 369–424.

Diamond, Jared M. *Guns, Germs, and Steel*. New York: W.W. Norton & Company, 1997.

Dickman, Paul W., *et al.* "Survival of Cancer Patients in Finland 1955–1994." *Acta Oncologica* 38, no. 12 (1999): 1–103.

Dittmann, Sieghart, *et al.* "Successful Control of Epidemic Diphtheria in the States of the Former USSR." *Journal of Infectious Diseases* 181, no. Supplement 1 (2000): S10-S22.

Doll, Richard. "Tobacco: A Medical History." *Journal of Urban Health* 76, no. 3 (1999): 289–313.

Doll, Richard, and Richard Peto. "The Causes of Cancer: Quantitative Estimates of Avoidable Risks of Cancer in the United States Today." *JNCI: Journal of the National Cancer Institute* 66, no. 6 (1981): 1192–308.

Doll, Richard, *et al.* "Mortality in Relation to Smoking: 50 Years' Observations on Male British Doctors." *British Medical Journal* 328, no. 7455 (2004): 1519–28.

Domnich, Alexander, *et al.* "Effectiveness of Mf59-Adjuvanted Seasonal Influenza Vaccine in the Elderly." *Vaccine* 35, no. 4 (2017): 513–20.

Donaldson, G. C., and W. R. Keatinge. "Excess Winter Mortality: Influenza or Cold Stress?" [In eng]. *British Medical Journal* 324, no. 7329 (2002): 89–90.

Drancourt, Michel. "Finally, Plague Is Plague." *Clinical Microbiology and Infection* 18, no. 2 (2012): 105–06.

Drancourt, Michel, *et al.* "Detection of 400-Year-Old Yersinia Pestis DNA in Human Dental Pulp." *Proceedings of the National Academy of Sciences* 95, no. 21 (1998): 12637–40.

Drolet, Godias J. "World War I and Tuberculosis. A Statistical Summary and Review." *American Journal of Public Health and the Nations Health* 35, no. 7 (1945): 689–97.

Drukker, J.W., and Vincent Tassenaar. "Paradoxes of Modernization and Material Well-Being in the Netherlands During the Nineteenth Century." In *Health and Welfare During Industrialization*, edited by R.H. Steckel and R. Floud, 331–78. Chicago & London: Chicago University Press, 1997.

Dubos, René J. *Mirage of Health.* New York: Harper & Brothers, 1959.

Dubos, René J. *Man Adapting.* New Haven and London: Yale University Press, 1965.

Dubos, René J., and Jean Dubos. *The White Plague.* Boston: Little, Brown & Company, 1952.

Duffin, Jacalyn. "Pneumonia." In *Cambridge World History of Human Disease*, edited by Kenneth F. Kiple, 938–42. Cambridge etc.: Cambridge University Press, 1993.

Dugac, Zeljko. "New Public Health for a New State." In *Facing Illness in Troubled Times*, edited by Iris Borowy and Wolf Gruner, 277–304. Frankfurt am Main: Peter Lang, 2005.

Dugac, Zeljko. "Andrija Stampar (1888–1958): Resolute Fighter for Health and Social Justice." In *Of Medicine and Men*, edited by Iris Borowy and Anne Hardy, 73–102. Frankfurt am Main etc.: Peter Lang, 2008.

Duncan, C.J., S.R. Duncan, and Susan Scott. "The Dynamics of Measles Epidemics." *Theoretical Population Biology* 52, no. 2 (1997): 155–63.

Durkheim, Emile. *Suicide: Étude de Sociologie.* Paris: Félix Alcan, 1897.

Easterly, William. "Life During Growth." *Journal of Economic Growth* 4, no. 3 (1999): 239–76.

Edvinsson, Sören, Ólöf Garðarsdóttir, and Gunnar Thorvaldsen. "Infant Mortality in the Nordic Countries, 1780–1930." *Continuity and Change* 23, no. 3 (2008): 457–85.

Eisner, Manuel P. "Modernization, Self-Control and Lethal Violence." *British Journal of Criminology* 41 (2001): 618–38.

Eisner, Manuel P. "Modernity Strikes Back?." *International Journal of Conflict and Violence* 2, no. 2 (2008): 288 – 316.

Eisner, Manuel P. "From Swords to Words." *Crime and Justice* 43, no. 1 (2014): 65–134.

Elias, Norbert. *Uber den Prozess der Zivilisation.* Basel: Verlag Haus zum Falken, 1939.

Ellaway, Anne, *et al.* "In the Driving Seat." *Transportation Research Part F: Traffic Psychology and Behaviour* 6, no. 3 (2003): 217–31.

Esping-Andersen, Gøsta. *The Three Worlds of Welfare Capitalism.* Cambridge: Polity Press, 1990.

Etheridge, Elisabeth W. "Pellagra." In *Cambridge World History of Human Disease*, edited by Kenneth F. Kiple, 918–24. Cambridge etc.: Cambridge University Press, 1993.

EURO-Peristat Project. *European Perinatal Health Report.* n.p.: EURO-Peristat Project, 2018.

Eurodiab ACE Study Group. "Variation and Trends in Incidence of Childhood Diabetes in Europe." *Lancet* 355, no. 9207 (2000): 873–76.

European Centers for Disease Control. *HIV/AIDS Surveillance in Europe: 2017 Data.* Copenhagen: World Health Organization, 2018.

European Centers for Disease Control. *Tuberculosis Surveillance and Monitoring in Europe 2019.* Copenhagen: WHO Regional Office for Europe, 2019.

Evans, Alun, *et al.* "Trends in Coronary Risk Factors in the WHO MONICA Project." *International Journal of Epidemiology* 30, no. Supplement 1 (2001): S35-S40.

Evans, Richard J. *Death in Hamburg.* Oxford: Clarendon Press, 1987.

Evans, Richard J. "Epidemics and Revolutions: Cholera in Nineteenth-Century Europe." *Past & Present*, no. 120 (1988): 123–46.

Evers, Johannes C.G. *Bijdrage tot de Bevolkingsleer van Nederland.* 's-Gravenhage: Gebr. Belinfante, 1882.

Eyler, John M. *Sir Arthur Newsholme and State Medicine, 1885–1935.* Cambridge etc.: Cambridge University Press, 2002.

Ezzati, Majid, *et al.* "Contributions of Risk Factors and Medical Care to Cardiovascular Mortality Trends." *Nature Reviews Cardiology* 12, no. 9 (2015): 508–30.

Ezzati, Majid, *et al.* "Rethinking the "Diseases of Affluence" Paradigm." *PLoS Medicine* 2, no. 5 (2005): e133.

Fagan, Brian. *The Little Ice Age.* New York: Basic Books, 2000.

Fairchild, Amy L., and Gerald M. Oppenheimer. "Public Health Nihilism Vs Pragmatism." *American Journal of Public Health* 88, no. 7 (1998): 1105–17.

Falaschetti, Emanuela, *et al.* "Continued Improvement in Hypertension Management in England." *Hypertension* 53, no. 3 (2009): 480–86.

Farley, John. *To Cast out Disease.* Oxford etc.: Oxford University Press, 2004.

Farmer, Paul. "Social Inequalities and Emerging Infectious Diseases." *Emerging Infectious Diseases* 2, no. 4 (1996): 259–69.

Fee, Elizabeth. "Henry E. Sigerist." *Milbank Quarterly* 67, no. Suppl. 1 (1989): 127–50.

Feigin, Valery L., *et al.* "Worldwide Stroke Incidence and Early Case Fatality Reported in 56 Population-Based Studies." *Lancet Neurology* 8, no. 4 (2009): 355–69.

Ferguson, Niall. *Civilization: The West and the Rest.* London: Allen Lane, 2011.

Ferlay, J., *et al.* "Cancer Incidence and Mortality Patterns in Europe." *European Journal of Cancer* 103 (2018): 356–87.

Ferreira, F. A. Gonçalves. *História da Saúde e dos Serviços de Saúde em Portugal.* Lisbon: Edição da Fundação Calouste Gulbenkian, 1990.

Feudtner, Chris. *Bittersweet.* Chapel Hill & London: University of North Carolina Press, 2004.

Field, Mark G. *Soviet Socialized Medicine: An Introduction.* New York: Free Press, 1967.

Figes, Orlando. *Natasha's Dance.* London: Allen Lane, 2002.

Fildes, Valerie. *Breasts, Bottles and Babies.* Edinburgh: Edinburgh University Press, 1986.

Filtzer, Donald. *The Hazards of Urban Life in Late Stalinist Russia.* Cambridge etc.: Cambridge University Press, 2010.

Finlayson, Rodney. "Ischaemic Heart Disease, Aortic Aneurysms, and Atherosclerosis in the City of London, 1868–1982." *Medical History* 29, no. S5 (1985): 151–68.

Fiorino, Daniel J. *Can Democracy Handle Climate Change.* Cambridge: Polity, 2018.

Floud, Roderick, *et al. The Changing Body*. Cambridge etc.: Cambridge University Press, 2011.

Floud, Roderick, and Bernard Harris. "Health, Height and Welfare: Britain 1700–1980." In *Health and Welfare During Industrialization*, edited by R.H. Steckel and R. Floud, 91–126. Chicago & London: Chicago University Press, 1997.

Fogel, Robert W. *The Escape from Hunger and Premature Death, 1700–2100*. Cambridge etc.: Cambridge University Press, 2004.

Fogel, Robert W., *et al.* "Secular Changes in American and British Stature and Nutrition." *Journal of Interdisciplinary History* 14, no. 2 (1983): 445–81.

Fombonne, Eric. "Increased Rates of Depression." *Acta Psychiatrica Scandinavica* 90, no. 3 (1994): 145–56.

Ford, Earl S., and Simon Capewell. "Proportion of the Decline in Cardiovascular Mortality Disease Due to Prevention Versus Treatment." *Annual Review of Public Health* 32 (2011): 5–22.

Forey, Barbara, *et al. International Smoking Statistics*. Oxford etc.: Oxford University Press, 2009.

Forouzanfar, Mohammad H., *et al.* "Global Burden of Hypertension and Systolic Blood Pressure of at Least 110 to 115 Mm Hg, 1990–2015." *Journal of the American Medical Association* 317, no. 2 (2017): 165–82.

Foucault, Michel. "Les Mots et les Choses." Paris: Gallimard, 1966.

Foulds, Jonathan, *et al.* "Effect of Smokeless Tobacco (Snus) on Smoking and Public Health in Sweden." *Tobacco Control* 12, no. 4 (2003): 349–59.

Franco, Giuliano. "Ramazzini and Workers' Health." *Lancet* 354, no. 9181 (1999): 858–61.

Frenk, Julio, *et al.* "Elements for a Theory of the Health Transition." *Health Transition Review* 1, no. 1 (1991): 21–38.

Fries, James F. "Aging, Natural Death, and the Compression of Morbidity." *New England Journal of Medicine* 303 (1980): 130–35.

Fye, W. Bruce. "The Delayed Diagnosis of Myocardial Infarction: It Took Half a Century!." *Circulation* 72, no. 2 (1985): 262–71.

Gageldonk-Lafeber, A.B. van, *et al.* "Time Trends in Primary-Care Morbidity, Hospitalization and Mortality Due to Pneumonia." *Epidemiology & Infection* 137, no. 10 (2009): 1472–78.

Galanti, Maria R., *et al.* "Use of Snus and Lung Cancer Mortality: Unwarranted Claim of Causal Association." *Scandinavian Journal of Public Health* 38 (2010): 332–33.

Galbraith, Spence, and Anna McCormack. "Infection in England and Wales, 1838–1993." In *The Health of Adult Britain 1841–1994. Volume 2*, edited by J. Charlton and M. Murphy, 1–20. London: The Stationery Office, 1997.

Gale, Edwin A.M. "The Rise of Childhood Type 1 Diabetes in the 20th Century." *Diabetes* 51, no. 12 (2002): 3353–61.

Garnel, Rita. "Disease and Public Health (Portugal)." In *International Encyclopedia of the First World War*, edited by Ute Daniel, Peter Gatrell, Oliver Janz, Heather Jones, Jennifer Keene, Alan Kramer and Bill Nasson. Berlin: Freie Universitat Berlin, 2014.

Garraway, W. Michael, Jack P. Whisnant, and Ivo Drury. "The Changing Pattern of Survival Following Stroke." *Stroke* 14, no. 5 (1983): 699–703.

GBD 2017 Collaborators. "Global, Regional, and National Comparative Risk Assessment of 84 Behavioural, Environmental and Occupational, and Metabolic Risks." *Lancet* 392 (2018): 1923–94.

GBD 2017 Collaborators. "Global, Regional, and National Disability-Adjusted Life-Years (Dalys) for 359 Diseases and Injuries and Healthy Life Expectancy (Hale)." *Lancet* 392, no. 10159 (2018): 1859–922.

GBD 2017 Collaborators. "Global, Regional, and National Incidence, Prevalence, and Years Lived with Disability for 354 Diseases and Injuries." *Lancet* 392, no. 10159 (2018): 1789–858.

Geus, Marius de. *Ecological Utopias*. Utrecht: International Books, 1999.

Gilbert, Paul. *Depression: The Evolution of Powerlessness*. London: Routledge, 1992.

Gilbert, Paul, and Steven Allan. "The Role of Defeat and Entrapment (Arrested Flight) in Depression: An Exploration of an Evolutionary View." *Psychological Medicine* 28, no. 3 (1998): 585–98.

Gille, Halvor. "The Demographic History of the Northern European Countries in the Eighteenth Century." *Population Studies* 3, no. 1 (1949): 3–65.

Gilman, Sander L., and Xun Zhou. *Smoke: A Global History of Smoking*. London: Reaktion Books, 2004.

Gilmore, Anna B., and Martin McKee. "Tobacco and Transition: An Overview of Industry Investments, Impact and Influence in the Former Soviet Union." *Tobacco Control* 13, no. 2 (2004): 136–42.

Ginnaio, Monica, and Amy Jacobs. "Pellagra in Late Nineteenth Century Italy: Effects of a Deficiency Disease." *Population (French edition)* 66, no. 3 (2011): 583–609.

Gissler, Mika, *et al.* "Perinatal Health Monitoring in Europe: Results from the Euro-Peristat Project." *Informatics for Health and Social Care* 35, no. 2 (2010): 64–79.

Gjonca, Arjan. "Mortality Transition in Albania, 1950–1990." University of London, 1999.

Gjonca, Arjan, Chris Wilson, and Jane Falkingham. "Paradoxes of Health Transition in Europe's Poorest Country: Albania 1950–90." *Population and Development Review* 23, no. 3 (1997): 585–609.

Glaziou, Philippe, Katherine Floyd, and Mario Raviglione. "Trends in Tuberculosis in the UK." *Thorax* 73 (2018): 702–03.

Glenny, Misha. *The Balkans, 1804–1999*. New York etc.: Viking Penguin, 2000.

Glynn, Liam G., *et al.* "Interventions Used to Improve Control of Blood Pressure in Patients with Hypertension." *Cochrane Database of Systematic Reviews*, no. 3 (2010).

Goldacre, Michael J., *et al.* "Trends in Death Certification for Multiple Sclerosis, Motor Neuron Disease, Parkinson's Disease and Epilepsy." *Journal of Neurology* 257, no. 5 (2010): 706–15.

Gomes, M.C., J.J. Gomes, and A.C. Paulo. "Diphtheria, Pertussis, and Measles in Portugal before and after Mass Vaccination." *European Journal of Epidemiology* 15, no. 9 (1999): 791–98.

Gordis, Leon. "The Virtual Disappearance of Rheumatic Fever in the United States." *Circulation* 72, no. 6 (1985): 1155–62.

Gorsky, Martin, *et al.* "The 'Cultural Inflation of Morbidity' During the English Mortality Decline." *Social Science & Medicine* 73, no. 12 (2011): 1775–83.

Gortmaker, Steven L., and Paul H. Wise. "The First Injustice: Socioeconomic Disparities, Health Services Technology, and Infant Mortality." *Annual Review of Sociology* 23, no. 1 (1997): 147–70.

Goudsblom, Johan. "Public Health and the Civilizing Process." *Milbank Quarterly* 64, no. 2 (1986): 161–88.

Gourbin, G., and Godelieve Masuy-Stroobant. "Registration of Vital Data: Are Live Births and Stillbirths Comparable All over Europe?." *Bulletin of the World Health Organization* 73, no. 4 (1995): 449–60.

Graaf, Ron de , *et al.* "Prevalence of Mental Disorders and Trends from 1996 to 2009." *Social Psychiatry and Psychiatric Epidemiology* 47, no. 2 (2012): 203–13.

Graafmans, Wilco C., *et al.* "Comparability of Published Perinatal Mortality Rates in Western Europe." *BJOG: An International Journal of Obstetrics & Gynaecology* 108, no. 12 (2001): 1237–45.

Graça, Luis. "História e Memória da Saúde Pública." *Revista Portuguesa de Saúde Pública* 33, no. 2 (2015): 125–27.

Green, Tana, M.D. Talbot, and R.S. Morton. "The Control of Syphilis, a Contemporary Problem: A Historical Perspective." *Sexually Transmitted Infections* 77, no. 3 (2001): 214–17.

Griffiths, Clare, and Anita Brock. "Twentieth Century Mortality Trends in England and Wales." *Health Statistics Quarterly* 18, no. 2 (2003): 5–17.

Grigoriev, Pavel, *et al.* "The Recent Mortality Decline in Russia: Beginning of the Cardiovascular Revolution?." *Population and Development Review* 40, no. 1 (2014): 107–29.

Grigoriev, Pavel, and Markéta Pechholdová. "Health Convergence between East and West Germany as Reflected in Long-Term Cause-Specific Mortality Trends." *European Journal of Population* 33, no. 5 (2017): 701–31.

Grin, E.I., and T. Guthe. "Evaluation of a Previous Mass Campaign against Endemic Syphilis in Bosnia and Herzegovina." *British Journal of Venereal Diseases* 49, no. 1 (1973): 1–19.

Griskevica, Aija, *et al.* "Diphtheria in Latvia, 1986–1996." *Journal of Infectious Diseases* 181, no. Supplement 1 (2000): S60-S64.

Grmek, Mirko D. "Préliminaires d'une Étude Historique des Maladies." *Annales. Histoire, sciences sociales* 24, no. 6 (1969): 1473–83.

Grmek, Mirko D. *Histoire Du Sida.* Paris: Payot, 1989.

Gross Solomon, Susan. "The Expert and the State in Russian Public Health." In *The History of Public Health and the Modern State*, edited by D. Porter, 183–223. Amsterdam - Atlanta: Rodopi, 1994.

Gross Solomon, Susan. "A Matter of 'Reach'. Fact Finding in the Wake of World War I." In *Shifting Boundaries of Public Health*, edited by S. Gross Salomon, L. Murard and P. Zylberman, 231–68. Rochester: University of Rochester Press, 2008.

Gross Solomon, Susan, and John F. Hutchinson, eds. *Health and Society in Revolutionary Russia.* Bloomington: Indiana University Press, 1990.

Gruenberg, Ernest M. "Epidemiology of Senile Dementia." *Advances in Neurology* 19 (1978): 437–57.

Grundy, Emily. "Commentary: The McKeown Debate: Time for Burial." *International Journal of Epidemiology* 34, no. 3 (2004): 529–33.

Guehne, Uta, Steffi Riedel-Heller, and Matthias C. Angermeyer. "Mortality in Dementia." *Neuroepidemiology* 25, no. 3 (2005): 153–62.

Gunnell, David J. "The Epidemiology of Suicide." *International Review of Psychiatry* 12, no. 1 (2000): 21–26.

Gunnell, David J., *et al.* "Why Are Suicide Rates Rising in Young Men but Falling in the Elderly?" *Social Science & Medicine* 57, no. 4 (2003): 595–611.

Guthe, Thorstein. *Worldwide Epidemiological Trends in Syphilis and Gonorrhea.* Washington: World Health Organization, 1970.

Guthe, Thorstein, and O. Idsoe. "The Rise and Fall of the Treponematoses. II. Endemic Treponematoses of Childhood." *British Journal of Venereal Diseases* 44, no. 1 (1968): 35–48.

Gutierrez, Hector, and Jacques Houdaille. "La Mortalité Maternelle en France au XVIIIe Siecle." *Population (French Edition)* 36, no. 6 (1983): 975–94.

Guttormsson, Loftur, and Ólöf Garðarsdóttir. "The Development of Infant Mortality in Iceland, 1800–1920." *Hygiea Internationalis* 3, no. 1 (2002): 151–76.

Haas-Posthuma, J.H. de, and J.H. de Haas. *Infant Loss in the Netherlands.* Washington: National Center for Health Statistics, 1968.

Haddon, William. "Options for the Prevention of Motor Vehicle Crash Injury." *Israel Journal of Medical Sciences* 16, no. 1 (1980): 45–65.

Hagen, Edward H. "Evolutionary Theories of Depression: A Critical Review." *Canadian Journal of Psychiatry* 56, no. 12 (2011): 716–26.

Hakulinen, T., *et al.* "Trends in Cancer Incidence in the Nordic Countries." *Acta Pathologica, Microbiologica, et Immunologica Scandinavica* 94 no. S288 (1986): 1–151.

Hamlin, Christopher. "Public Health in Great Britain." In *The History of Public Health and the Modern State*, edited by D. Porter, 132–64. Amsterdam: Editions Rodopi, 1994.

Hamlin, Christopher. *Public Health and Social Justice in the Age of Chadwick: Britain, 1800–1854.* Cambridge etc.: Cambridge University Press, 1998.

Hamlin, Christopher. *Cholera: The Biography.* Oxford etc.: Oxford University Press, 2009.

Hamlin, Christopher, and Pat Sidley. "Revolutions in Public Health: 1848, and 1998?." *British Medical Journal* 317, no. 7158 (1998): 587–91.

Hancock, Trevor. "Lalonde and Beyond: Looking Back at 'a New Perspective on the Health of Canadians'." *Health Promotion International* 1, no. 1 (1986): 93–100.

Hardy, Anne. *The Epidemic Streets: Infectious Disease and the Rise of Preventive Medicine, 1856–1900.* Oxford etc.: Oxford University Press, 1993.

Hardy, Anne. "Scarlet Fever." In *Cambridge World History of Human Disease*, edited by Kenneth F. Kiple, 990–92. Cambridge etc.: Cambridge University Press, 1993.

Hardy, Anne. "Whooping Cough." In *Cambridge World History of Human Disease*, edited by Kenneth F. Kiple, 1094–96. Cambridge etc.: Cambridge University Press, 1993.

Harper, Kristin N., *et al.* "On the Origin of the Treponematoses: A Phylogenetic Approach." *PLoS Neglected Tropical Diseases* 2, no. 1 (2008): e148.

Harris, Bernard. "Public Health, Nutrition, and the Decline of Mortality." *Social History of Medicine* 17, no. 3 (2004): 379–407.

Harris, Bernard, *et al.* "Long-Term Changes in Sickness and Health." *Economic History Review* 65, no. 2 (2012): 719–45.

Harrison, Brian. *Drink and the Victorians.* London: Faber and Faber, 1971.

Harrison, Mark. *Disease and the Modern World.* Cambridge: Polity, 2004.

Harrison, Mark. "Disease, Diplomacy and International Commerce." *Journal of Global History* 1, no. 2 (2006): 197–217.

Harrison, Mark. *Contagion.* New Haven and London: Yale University Press, 2012.

Hatton, Timothy J. "How Have Europeans Grown So Tall?." *Oxford Economic Papers* 66, no. 2 (2014): 349–72.

Hatton, Timothy J., and Bernice E. Bray. "Long Run Trends in the Heights of European Men, 19th–20th Centuries." *Economics & Human Biology* 8, no. 3 (2010): 405–13.

Hays, Jo N. *Epidemics and Pandemics: Their Impacts on Human History.* Santa Barbara etc.: Abc-clio, 2005.

Hemminki, Elina, and Anneli Paakkulainen. “The Effect of Antibiotics on Mortality from Infectious Diseases in Sweden and Finland.” *American Journal of Public Health* 66, no. 12 (1976): 1180–84.

Henschen, Folke. *The History and Geography of Diseases.* Translated by Joan Tate. London: Longmans, Green & Co., 1966.

Hermanides, J., *et al.* “Lagere Incidentie van Diabetes Mellitus Type 2 bij Verandering van Leefstijl.” *Nederlands Tijdschrift voor Geneeskunde* 152, no. 44 (2008): 2415–17.

Hilton, Matthew. *Smoking in British Popular Culture 1800–2000.* Manchester: Manchester University Press, 2000.

Hirsch, August. *Handbook of Geographical and Historical Pathology.* Translated by Charles Creighton. London: New Sydenham Society, 1883.

Hjellvik, Vidar, *et al.* “Dementia in the National Cause of Death Registry in Norway 1969–2010.” *Norsk Epidemiologi* 22, no. 2 (2012): 217–24.

Hodgson, Dennis. “Demography as Social Science and Policy Science.” *Population and Development Review* 9, no. 1 (1983): 1–34.

Hoesly, Rachel M., *et al.* “Historical (1750–2014) Anthropogenic Emissions of Reactive Gases and Aerosols.” *Geoscientific Model Development* 11 (2018): 369–408.

Hoffmann, David L. *Cultivating the Masses.* New York: Cornell University Press, 2011.

Hoffmann, Rasmus, *et al.* “Innovations in Health Care and Mortality Trends from Five Cancers.” *International Journal of Public Health* 59, no. 2 (2014): 341–50.

Hoffmann, Rasmus, *et al.* “Innovations in Medical Care and Mortality Trends from Four Circulatory Diseases.” *European Journal of Public Health* 23, no. 5 (2013): 852–57.

Hofstede, Geert. *Culture's Consequences.* Thousand Oaks etc.: Sage, 2001.

Hofstee, Evert W. *De Demografische Ontwikkeling van Nederland in de Eerste Helft van de 19de Eeuw.* Deventer: Van Loghum Slaterus, 1978.

Hofstee, Evert W. *Korte Demografische Geschiedenis van Nederland van 1800* tot Heden Haarlem: Fibula-Van Dishoeck, 1981.

Högberg, Ulf. “The Decline in Maternal Mortality in Sweden: The Role of Community Midwifery.” *American Journal of Public Health* 94, no. 8 (2004): 1312–20.

Högberg, Ulf, Stig Wall, and Göran Broström. “The Impact of Early Medical Technology on Maternal Mortality in Late 19th Century Sweden.” *International Journal of Gynecology & Obstetrics* 24, no. 4 (1986): 251–61.

Holland, Walter W. “The ‘Avoidable Death’ Guide to Europe.” *Health Policy* 6, no. 6 (1986): 115–17.

Holmgren, Anton, *et al.* “Nordic Populations Are Still Getting Taller–Secular Changes in Height from the 20th to 21st Century.” *Acta Paediatrica* 108 (2019): 1311–20.

Hoogendoorn, Dick. *Over de Diphtherie in Nederland.* Zwolle: Tijl, 1948.

Hord, Charlotte, *et al.* “Reproductive Health in Romania: Reversing the Ceausescu Legacy.” *Studies in Family Planning* 22, no. 4 (1991): 231–40.

Horkheimer, Max, and Theodor W. Adorno. *Dialektik der Aufklärung*. Amsterdam: Querido, 1947.

Houston, Robert A. *Literacy in Early Modern Europe*. Edinburgh etc.: Pearson Education Limited, 2002.

Houwaart, Eduard S. *De Hygiënisten*. Groningen: Historische Uitgeverij Groningen, 1991.

Howson, Christopher P., Tomohiko Hiyama, and Ernst L. Wynder. "The Decline in Gastric Cancer: Epidemiology of an Unplanned Triumph." *Epidemiologic Reviews* 8, no. 1 (1986): 1–27.

Hoyle, Richard. "Britain." In *Famine in European History*, edited by Guido Alfani and Cormac Ó Gráda, 141–65. Cambridge etc.: Cambridge University Press, 2017.

Huber, Evelyne, and John D. Stephens. *Development and Crisis of the Welfare State*. Chicago: University of Chicago Press, 2001.

Hunt, John A. "A Short History of Soap." *Pharmaceutical Journal* 263, no. 7076 (1999): 985–89.

Huntington, Samuel P. *The Clash of Civilizations and the Remaking of World Order*. New York etc.: Simon & Schuster, 1996.

Huss, Anke, *et al.* "Efficacy of Pneumococcal Vaccination in Adults: A Meta-Analysis." *Canadian Medical Association Journal* 180, no. 1 (2009): 48–58.

Idsoe, O., and Thorstein Guthe. "The Rise and Fall of the Treponematoses. I. Ecological Aspects and International Trends. In Venereal Syphilis." *British Journal of Venereal Diseases* 43, no. 4 (1967): 227–43.

Iliffe, John. *The African AIDS Epidemic: A History*. Athens: Ohio University Press, 2006.

Illich, Ivan. *Medical Nemesis: The Expropriation of Health*. London: Calder & Boyars, 1975.

Im Hof, Ulrich. *The Enlightenment: An Historical Introduction*. Oxford: Blackwell, 1994.

Inglehart, Ronald. *Modernization and Postmodernization*. Princeton: Princeton University Press, 1997.

Inglehart, Ronald, and Wayne E. Baker. "Modernization, Cultural Change, and the Persistence of Traditional Values." *American Sociological Review* 65, no. 1 (2000): 19–51.

Israel, Jonathan I. *The Dutch Republic: Its Rise, Greatness, and Fall, 1477–1806*. Oxford etc.: Clarendon Press Oxford, 1995.

Jackson, Douglas W., and Pejman Rohani. "Perplexities of Pertussis." *Epidemiology & Infection* 142, no. 4 (2014): 672–84.

Jakopanec, Irena, *et al.* "Syphilis Epidemiology in Norway, 1992–2008." *BMC Infectious Diseases* 10, no. 1 (2010): 105.

Jakszyn, Paula, and Carlos Alberto González. "Nitrosamine and Related Food Intake and Gastric and Oesophageal Cancer Risk." *World Journal of Gastroenterology* 12, no. 27 (2006): 4296–303.

Jansen, Angelique G., *et al.* "Decline in Influenza-Associated Mortality among Dutch Elderly." *Vaccine* 26, no. 44 (2008): 5567–74.

Janssen, Fanny, Johan P. Mackenbach, and Anton E. Kunst. "Trends in Old-Age Mortality in Seven European Countries, 1950–1999." *Journal of Clinical Epidemiology* 57, no. 2 (2004): 203–16.

Järvholm, Bengt, and Alex Burdorf. "Emerging Evidence That the Ban on Asbestos Use Is Reducing the Occurrence of Pleural Mesothelioma in Sweden." *Scandinavian Journal of Public Health* 43, no. 8 (2015): 875–81.

Jenner, Edward. *An Inquiry into Causes and Effects of the Variolae Vaccinae.* London: Sampson Low, 1798.

Jernigan, David H. "The Global Alcohol Industry: An Overview." *Addiction* 104, no. Suppl. 1 (2009): 6–12.

Jernigan, David H., *et al.* "Alcohol Marketing and Youth Alcohol Consumption." *Addiction* 112, no. Suppl. 1 (2017): 7–20.

Jeuring, Hans W., *et al.* "Secular Trends in the Prevalence of Major and Subthreshold Depression among 55–64-Year Olds over 20 Years." *Psychological Medicine* 48, no. 11 (2018): 1824–34.

Johannisson, Karin. "The People's Health: Public Health Policies in Sweden." In *The History of Public Health and the Modern State*, edited by D. Porter, 165–82. Amsterdam & Atlanta: Editions Rodopi, 1994.

Johansson, Egil. *The History of Literacy in Sweden: In Comparison with Some Other Countries*. Educational Reports Umeå. Vol. 12, Umeå: Umeå universitet, 1977.

Johansson, S. Ryan. "The Health Transition: The Cultural Inflation of Morbidity During the Decline of Mortality." *Health Transition Review* 1, no. 1 (1991): 39–68.

Johansson, S. Ryan. "Macro and Micro Perspectives on Mortality History." *Historical Methods* 33, no. 2 (2000): 59–72.

Johansson, S. Ryan, and Alice B. Kasakoff. "Mortality History and the Misleading Mean." *Historical Methods* 33, no. 2 (2000): 56–58.

Johnson, Niall P.A.S., and Juergen Mueller. "Updating the Accounts: Global Mortality of the 1918–1920 'Spanish' Influenza Pandemic." *Bulletin of the History of Medicine* 76, no. 1 (2002): 105–15.

Jones, David S. *Broken Hearts.* Baltimore: Johns Hopkins University Press, 2013.

Jones, David S., and Jeremy A. Greene. "The Contributions of Prevention and Treatment to the Decline in Cardiovascular Mortality." *Health Affairs* 31, no. 10 (2012): 2250–58.

Jones, Ellen, and Fred W. Grupp. "Infant Mortality Trends in the Soviet Union." *Population and Development Review* 9, no. 2 (1983): 213–46.

Jones, Harold B. "The Protestant Ethic: Weber's Model and the Empirical Literature." *Human Relations* 50, no. 7 (1997): 757–78.

Joossens, Luk, and Martin Raw. *The Tobacco Control Scale 2016 in Europe.* Brussels: Association of the European Cancer Leagues, 2017.

Jorland, Gérard. *Une Société à Soigner.* Paris: Gallimard, 2010.

Józan, Peter "Main Features of Epidemiological Development in Hungary after the Second World War." *Hungarian Statistical Review* 86, no. 12 (2008): 1–78.

Juel, Knud, Peter Bjerregaard, and Mette Madsen. "Mortality and Life Expectancy in Denmark and in Other European Countries." *European Journal of Public Health* 10, no. 2 (2000): 93–100.

Kaiser, Sanja, and Johan P. Mackenbach. "Public Health in Eight European Countries: An International Comparison of Terminology." *Public Health* 122, no. 2 (2008): 211–16.

Kameda, Takashi, *et al.* "Asbestos: Use, Bans and Disease Burden in Europe." *Bulletin of the World Health Organization* 92 (2014): 790–97.

Karabchuk, T., *et al.* "как оценить стоимость человеческой жизни? [How to Evaluate the Value of Human Life?]." *Economic Sociology* 15, no. 1 (2014): 89–106.

Karim-Kos, Henrike E., *et al.* "Recent Trends of Cancer in Europe." *European Journal of Cancer* 44, no. 10 (2008): 1345–89.

Kasekamp, Andres. *A History of the Baltic States.* London: Palgrave Macmillan 2017.

Kazan-Allen, Laurie. "Asbestos and Mesothelioma: Worldwide Trends." *Lung Cancer* 49 (2005): S3-S8.

Keene, Janet, *et al.* "Death and Dementia." *International Journal Geriatric Psychiatry* 16, no. 10 (2001): 969–74.

Kelly, Morgan, and Cormac Ó Gráda. "The Waning of the Little Ice Age: Climate Change in Early Modern Europe." *Journal of Interdisciplinary History* 44, no. 3 (2013): 301–25.

Kersbergen, Kees van, and Barbara Vis. *Comparative Welfare State Politics.* Cambridge etc.: Cambridge University Press, 2014.

Kessler, Ronald C., and Evelyn J. Bromet. "The Epidemiology of Depression across Cultures." *Annual Review of Public Health* 34 (2013): 119–38.

Kesztenbaum, Lionel, and Jean-Laurent Rosenthal. "Sewers' Diffusion and the Decline of Mortality: The Case of Paris, 1880–1914." *Journal of Urban Economics* 98 (2017): 174–86.

Keys, Ancel. "Coronary Heart Disease in Seven Countries." *Circulation* 41, no. 1 (1970): 186–95.

Khalil, Charbel Abi, *et al.* "Cause-Specific Mortality in Diabetes: Recent Changes in Trend Mortality." *European Journal of Preventive Cardiology* 19, no. 3 (2012): 374–81.

Kim-Farley, Robert J. "Measles." In *Cambridge World History of Human Disease*, edited by Kenneth F. Kiple, 871–75. Cambridge etc.: Cambridge University Press, 1993.

Kiple, Kenneth F., ed. *Cambridge World History of Human Disease*. Cambridge etc.: Cambridge University Press, 1993.

Kirk, Dudley. *Europe's Population in the Interwar Years.* Geneva: League of Nations, 1946.

Kirk, Dudley. "Demographic Transition Theory." *Population Studies* 50, no. 3 (1996): 361–87.

Kirkwood, Thomas B.L. *Time of Our Lives.* Oxford etc.: Oxford University Press, 1999.

Kirkwood, Thomas B.L., and Steven N. Austad. "Why Do We Age?." *Nature* 408, no. 6809 (2000): 233–38.

Klomp, Jeroen, and Jakob de Haan. "Is the Political System Really Related to Health?" *Social Science and Medicine* 69, no. 1 (2009): 36–46.

Klüsener, Sebastian, *et al.* "Spatial Inequalities in Infant Survival at an Early Stage of the Longevity Revolution." *Demographic Research* 30 (2014): 1849–64.

Kodaman, Nuri, *et al.* "Human and Helicobacter Pylori Coevolution Shapes the Risk of Gastric Disease." *Proceedings of the National Academy of Sciences* 111, no. 4 (2014): 1455–60.

Kohn, Kurt, Hans H. Jansen, and Karl Freudenberg. *Gestaltwandel Klassischer Krankheitsbilder.* Edited by Wilhelm Doerr. Berlin etc.: Springer-Verlag, 1957.

Komlos, John. "The Secular Trend in the Biological Standard of Living in the United Kingdom, 1730–1860." *Economic History Review* 46, no. 1 (1993): 115–44.

Kopits, Elizabeth, and Maureen Cropper. "Traffic Fatalities and Economic Growth." *Accident Analysis and Prevention* 37 (2005): 169–78.

Kôrv, Janika, Mai Roose, and Ain-Elmar Kaasik. "Changed Incidence and Case-Fatality Rates of First-Ever Stroke between 1970 and 1993 in Tartu, Estonia." *Stroke* 27, no. 2 (1996): 199–203.

Kramer, M. "The Rising Pandemic of Mental Disorders and Associated Chronic Diseases and Disabilities." *Acta Psychiatrica Scandinavica* 62, no. Suppl. 285 (1980): 282–97.

Kreitman, Norman. "The Coal Gas Story. United Kingdom Suicide Rates, 1960–71." *Journal of Epidemiology & Community Health* 30, no. 2 (1976): 86–93.

Krieger, Nancy. *Epidemiology and the People's Health.* Oxford etc.: Oxford University Press, 2011.

Kromhout, Daan, Alessandro Menotti, and Henry Blackburn. *Prevention of Coronary Heart Disease.* Dordrecht: Kluwer Academic Publishers, 2002.

Krose, Hermann A. *Der Selbstmord im 19. Jahrhundert nach Seiner Verteilung auf Staaten und Verwaltungsbezirke.* Freiburg im Breisgau: Herdersche Verlagshandlung, 1906.

Kruijt, Cornelis S. *Zelfmoord: Statistisch-Sociologische Verkenningen.* Assen Van Gorcum, 1960.

Kuagbenou, Victor K., and Jean-Noel Biraben. *Introduction à l'Etude de la Mortalité par Cause de Décès à Paris dans la Première Moitié du XIXème Siècle.* Paris: Institut National d'Études Démographiques, 1998.

Kubik, Antonin K., *et al.* "Patterns of Cigarette Sales and Lung Cancer Mortality in Some Central and Eastern European Countries." *Cancer* 75, no. 10 (1995): 2452–60.

Kuhn, Thomas S. *The Structure of Scientific Revolutions.* Chicago: University of Chicago Press, 1962.

Kulhanova, Ivana, *et al.* "Why Does Spain Have Smaller Inequalities in Mortality?" *European Journal of Public Health* 24, no. 3 (2014): 370–77.

Kumar, Krishan. "The Ends of Utopia." *New Literary History* 41, no. 3 (2010): 549–69.

Kunitz, Stephen J. "Explanations and Ideologies of Mortality Patterns." *Population and Development Review* 13, no. 3 (1987): 379–408.

Kunitz, Stephen J. "The Making and Breaking of Yugoslavia and Its Impact on Health." *American Journal of Public Health* 94, no. 11 (2004): 1894–904.

Kuulasmaa, Kari, *et al.* "Estimation of Contribution of Changes in Classic Risk Factors to Trends in Coronary-Event Rates." *Lancet* 355, no. 9205 (2000): 675–87.

Kytir, Josef, Christian Köck, and Rainer Münz. "Historical Regional Patterns of Infant Mortality in Austria." *European Journal of Population/Revue européenne de Démographie* 11, no. 3 (1995): 243–59.

La Berge, Ann E.F. *Mission and Method.* Cambridge etc.: Cambridge University Press, 2002.

La Vecchia, Carlo, *et al.* "The Impact of Therapeutic Improvements in Reducing Peptic Ulcer Mortality in Europe." *International Journal of Epidemiology* 22, no. 1 (1993): 96–106.

La Vecchia, Carlo, *et al.* "Cancer Mortality in Europe, 2000–2004, and an Overview of Trends since 1975." *Annals of Oncology* 21, no. 6 (2009): 1323–60.

Laatikainen, Tiina, *et al.* "Explaining the Decline in Coronary Heart Disease Mortality in Finland between 1982 and 1997." *American Journal of Epidemiology* 162, no. 8 (2005): 764–73.

Lafortune, Gaetan, and Gaëlle Balestat. *Trends in Severe Disability among Elderly People.* OECD Health Working Papers. Vol. 26, Paris: Organisation for Economic Cooperation and Development, 2007.

Laisaar, Kaja-Triin, *et al.* "Estonia at the Threshold of the Fourth Decade of the AIDS Era in Europe." *AIDS Research and Human Retroviruses* 27, no. 8 (2011): 841–51.

Lamarque, J.-F., *et al.* "Historical (1850–2000) Gridded Anthropogenic and Biomass Burning Emissions of Reactive Gases and Aerosols." *Atmospheric Chemistry and Physics* 10, no. 15 (2010): 7017–39.

Lasky, Melvin J. *Utopia and Revolution.* Chicago: University of Chicago Press, 1976.

Lawlor, Clark. *From Melancholia to Prozac.* Oxford etc.: Oxford University Press 2012.

Lawlor, Debbie A., *et al.* "Secular Trends in Mortality by Stroke Subtype in the 20th Century." *Lancet* 360, no. 9348 (2002): 1818–23.

Lawn, Joy E., *et al.* "Stillbirths: Rates, Risk Factors, and Acceleration Towards 2030." *Lancet* 387, no. 10018 (2016): 587–603.

Lazarus, John H. “Iodine Status in Europe in 2014.” *European Thyroid Journal* 3, no. 1 (2014): 3–6.

Lazuka, Volha, Luciana Quaranta, and Tommy Bengtsson. “Fighting Infectious Disease: Evidence from Sweden 1870–1940.” *Population and Development Review* 42, no. 1 (2016): 27–52.

Le Fanu, James. *The Rise and Fall of Modern Medicine.* London: Little Brown & Co, 1999.

Learmonth, Andrew T.A. “Malaria.” In *World Geography of Human Diseases*, edited by G. Melvyn Howe, 61–108. London etc.: Academic Press, 1977.

Leitz, Christian. *Nazi Germany and Neutral Europe During the Second World War.* Manchester: Manchester University Press, 2000.

Leon, David A. “Trends in European Life Expectancy: A Salutary View.” *International Journal of Epidemiology* 40, no. 2 (2011): 271–77.

Leon, David A., *et al.* “Huge Variation in Russian Mortality Rates 1984–94: Artefact, Alcohol, or What?.” *Lancet* 350, no. 9075 (1997): 383–88.

Leon, David A., Dmitry A. Jdanov, and Vladimir M. Shkolnikov. “Trends in Life Expectancy and Age-Specific Mortality in England and Wales, 1970–2016.” *Lancet Public Health* 4, no. 11 (2019): e575-e82.

Levi, Fabio, *et al.* “Cancer Mortality in Europe, 1990–1994, and an Overview of Trends from 1955 to 1994.” *European Journal of Cancer* 35, no. 10 (1999): 1477–516.

Levi, Fabio, *et al.* “Trends in Mortality from Hodgkin’s Disease in Western and Eastern Europe.” *British Journal of Cancer* 87, no. 3 (2002): 291–93.

Levine, Harry G. “Temperance Cultures: Alcohol as a Problem in Nordic and English-Speaking Cultures.” In *The Nature of Alcohol and Drug Related Problems*, edited by M. Lader, G. Edwards and D.C. Drummond, 16–36: New York, 1993.

Lévy, F.M. “The Fiftieth Anniversary of Diphtheria and Tetanus Immunization.” *Preventive Medicine* 4, no. 2 (1975): 226–37.

Levy, Jack S., and William R. Thompson. *The Arc of War.* Chicago: University of Chicago Press, 2011.

Levy, Jack S. *Causes of War.* Chichester: Wiley-Blackwell, 2011.

Levy, Sharon. “The Evolution of Tuberculosis.” *BioScience* 62, no. 7 (2012): 625–29.

Lewis, Jane. “The Prevention of Diphtheria in Canada and Britain 1914–1945.” *Journal of Social History* 20, no. 1 (1986): 163–76.

Lewontin, Richard C. *The Triple Helix.* Boston: Harvard University Press, 2001.

Lieburg, Mart J. van, and Hilary Marland. “Midwife Regulation, Education, and Practice in the Netherlands During the Nineteenth Century.” *Medical History* 33, no. 3 (1989): 296–317.

Lilienfeld, Abraham M., and David E. Lilienfeld. *Foundations of Epidemiology.* Second ed. Oxford etc.: Oxford University Press, 1981.

Lind, Inga, and Steen Hoffmann. “Recorded Gonorrhoea Rates in Denmark, 1900–2010.” *BMJ Open* 5, no. 11 (2015): e008013.

Link, Bruce G., and Jo Phelan. "Social Conditions as Fundamental Causes of Disease." *Journal of Health and Social Behavior* Spec No (1995): 80–94.

Livi Bacci, Massimo. *The Population of Europe: A History.* Oxford: Blackwell, 1999.

Løkke, Anne. "The Antibiotic Transformation of Danish Obstetrics." *Annales de Démographie Historique*, no. 1 (2012): 205–24.

Lopez, Alan D., Neil E. Collishaw, and Tapani Piha. "A Descriptive Model of the Cigarette Epidemic in Developed Countries." *Tobacco Control* 3, no. 3 (1994): 242–47.

Lopez, Alan D., *et al.* "Chronic Obstructive Pulmonary Disease: Current Burden and Future Projections." *European Respiratory Journal* 27, no. 2 (2006): 397–412.

Loudon, Irvine. "Maternal Mortality: 1880–1950. Some Regional and International Comparisons." *Social History of Medicine* 1, no. 2 (1988): 183–228.

Loudon, Irvine. *Death in Childbirth.* Oxford etc.: Oxford University Press, 1992.

Loudon, Irvine. "The Transformation of Maternal Mortality." *British Medical Journal* 305, no. 6868 (Dec 19–26 1992): 1557–60.

Loudon, Irvine. *The Tragedy of Childbed Fever.* Oxford etc.: Oxford University Press, 2000.

Luckin, Bill. "War on the Roads: Traffic Accidents and Social Tension in Britain, 1939–45." In *Accidents in History*, edited by R. Cooter and B. Luckin, 234–54. Amsterdam & Atlanta: Editions Rodopi, 1997.

Maçães, Bruno. *The Dawn of Eurasia.* London: Allen Lane, 2018.

MacDonald, Michael. "The Medicalization of Suicide in England: Laymen, Physicians, and Cultural Change, 1500–1870." *Milbank Quarterly* 67, no. Suppl. 1 (1989): 69–91.

Macedo, Mário Espiga, *et al.* "Prevalence, Awareness, Treatment and Control of Hypertension in Portugal." *Journal of Hypertension* 23, no. 9 (2005): 1661–66.

Macintyre, Sally, *et al.* "Do Housing Tenure and Car Access Predict Health Because They Are Simply Markers of Income or Self Esteem?." *Journal of Epidemiology & Community Health* 52, no. 10 (1998): 657–64.

Mackenbach, Johan P., *et al.* "Socioeconomic Inequalities in Health in 22 European Countries." *New England Journal of Medicine* 358, no. 23 (2008): 2468–81.

Mackenbach, Johan P. *De Veren van Icarus.* Utrecht: Bunge, 1992.

Mackenbach, Johan P. "The Epidemiologic Transition Theory." *Journal of Epidemiology and Community Health* 48, no. 4 (1994): 329–32.

Mackenbach, Johan P. "The Contribution of Medical Care to Mortality Decline: Mckeown Revisited." *Journal of Clinical Epidemiology* 49, no. 11 (1996): 1207–13.

Mackenbach, Johan P. "Carl Von Linné, Thomas Mckeown, and the Inadequacy of Disease Classifications." *European Journal of Public Health* 14, no. 3 (2004): 225.

Mackenbach, Johan P. "Thomas More, Etienne Cabet and the Paradoxes of Utopian Thinking." *European Journal of Public Health* 14, no. 2 (2004): 113.

Mackenbach, Johan P. "The Origins of Human Disease: A Short Story on 'Where Diseases Come From'." *Journal of Epidemiology & Community Health* 60, no. 1 (2006): 81–86.

Mackenbach, Johan P. "Jean Calvin, Calvinism, and Population Health: Impressions from Switzerland." *European Journal of Public Health* 17, no. 1 (2007): 1.

Mackenbach, Johan P. "The Mediterranean Diet Story Illustrates That 'Why' Questions Are as Important as 'How' Questions." *Journal of Clinical Epidemiology* 60, no. 2 (2007): 105–09.

Mackenbach, Johan P. "Bacalhao under the Ponte 25 De Abril: Impressions from Lisbon." *European Journal Public Health* 19, no. 1 (2009): 1.

Mackenbach, Johan P. "Politics Is Nothing but Medicine at a Larger Scale: Reflections on Public Health's Biggest Idea." *Journal of Epidemiology & Community Health* 63, no. 3 (2009): 181–84.

Mackenbach, Johan P. "Convergence and Divergence of Life Expectancy in Europe: A Centennial View." *European Journal of Epidemiology* 28, no. 3 (2013): 229–40.

Mackenbach, Johan P. "Political Conditions and Life Expectancy in Europe, 1900–2008." *Social Science & Medicine* 82 (2013): 134–46.

Mackenbach, Johan P. "Cultural Values and Population Health." *Health & Place* 28 (2014): 116–32.

Mackenbach, Johan P. "Persistence of Social Inequalities in Modern Welfare States." *Scandinavian Journal of Public Health* 45, no. 2 (2017): 113–20.

Mackenbach, Johan P. *Health Inequalities: Persistence and Change in European Welfare States*. Oxford etc.: Oxford University Press, 2019.

Mackenbach, Johan P. , *et al.* "Sharp Upturn of Life Expectancy in the Netherlands." *European Journal of Epidemiology* 26, no. 12 (2011): 903–14.

Mackenbach, Johan P., *et al.* "Using 'Amenable Mortality' as Indicator of Healthcare Effectiveness in International Comparisons." *Journal of Epidemiology and Community Health* 67, no. 2 (2013): 139–46.

Mackenbach, Johan P., Yannan Hu, and Caspar W.N. Looman. "Democratization and Life Expectancy in Europe, 1960–2008." *Social Science & Medicine* 93 (2013): 166–75.

Mackenbach, Johan P., Marina Karanikolos, and Caspar W.N. Looman. "The Rise of Mortality from Mental and Neurological Diseases in Europe, 1979–2009." *BMC Public Health* 14, no. 1 (2014): 840.

Mackenbach, Johan P., *et al.* "Changes in Mortality Inequalities over Two Decades." *British Medical Journal* 353 (2016): i1732.

Mackenbach, Johan P., *et al.* "The Population and High-Risk Approaches to Prevention." *European Journal of Public Health* 23, no. 6 (2012): 909–15.

Mackenbach, Johan P., and Caspar W.N. Looman. "Secular Trends of Infectious Disease Mortality in the Netherlands, 1911–1978." *International Journal of Epidemiology* 17, no. 3 (1988): 618–24.

Mackenbach, Johan P., and Caspar W.N. Looman. "Life Expectancy and National Income in Europe, 1900–2008." *International Journal of Epidemiology* 42, no. 4 (2013): 1100–10.

Mackenbach, Johan P., *et al.* "Fundamental Causes of Inequalities in Mortality." *Sociology of Health and Illness* 39, no. 7 (2017): 1117–33.

Mackenbach, Johan P., *et al.* "Post-1950 Mortality Trends and Medical Care." *Social Science & Medicine* 27, no. 9 (1988): 889–94.

Mackenbach, Johan P., and Martin McKee. "Social-Democratic Government and Health Policy in Europe." *International Journal of Health Services* 43, no. 3 (2013): 389–413.

Mackenbach, Johan P., and Martin McKee, eds. *Successes and Failures of Health Policy in Europe*. Maidenhead: Open University Press, 2013.

Mackenbach, Johan P., Adrianna Murphy, and Martin McKee. "Ukraine: Not Only a Matter of Geopolitics." *Lancet* 383, no. 9920 (2014): 848–50.

Mackenbach, Johan P., *et al.* "Recent Trends in Health Inequalities in 27 European Countries." *Proceedings of the National Academy of Sciences* 115, no. 25 (2018): 6440–45.

MacMahon, Brian, and Thomas F. Pugh. *Epidemiology: Principles and Methods.* Boston: Little, Brown & Company, 1970.

Maddison, Angus. *The World Economy.* Paris: Organization for Economic Cooperation and Development, 2001.

Madsen, Thorvald. "Diphtheria in Denmark from 23,695 to 1 Case: Post or Propter? I. Serum Therapy." *Danish Medical Bulletin* 3, no. 4 (1956): 112–15.

Malik, Khalid. *Human Development Report 2014.* New York: United Nations Development Programme, 2014.

Manton, Kenneth G. "Changing Concepts of Morbidity and Mortality in the Elderly Population." *Milbank Memorial Fund Quarterly. Health and Society* 60, no. 2 (1982): 183–244.

Mariani-Costantini, Renato, and Aldo Mariani-Costantini. "An Outline of the History of Pellagra in Italy." *Journal of Anthropological Sciences* 85 (2007): 163–71.

Mark, L., A. Katona, and L. Deli. "An Attempt to Evaluate the Risk Factors Related to Coronary Heart Disease in Hungary." *Cor et Vasa* 33, no. 4 (1991): 265–72.

Markowitz, Gerald, and David Rosner. "The Illusion of Medical Certainty: Silicosis and the Politics of Industrial Disability, 1930–1960." *Milbank Quarterly* 67, no. Suppl. 2 (1989): 228–53.

Marks, Herbert H. "Longevity and Mortality of Diabetics." *American Journal of Public Health and the Nations Health* 55, no. 3 (1965): 416–23.

Marmot, Michael, *et al.* "WHO European Review of Social Determinants of Health and the Health Divide." *Lancet* 380, no. 9846 (2012): 1011–29.

Martino, Laurenzi, *et al.* "Is Italy Losing the 'Mediterranean Advantage'?." *Preventive Medicine* 18, no. 1 (1989): 35–44.

Mason, Karen Oppenheim. "Explaining Fertility Transitions." *Demography* 34, no. 4 (1997): 443–54.

Masuy-Stroobant, Godelieve. "Infant Health and Infant Mortality in Europe." In *The Decline of Infant and Child Mortality*, edited by C.A. Corsini and P.P. Viazzo, 1–34. Dordrecht: Martinus Nijhoff, 1997.

Mathers, Colin D., *et al.* "Causes of International Increases in Older Age Life Expectancy." *Lancet* 385, no. 9967 (2015): 540–48.

Mattisson, Cecilia, *et al.* "First Incidence Depression in the Lundby Study." *Journal of Affective Disorders* 87, no. 2–3 (2005): 151–60.

Mayr, Ernst. "Cause and Effect in Biology." *Science* 134, no. 3489 (1961): 1501–06.

Mazower, Mark. *Dark Continent.* London: Allen Lane, 1998.

Mazower, Mark. *The Balkans: From the End of Byzantium to the Present Day.* London: Weidenfeld & Nicolson, 2000.

McAlister, Finlay A., *et al.* "Randomised Trials of Secondary Prevention Programmes in Coronary Heart Disease." *British Medical Journal* 323, no. 7319 (2001): 957–62.

McCarron, Mark O., George Davey Smith, and P. McCarron. "Secular Stroke Trends: Early Life Factors and Future Prospects." *Quarterly Journal of Medicine* 99, no. 2 (2006): 117–22.

McKee, Martin. "Alcohol in Russia." *Alcohol and Alcoholism* 34, no. 6 (1999): 824–29.

McKee, Martin. "Cochrane on Communism." *International Journal of Epidemiology* 36, no. 2 (2007): 269–73.

McKee, Martin, *et al.* "Patterns of Smoking in Russia." *Tobacco Control* 7, no. 1 (1998): 22–26.

McKee, Martin, and Johan P. Mackenbach. "Hypertension." In *Successes and Failures of Health Policy in Europe*, edited by Johan P. Mackenbach and Martin McKee, 161–78. Maidenhead: Open University Press, 2013.

McKee, Martin, *et al.* "Health Policy-Making in Central and Eastern Europe: Lessons from the Inaction on Injuries?." *Health Policy and Planning* 15, no. 3 (2000): 263–69.

McKeown, Thomas. *The Modern Rise of Population.* London: Edward Arnold, 1976.

McKeown, Thomas. *The Role of Medicine: Dream, Mirage, or Nemesis?* London: Nuffield Provincial Hopsitals Trust, 1976.

McKeown, Thomas. *The Origins of Human Disease.* Oxford: Basil Blackwell, 1988.

McKeown, Thomas, and Robert G. Brown. "Medical Evidence Related to English Population Changes in the Eighteenth Century." *Population Studies* 9, no. 2 (1955): 119–41.

McKeown, Thomas, and Robert G. Record. "Reasons for the Decline of Mortality in England and Wales During the Nineteenth Century." *Population Studies* 16, no. 2 (1962): 94–122.

McKeown, Thomas, Robert G. Record, and R.D. Turner. "An Interpretation of the Decline of Mortality in England and Wales During the Twentieth Century." *Population Studies* 29, no. 3 (1975): 391–422.

McMichael, Anthony J. *Human Frontiers, Environments and Disease.* Cambridge etc.: Cambridge University Press, 2001.

McNeill, John R. *Something New under the Sun.* London: Allen Lane, 2000.

McNeill, John R. *Mosquito Empires.* Cambridge etc.: Cambridge University Press, 2010.

McNeill, William H. *The Rise of the West.* Chicago etc.: University of Chicago Press, 1963.

McNeill, William H. *Plagues and Peoples.* New York: Anchor Press/Doubleday, 1976.

Meerding, Willem J., *et al. Hoe Gezond Zijn de Zorguitgaven?* Zorg Voor Euro's. Vol. 6, Bilthoven: Rijksinstituut voor Volksgezondheid en Milieu, 2007.

Meiklejohn, Andrew. "History of Lung Diseases of Coal Miners in Great Britain: Part I, 1800–1875." *Occupational and Environmental Medicine* 8, no. 3 (1951): 127–37.

Meiklejohn, Andrew. "History of Lung Diseases of Coal Miners in Great Britain. Part III, 1920–1952." *Occupational and Environmental Medicine* 9, no. 3 (1952): 208–20.

Mercer, Alex. "Relative Trends in Mortality from Related Respiratory and Airborne Infectious Diseases." *Population Studies* 40, no. 1 (1986): 129–45.

Mercer, Alex. *Disease, Mortality, and Population in Transition.* Leicester etc.: Leicester University Press, 1990.

Mercer, Alex. *Infections, Chronic Disease, and the Epidemiological Transition.* Cambridge: Boydell & Brewer, 2014.

Meslé, France, and Jacques Vallin. "Reconstructing Long-Term Series of Causes of Death: The Case of France." *Historical Methods* 29, no. 2 (1996): 72–87.

Meslé, France. "Diverging Trends in Female Old-Age Mortality." *Population and Development Review* 32, no. 1 (2006): 123–45.

Milanovic, Branko. *Global Inequality.* Cambridge & London: Belknap Press, 2016.

Millward, Robert, and Joerg Baten. "Population and Living Standards, 1914–1945." In *Cambridge Economic History of Europe. Volume 2*, edited by Stephen Broadberry and Kevin H. O'Rourke, 232–63. Cambridge etc.: Cambridge University Press, 2010.

Minkov, Michael. *Cultural Differences in a Globalizing World.* Bingley: Emerald Group Publishing, 2011.

Minois, Georges. *Histoire du Suicide.* Paris: Fayard, 1995.

Mironov, Boris N. "The Development of Literacy in Russia and the USSR from the Tenth to the Twentieth Centuries." *History of Education Quarterly* 31, no. 2 (1991): 229–52.

Mirzaei, Masoud, *et al.* "Cerebrovascular Disease in 48 Countries: Secular Trends in Mortality 1950–2005." *Journal Neurology Neurosurgery Psychiatry* 83, no. 2 (2012): 138–45.

Mirzaei, Masoud, *et al.* "Coronary Heart Disease Epidemics: Not All the Same." *Heart* 95, no. 9 (2009): 740–46.

Mokyr, Joel. *The Gifts of Athena.* Princeton: Princeton University Press, 2002.

Mokyr, Joel, and Hans-Joachim Voth. "Understanding Growth in Europe, 1700–1870: Theory and Evidence." In *Cambridge Economic History of Europe. Volume 1: 1700–1870*, edited by Stephen Broadberry and Kenneth H. O'Rourke, 7–42. Cambridge etc.: Cambridge University Press, 2010.

Montanaro, Fabio, *et al.* "Pleural Mesothelioma Incidence in Europe." *Cancer Causes & Control* 14, no. 8 (2003): 791–803.

Mooij, Annet. *Geslachtsziekten en Besmettingsangst.* Amsterdam: Boom, 1993.

Mooney, Graham. *Intrusive Interventions.* Rochester: Rochester University Press, 2015.

Morabia, Alfredo. "Epidemiologic Interactions, Complexity, and the Lonesome Death of Max Von Pettenkofer." *American Journal of Epidemiology* 166, no. 11 (2007): 1233–38.

Moran, Andrew E., *et al.* "Temporal Trends in Ischemic Heart Disease Mortality in 21 World Regions, 1980 to 2010." *Circulation* 129, no. 14 (2014): 1483–92.

More, Thomas. *De Optimo Rei Publicae Statu Deque Nova Insula Utopia* [*On the Best State of a Republic and on the New Island Utopia*]. Leuven, 1516.

Moreda, Vicente Pérez, David S. Reher, and Alberto Sanz Gimeno. *La Conquista de la Salud.* Madrid: Marcial Pons, Ediciones de Historia, 2015.

Morel, Marie-France. "Les Soins Prodigués aux Enfants: Influence des Innovations Médicales et des Institutions Médicalisées (1750–1914)." *Annales de Démographie Historique* (1989): 157–81.

Morris, Ian. *Why the West Rules - for Now.* London: Profile Books, 2010.

Morris, Jerry N. "Recent History of Coronary Disease." *Lancet* 257, no. 6645 (1951): 1–7.

Morse, Stephen S. "Pandemic Influenza: Studying the Lessons of History." *Proceedings of the National Academy of Sciences* 104, no. 18 (2007): 7313–14.

Mortensen, Eric M., *et al.* "Causes of Death for Patients with Community-Acquired Pneumonia." *Archives of Internal Medicine* 162, no. 9 (2002): 1059–64.

Mortimer Jr, Edward A., and Paul K. Jones. "An Evaluation of Pertussis Vaccine." *Reviews of Infectious Diseases* 1, no. 6 (1979): 927–34.

Mukherjee, Siddhartha. *The Emperor of All Maladies.* New York etc.: Scribner, 2010.

Musini, Vijaya M., *et al.* "Pharmacotherapy for Hypertension in the Elderly." *Cochrane Database of Systematic Reviews*, no. 4 (2009): CD000028.

Musk, Arthur W., and Nicholas H. De Klerk. "History of Tobacco and Health." *Respirology* 8, no. 3 (2003): 286–90.

Navarro, Vicente. "Has Socialism Failed? An Analysis of Health Indicators under Socialism." *International Journal of Health Services* 22, no. 4 (1992): 583–601.

Navarro, Vicente, *et al.* "Politics and Health Outcomes." *Lancet* 368, no. 9540 (2006): 1033–37.

NCD Risk Factor Collaboration. "Worldwide Trends in Diabetes since 1980." *Lancet* 387, no. 10027 (2016): 1513–30.

Neligan, Aidan, *et al.* "Temporal Trends in the Mortality of People with Epilepsy." *Epilepsia* 51, no. 11 (2010): 2241–46.

Nelson, Martha I., and Michael Worobey. "Origins of the 1918 Pandemic: Revisiting the Swine "Mixing Vessel" Hypothesis." *American Journal of Epidemiology* 187, no. 12 (2018): 2498–502.

Nesse, Randolph M. "Is Depression an Adaptation?." *Archives of General Psychiatry* 57, no. 1 (2000): 14–20.

Nesse, Randolph M., and George C. Williams. *Why We Get Sick.* New York: Times Books, 1995.

Neushul, Peter. "Fighting Research." In *War, Medicine and Modernity*, edited by Roger Cooter, Mark Harrison and Steve Sturdy, 203–24. Phoenix Mill: Sutton Publishing Limited, 1998.

Newman, Lori, *et al.* "Global Estimates of Syphilis in Pregnancy and Associated Adverse Outcomes." *PLoS Medicine* 10, no. 2 (2013): e1001396.

Newsholme, Arthur. "An Inquiry into the Principal Causes of the Reduction in the Death-Rate from Phthisis During the Last Forty Years." *Journal of Hygiene (Camb.)* 6 (1906): 304–84.

Newsholme, Arthur, and John Adams Kingsbury. *Red Medicine.* London: Heinemann, 1934.

Nolte, Ellen, and Martin McKee. *Does Health Care Save Lives? Avoidable Mortality Revisited.* London: The Nuffield Trust, 2004.

Noordt, Maaike van der, *et al.* "Health Effects of Employment: A Systematic Review of Prospective Studies." *Occupational Environmental Medicine* 71, no. 10 (2014): 730–36.

Norman, Leslie G. *Road Traffic Accidents: Epidemiology, Control, and Prevention.* Geneva: World Health Organization, 1962.

Nunes, B., *et al.* "The 1918–1919 Influenza Pandemic in Portugal." *American Journal of Epidemiology* 187, no. 12 (2018): 2541–49.

Nusselder, Wilma J., and Johan P. Mackenbach. "Rectangularization of the Survival Curve in the Netherlands, 1950–1992." *Gerontologist* 36, no. 6 (1996): 773–82.

Ó Gráda, Cormac. "Ireland." In *Famine in European History*, edited by Guido Alfani and Cormac Ó Gráda, 166–84. Cambridge etc.: Cambridge University Press, 2017.

Ocaña, Esteban Rodriguez. "El Informe sobre la Sanidad Espanola (1926) de Charles A. Bailey." *Cronos* 4, no. 1–2 (2001): 63–79.

Ocaña, Esteban Rodriguez. "International Health Goals and Social Reform." In *Facing Illness in Troubled Times*, edited by Iris Borowy and Wolf Gruner, 247–76. Frankfurt am Main: Peter Lang, 2005.

Ocaña, Esteban Rodríguez. *Salud Pública en España: Ciencia, Profesión y Política, Siglos XVIII-XX.* Granada: Unversidad de Granada, 2005.

Ocaña, Esteban Rodríguez, and Ferran Martinez Navarro. *La Salud Pública en España. De la Edad Media al Siglo XX.* Vol. 68, Granada: Escuela Andaluza de Salud Publica, n.d.

Oeppen, Jim, and James W. Vaupel. "Broken Limits to Life Expectancy." *Science* 296 (2002): 1029–31.

Office for National Statistics. *Results from the ICD–10 V2010 Bridge Coding Study*. Statistical Bulletin. Newport: Office for National Statistics, 2011.

Olshansky, S. Jay, and A. Brian Ault. "The Fourth Stage of the Epidemiologic Transition: The Age of Delayed Degenerative Diseases." *Milbank Quarterly* 64, no. 3 (1986): 355–91.

Olshansky, S. Jay, *et al.* "Emerging Infectious Diseases: The Fifth Stage of the Epidemiologic Transition?." *World Health Statistics Quarterly* 51, no. 2–4 (1998): 207–17.

Omran, Abdel R. "The Epidemiologic Transition: A Theory of the Epidemiology of Population Change." *Milbank Memorial Fund Quarterly* 49 (1971): 509–38.

Omran, Abdel R. "The Epidemiologic Transition Theory. A Preliminary Update." *Journal of Tropical Pediatrics* 29 (1983): 305–16.

Omran, Abdel R. "The Epidemiologic Transition Theory Revisited Thirty Years Later." *World Health Statistics Quarterly* 51, no. 2–4 (1998): 99–119.

Otte, Christian, *et al.* "Major Depressive Disorder." *Nature Reviews Disease primers* 2 (2016): 16065.

Overton, Mark. *Agricultural Revolution in England.* Cambridge etc.: Cambridge University Press, 1996.

Packard, Randall M. *The Making of a Tropical Disease.* Baltimore: Johns Hopkins University Press, 2007.

Pampel, Fred C. "Cigarette Diffusion and Sex Differences in Smoking." *Journal of Health and Social Behavior* 42, no. 4 (2001): 388–404.

Pamuk, Elsie R. "Social Class Inequality in Mortality from 1921 to 1972 in England and Wales." *Population Studies (Cambridge)* 39, no. 1 (1985): 17–31.

Pamuk, Elsie R. "Social-Class Inequality in Infant Mortality in England and Wales from 1921 to 1980." *European Journal of Population/Revue Européenne de Démographie* 4, no. 1 (1988): 1–21.

Pamuk, Şevket. *Uneven Centuries: Economic Development of Turkey since 1820.* Princeton: Princeton University Press, 2018.

Panum, Peter L. *Lagttagelser, Anstillede under Maesllinge-Epidemien Paa Faeroerne I Aaret 1846* [*Observations Made During the Epidemic of Measles on the Faroe Islands in the Year 1846*]. Copenhagen: Bibiliothek for Laeger, 1847.

Parent-Duchâtelet, Alexandre. *De la Prostitution dans la Ville de Paris, Considérée sous le Rapport de l'Hygiène Publique, de la Morale et de l'Administration.* Paris: J.-B. Baillière et fils, 1836.

Park, Boyoung, *et al.* "Ecological Study for Refrigerator Use, Salt, Vegetable, and Fruit Intakes, and Gastric Cancer." *Cancer Causes & Control* 22, no. 11 (2011): 1497–503.

Park, Youngmee K., *et al.* "Effectiveness of Food Fortification in the United States: The Case of Pellagra." *American Journal of Public Health* 90, no. 5 (2000): 727–38.

Patterson, Christopher C., *et al.* "Incidence Trends for Childhood Type 1 Diabetes in Europe During 1989–2003 and Predicted New Cases 2005–20." *Lancet* 373, no. 9680 (2009): 2027–33.

Patterson, K. David. *Pandemic Influenza, 1700–1900.* Totowa: Rowman & Littlefield 1986.

Patterson, K. David. "Bacillary Dysentery." In *Cambridge World History of Human Disease*, edited by Kenneth F. Kiple, 604–06. Cambridge etc.: Cambridge University Press, 1993.

Patterson, K. David. "Cholera Diffusion in Russia, 1823–1923." *Social Science & Medicine* 38, no. 9 (1994): 1171–91.

Patterson, K. David. "Mortality in Late Tsarist Russia: A Reconnaissance." *Social History of Medicine* 8, no. 2 (1995): 179–210.

Peden, Margie, *et al. World Report on Road Traffic Injury Prevention.* Geneva: World Health Organization, 2004.

Peltola, Heikki, *et al.* "Measles, Mumps, and Rubella in Finland." *Lancet Infectious Diseases* 8, no. 12 (2008): 796–803.

Perrenoud, Alfred. "The Attenuation of Mortality Crises and the Decline of Mortality." In *The Decline of Mortality in Europe*, edited by Roger S. Schofield, David Reger and Alain Bideau, 18–37. Oxford: Clarendon Press, 1991.

Peto, Julian. "Cancer Epidemiology in the Last Century and the Next Decade." *Nature* 411, no. 6835 (2001): 390–95.

Peto, Julian, *et al.* "Continuing Increase in Mesothelioma Mortality in Britain." *Lancet* 345, no. 8949 (1995): 535–39.

Peto, Richard, *et al.* "Mortality from Tobacco in Developed Countries: Indirect Estimation from National Vital Statistics." *Lancet* 339, no. 8804 (1992): 1268–78.

Pharris, Anastasia, *et al.* "Human Immunodeficiency Virus in Injecting Drug Users in Europe." *Eurosurveillance* 16, no. 48 (2011): 20032.

Piana, Francesca. "Humanitaire et Politique, in Medias Res." *Relations Internationales* 2, no. 138 (2009): 23–38.

Piazuelo, M. Blanca, Meira Epplein, and Pelayo Correa. "Gastric Cancer: An Infectious Disease." *Infectious Disease Clinics* 24, no. 4 (2010): 853–69.

Piketty, Thomas. *Capital in the Twenty-First Century.* Cambridge (Mass): Harvard University Press, 2014.

Pimm, Stuart L., *et al.* "The Biodiversity of Species and Their Rates of Extinction, Distribution, and Protection." *Science* 344, no. 6187 (2014): 1246752-1-10.

Pinker, Steven. *The Better Angels of Our Nature.* London: Allen Lane, 2011.

Pinker, Steven. *Enlightenment Now.* London: Allen Lane, 2018.

Pitkänen, Kari J., James H. Mielke, and Lynn B. Jorde. "Smallpox and Its Eradication in Finland: Implications for Disease Control." *Population Studies* 43, no. 1 (1989): 95–111.

Pomeranz, Kenneth. *The Great Divergence.* Princeton & Oxford: Princeton University Press, 2000.

Poppel, Frans van, and Cor van der Heijden. "The Effects of Water Supply on Infant and Childhood Mortality." *Health Transition Review* 7, no. 2 (1997): 113–48.

Porter, Dorothy. *The History of Public Health and the Modern State.* Amsterdam: Editions Rodopi, 1994.

Porter, Dorothy. *Health, Civilization and the State.* London and New York: Routledge, 2005.

Porter, Dorothy. *Health Citizenship.* Berkeley etc.: University Of California Medical Humanities Press, 2011.

Porter, Roy. "Cleaning up the Great Wen: Public Health in Eighteenth-Century London." *Medical History* 35, no. S11 (1991): 61–75.

Porter, Roy. *The Greatest Benefit to Mankind.* London: HarperCollins, 1997.

Porter, Roy. *Enlightenment: Britain and the Creation of the Modern World.* London: Allen Lane, 2000.

Post, John D. *Food Shortage, Climatic Variability, and Epidemic Disease in Preindustrial Europe.* New York: Cornell University Press, 1985.

Potter, Christopher W. "A History of Influenza." *Journal of Applied Microbiology* 91, no. 4 (2001): 572–79.

Poulain, Michel, Anne Herm, and Gianni Pes. "Blue Zones: Areas of Exceptional Longevity around the World." *Vienna Yearbook of Population Research* 11 (2013): 87–108.

Pound, Pandora, Michael Bury, and Shah Ebrahim. "From Apoplexy to Stroke." *Age and Ageing* 26, no. 5 (1997): 331–37.

Pozzi, Lucia, and Diego Ramiro Fariñas. "Infant and Child Mortality in the Past." *Annales de Démographie Historique*, no. 1 (2015): 55–75.

Preston, Samuel H. "The Changing Relation between Mortality and Level of Economic Development." *Population Studies* 29, no. 2 (1975): 231–48.

Preston, Samuel H., Dana A. Glei, and John R. Wilmoth. "A New Method for Estimating Smoking-Attributable Mortality in High-Income Countries." *International Journal of Epidemiology* 39, no. 2 (2009): 430–38.

Preston, Samuel H., and Michael R. Haines. *Fatal Years.* Princeton: Princeton University Press, 1991.

Preston, Samuel H., N. Keyfitz, and R. Schoen. *Causes of Death: Life Tables for National Populations.* New York: Seminar Press, 1972.

Pridemore, William A., *et al.* "The Impact of a National Alcohol Policy on Deaths Due to Transport Accidents in Russia." *Addiction* 108, no. 12 (2013): 2112–18.

Primatesta, Paola, and Neil R. Poulter. "Improvement in Hypertension Management in England." *Journal of Hypertension* 24, no. 6 (2006): 1187–92.

Prince, Martin, *et al.* "Recent Global Trends in the Prevalence and Incidence of Dementia, and Survival with Dementia." *Alzheimer's Research & Therapy* 8, no. 1 (2016): 23.

Pritchard, Colin W., David S. Baldwin, and Andrew G. Mayers. "Changing Patterns of Adult Neurological Deaths in the Major Western World Countries." *Public Health* 118, no. 4 (2004): 268–83.

Pritchett, Lant, and Lawrence H. Summers. "Wealthier Is Healthier." *Journal of Human Resources* 31, no. 4 (1996): 841–68.

Proctor, Robert N. *Cancer Wars*. New York: Basic Books, 1995.

Proctor, Robert N. *The Nazi War on Cancer*. Princeton: Princeton University Press, 2000.

Proctor, Robert N. *Golden Holocaust*. Berkeley etc.: Univ of California Press, 2011.

Proctor, Robert N. "The History of the Discovery of the Cigarette–Lung Cancer Link." *Tobacco Control* 21, no. 2 (2012): 87–91.

Puranen, Britt-Inger. *Tuberkulos: En Sjukdoms Förekomst och dess Orsaker: Sverige 1750–1980*. Umeå Studies in Economic History. Vol. 7, Umeå: Umeå Universitet, 1984.

Puranen, Britt-Inger. "Tuberculosis and the Decline of Mortality in Sweden." In *The Decline of Mortality in Europe*, edited by Roger S. Schofield, David S. Reher and Alain Bideau, 97–117. Oxford etc.: Clarendon Press, 1991.

Rabson, S. Milton. "Alfred Grotjahn, Founder of Social Hygiene." *Bulletin of the New York Academy of Medicine* 12, no. 2 (1936): 43–58.

Ramiro Fariñas, Diego, and Alberto G. Sanz. "Childhood Mortality in Central Spain, 1790–1960." *Continuity and Change* 15, no. 2 (2000): 235–67.

Ramsey, Matthew. "Public Health in France." In *The History of Public Health and the Modern State*, edited by D. Porter, 45–118. Amsterdam: Editions Rodopi, 1994.

Ramstedt, Mats. "Alcohol-Related Mortality in 15 European Countries in the Postwar Period." *European Journal of Population/Revue Européenne de Démographie* 18, no. 4 (2002): 307–23.

Raoult, Didier, *et al.* "Evidence for Louse-Transmitted Diseases in Soldiers of Napoleon's Grand Army in Vilnius." *Journal of Infectious Diseases* 193, no. 1 (2006): 112–20.

Raviglione, Mario C. "XDR-TB: Entering the Post-Antibiotic Era?." *International Journal of Tuberculosis and Lung Disease* 10, no. 11 (2006): 1185–87.

Raviglione, Mario C., *et al.* "Tuberculosis Trends in Eastern Europe and the Former USSR." *Tubercle and Lung disease* 75, no. 6 (1994): 400–16.

Raviglione, Mario C., *et al.* "Secular Trends of Tuberculosis in Western Europe." *Bulletin of the World Health Organization* 71, no. 3–4 (1993): 297–306.

Razvodovsky, Yury. "Homicide and Alcohol Intoxication in Russia, 1956–2005." *Alcoholism* 43, no. 1 (2007): 36–50.

Razzell, Peter. *The Conquest of Smallpox*. Firle: Caliban Books, 1977.

Rechel, Bernd. "HIV/AIDS in the Countries of the Former Soviet Union." *Central European Journal of Public Health* 18, no. 2 (2010): 110–15.

Rechel, Bernd, and Martin McKee. "Health Reform in Central and Eastern Europe and the Former Soviet Union." *Lancet* 374, no. 9696 (2009): 1186–95.

Rechel, Bernd, *et al.* "Health and Health Systems in the Commonwealth of Independent States." *Lancet* 381, no. 9872 (2013): 1145–55.

Regidor, Enrique, *et al.* "The Role of Political and Welfare State Characteristics in Infant Mortality." *International Journal of Epidemiology* 40, no. 5 (2011): 1187–95.

Regidor, Enrique, *et al.* "Major Reduction in AIDS-Mortality Inequalities after HAART." *Social Science & Medicine* 68, no. 3 (2009): 419–26.

Reid, Alice, and Eilidh Garrett. "Doctors and the Causes of Neonatal Death in Scotland in the Second Half of the Nineteenth Century." *Annales de Démographie Historique*, no. 1 (2012): 149–79.

Reseland, Svein, Isabelle Bray, and David Gunnell. "Relationship between Antidepressant Sales and Secular Trends in Suicide Rates in the Nordic Countries." *British Journal of Psychiatry* 188, no. 4 (2006): 354–58.

Reves, Randall. "Declining Fertility in England and Wales as a Major Cause of the Twentieth Century Decline in Mortality." *American Journal of Epidemiology* 122, no. 1 (1985): 112–26.

Ricklefs, Robert E., and Caleb E. Finch. *Aging: A Natural History.* New York: Scientific American Books, 1995.

Ridley, Matt. *Nature Via Nurture. Genes, Experience and What Makes Us Human.* London: Harper, 2004.

Rieder, H.L., *et al.* "Tuberculosis Control in Europe and International Migration." *European Respiratory Journal* 7, no. 8 (1994): 1545–53.

Riley, James C. *The Eighteenth Century Campaign to Avoid Disease.* New York: St. Martin's Press, 1987.

Riley, James C. *Sickness, Recovery, and Death.* London: MacMillan Press, 1989.

Riley, James C. *Rising Life Expectancy: A Global History.* Cambridge etc.: Cambridge University Press, 2001.

Rizzo, Caterina, *et al.* "Influenza-Related Mortality in the Italian Elderly." *Vaccine* 24, no. 42–43 (2006): 6468–75.

Roberts, Bayard, *et al.* "Changes in Smoking Prevalence in 8 Countries of the Former Soviet Union between 2001 and 2010." *American Journal of Public Health* 102, no. 7 (2012): 1320–28.

Roberts, Bayard, *et al.* "Irregular Treatment of Hypertension in the Former Soviet Union." *Journal Epidemiology Community Health* 66, no. 6 (2012): 482–88.

Roberts, John M. *The Penguin History of Europe.* London etc.: Penguin, 1996.

Robine, Jean-Marie, and Michel Allard. "The Oldest Human." *Science* 279, no. 5358 (1998): 1831–31.

Robine, Jean-Marie, *et al.* "The Real Facts Supporting Jeanne Calment as the Oldest Ever Human." *Journals of Gerontology: Series A* 74, no. S1 (2019): S13-S20.

Robine, Jean-Marie, and Emmanuelle Cambois. "Healthy Life Expectancy in Europe." *Population & Sociétés*, no. 499 (2013): 1–4.

Robinson, Paul. *The Modernization of Sex.* Oxford etc.: Harper & Row, 1976.

Roe, Daphne A. *A Plague of Corn.* London: Cornell University Press, 1973.

Rogers, Richard G., and Robert Hackenberg. "Extending Epidemiologic Transition Theory: A New Stage." *Social Biology* 34, no. 3–4 (1987): 234–43.

Rokholm, Benjamin, Jennifer L. Baker, and Thorkild I.A. Sørensen. "The Levelling Off of the Obesity Epidemic since the Year 1999." *Obesity Reviews* 11, no. 12 (2010): 835–46.

Rollet-Echalier, Catherine. "La Politique à l'Egard de la Petite Enfance sous la IIIe République." *Population (French Edition)* 46, no. 2 (1991): 349–58.

Rose, Geoffrey. *The Strategy of Preventive Medicine.* Oxford etc.: Oxford University Press, 1992.

Rosen, George. "What Is Social Medicine?." *Bulletin of the History of Medicine* 21, no. 5 (1947): 674–733.

Rosen, George. "Biography of Dr. Johann Peter Frank Written by Himself." *Journal of the History of Medicine and Allied Sciences* 3, no. 2 (1948): 279–314.

Rosen, George. "Cameralism and the Concept of Medical Police." *Bulletin of the History of Medicine* 27 (1953): 21–42.

Rosen, George. "The Fate of the Concept of Medical Police 1780–1890." *Centaurus* 5, no. 2 (1957): 97–113.

Rosen, George. *A History of Public Health.* Baltimore: Johns Hopkins University Press, 1958 [expanded edition 1993].

Rosner, David, and Gerald Markowitz. "Consumption, Silicosis, and the Social Construction of Industrial Disease." *Yale Journal of Biology and Medicine* 64, no. 5 (1991): 481–98.

Roth, Gregory A., *et al.* "Global, Regional, and National Burden of Cardiovascular Diseases for 10 Causes, 1990 to 2015." *Journal of the American College of Cardiology* 70, no. 1 (2017): 1–25.

Rothenberg, Gunther E. "The Austrian Sanitary Cordon and the Control of the Bubonic Plague: 1710–1871." *Journal of the History of Medicine and Allied Sciences* 28, no. 1 (1973): 15–23.

Rothschuh, Karl E. "Der Krankheitsbegriff (Was Ist Krankheit)." In *Was Ist Krankheit?*, edited by Karl E. Rothschuh, 397–420. Darmstadt: Wisenschaftliche Buchgesellschaft, 1975.

Rothwell, Peter M., *et al.* "Change in Stroke Incidence, Mortality, Case-Fatality, Severity, and Risk Factors in Oxfordshire." *Lancet* 363, no. 9425 (2004): 1925–33.

Roundtable, AHR. "Historians and the Question of 'Modernity'." *American Historical Review* 116, no. 3 (2011): 631–751.

Ruhm, Christopher J. "Are Recessions Good for Your Health?" *Quarterly Journal of Economics* 115, no. 2 (2000): 617–50.

Russell, W.T. "Epidemiology of Diphtheria During the Last Forty Years." London: His Majesty's Stationery Office, 1943.

Rutqvist, Lars E., *et al.* "Swedish Snus and the Gothiatek® Standard." *Harm Reduction Journal* 8, no. 1 (2011): 11.

Rutstein, David D., *et al.* "Measuring the Quality of Medical Care: A Clinical Method." *New England Journal of Medicine* 294, no. 11 (1976): 582–88.

Rutten, Willibrord. *"De Vreselijkste Aller Harpijen."* Wageningen: Afdeling Agrarische Geschiedenis, Landbouwuniversiteit Wageningen, 1997.

Saltman, Richard B., and Hans F.W. Dubois. "The Historical and Social Base of Social Health Insurance Systems." In *Social Health Insurance Systems in Western Europe*, edited by Richard B Saltman, R. Busse and J. Figueres, 21–32. Maidenhead: Open University Press, 2004.

Sandberg, Lars G., and Richard H. Steckel. "Was Industrialization Hazardous to Your Health? Not in Sweden!" In *Health and Welfare During Industrialization*, edited by Richard H. Steckel and R. Floud, 127–60. Chicago & London: University of Chicago Press, 1997.

Sant, Milena, *et al.* "EUROCARE-4. Survival of Cancer Patients Diagnosed in 1995–1999. Results and Commentary." *European Journal of Cancer* 45, no. 6 (2009): 931–91.

Santana, Paula, and Helena Nogueira. "AIDS/HIV Mortality in Portugal in the 90s." *Revista Portuguesa de Saúde Pública*, no. 1 (2005): 57–68.

Savolainen, Jukka, Martti Lehti, and Janne Kivivuori. "Historical Origins of a Cross-National Puzzle: Homicide in Finland, 1750 to 2000." *Homicide Studies* 12, no. 1 (2008): 67–89.

Sawin, Clark T. "Goiter." In *Cambridge World History of Human Disease*, edited by Kenneth F. Kiple, 750–56. Cambridge etc.: Cambridge University Press, 1993.

Schaefer Elinder, Liselotte, and Caroline Bollars. "Food and Nutrition." In *Successes and Failures of Health Policy in Europe*, edited by Johan P. Mackenbach and Martin McKee, 59–89. Maidenhead: Open University Press, 2013.

Schaufeli, Wilmar B., and Toon W. Taris. "A Critical Review of the Job Demands-Resources Model." In *Bridging Occupational, Organizational and Public Health*, edited by Georg F. Bauer and Oliver Hämmig, 43–68. Dordrecht: Springer, 2014.

Schmidt, Ida M., M.H. Jørgensen, and Kim Fleischer Michaelsen. "Height of Conscripts in Europe: Is Postneonatal Mortality a Predictor?" *Annals of Human Biology* 22, no. 1 (1995): 57–67.

Schmidt, James. "What Enlightenment Project?" *Political Theory* 28, no. 6 (2000): 734–57.

Schneider, Dona, and David E. Lilienfeld, eds. *Public Health: The Development of a Discipline*. New Brunswick etc.: Rutgers University Press, 2011.

Schönbeck, Yvonne, *et al.* "The World's Tallest Nation Has Stopped Growing Taller." *Pediatric Research* 73, no. 3 (2013): 371–77.

Schulze, Hagen. *States, Nations and Nationalism.* Oxford: Blackwell, 1996.

Sealey, Patricia A. "The League of Nations Health Organisation and the Evolution of Transnational Public Health." Doctor of Philosophy, Ohio State University, 2011.

Segura, O., Alex Burdorf, and Caspar Looman. "Update of Predictions of Mortality from Pleural Mesothelioma in the Netherlands." *Occupational and Environmental Medicine* 60, no. 1 (2003): 50–55.

Semashko, Nikolai A. "Karl Marx und die Sozialhygiene." In *Der Rote Oktober und der Sowjetische Gesundheitsschutz*, edited by Kurt Winter, Alfred Keck, Rolf Lother and Horst Spaar, 13–17. Jena: VEB Gustav Fischer Verlag, 1977 [1933].

Sethi, Dinesh. *Injuries and Violence in Europe: Why They Matter and What Can Be Done.* Copenhagen WHO Regional Office Europe, 2006.

Sethi, Dinesh, and Franco Mitis. "Road Traffic Injuries." In *Successes and Failures of Health Policy in Europe*, edited by Johan P. Mackenbach and Martin McKee, 215–38. Maidenhead: Open University Press.

Shkolnikov, Vladimir M., *et al.* "Mortality Reversal in Russia: The Story So Far." *Hygiea Internationalis* 4, no. 1 (2004): 29–80.

Shkolnikov, Vladimir M., *et al.* "Components and Possible Determinants of the Decrease in Russian Mortality in 2004–2010." *Demographic Research* 28 (2013): 917–50.

Shkolnikov, Vladimir M., *et al.* "Patterns in the Relationship between Life Expectancy and Gross Domestic Product in Russia in 2005–15." *Lancet Public Health* 4, no. 4 (2019): e181-e88.

Shkolnikov, Vladimir M., France Meslé, and Jacques Vallin. "Recent Trends in Life Expectancy and Causes of Death in Russia, 1970–1993." In *Premature Death in the New Independent States*, edited by J.A. Bobadilla, C.A. Costello and F. Mitchell, 34–65. Washington (DC): National Academies Press, 1997.

Siegelbaum, Lewis H. *Cars for Comrades.* Ithaca: Cornell University Press, 2008.

Sienkiewicz-Jarosz, Halina, *et al.* "Incidence and Case Fatality Rates of First-Ever Stroke." *Neurologia i Neurochirurgia Polska* 45, no. 3 (2011): 207–12.

Sigerist, Henry E. "Frank, Johann Peter. The People's Misery: Mother of Diseases." *Bulletin of the History of Medicine* 9 (1941): 81–100.

Sigerist, Henry E. *Civilization and Disease.* New York: Cornell University Press, 1943.

Sigerist, Henry E. *Medicine and Health in the Soviet Union.* Binghamton: Citadel Press, 1947.

Sijbrands, Eric J.G., *et al.* "Mortality over Two Centuries in Large Pedigree with Familial Hypercholesterolaemia." *British Medical Journal* 322, no. 7293 (2001): 1019–23.

Simmons, R.D., *et al.* "Ten-Year Mortality Trends among Persons Diagnosed with HIV Infection in England and Wales." *HIV Medicine* 14, no. 10 (2013): 596–604.

Singer, Peter. *The Expanding Circle.* Princeton: Princeton University Press, 1981.

Singh, Bruce, and Rachel Jenkins. "Suicide Prevention Strategies: An International Perspective." *International Review of Psychiatry* 12, no. 1 (2000): 7–14.

Sivenius, Juhani, *et al.* "Continuous 15-Year Decrease in Incidence and Mortality of Stroke in Finland." *Stroke* 35, no. 2 (2004): 420–25.

Slack, Paul. "The Black Death Past and Present. 2. Some Historical Problems." *Transactions of the Royal Society of Tropical Medicine and Hygiene* 83, no. 4 (1989): 461–63.

Smith, Dale. "Typhoid Fever." In *Cambridge World History of Human Disease*, edited by Kenneth F. Kiple, 1071–77. Cambridge etc.: Cambridge University Press, 1993.

Smith, Francis B. *The People's Health, 1830–1910*. Canberra: Australian National University Press, 1979.

Smith, George Davey. "Commentary: Behind the Broad Street Pump." *International Journal of Epidemiology* 31, no. 5 (2002): 920–32.

Smith, Kirk R., and Majid Ezzati. "How Environmental Health Risks Change with Development." *Annual Review Environmental Resources* 30 (2005): 291–333.

Smith, Steven J., *et al.* "Anthropogenic Sulfur Dioxide Emissions: 1850–2005." *Atmospheric Chemistry and Physics* 11, no. 3 (2011): 1101–16.

Snowden, Frank M. *Naples in the Time of Cholera, 1884–1911*. Cambridge etc.: Cambridge University Press, 1995.

Snowden, Frank M. *Epidemics and Society: From the Black Death to the Present.* New Haven: Yale University Press, 2019.

Snyder, John C. "Typhus Fever in the Second World War." *California Medicine* 66, no. 1 (1947): 3–10.

Snyder, Timothy. *Bloodlands: Europe between Hitler and Stalin.* London: Bodley Head, 2010.

Søgaard, Mette, *et al.* "Nationwide Trends in Pneumonia Hospitalization Rates and Mortality, Denmark 1997–2011." *Respiratory Medicine* 108, no. 8 (2014): 1214–22.

Sonnenberg, Amnon. "Causes Underlying the Birth-Cohort Phenomenon of Peptic Ulcer." *International journal of epidemiology* 35, no. 4 (2006): 1090–97.

Sonnenberg, Amnon. "Time Trends of Ulcer Mortality in Europe." *Gastroenterology* 132, no. 7 (2007): 2320–27.

Sontag, Susan. *Illness as Metaphor.* New York: Farrar, Straus & Giroux, 1978.

Sørensen, Kristine, *et al.* "Health Literacy in Europe: Comparative Results of the European Health Literacy Survey (HLS-EU)." *European Journal of Public Health* 25, no. 6 (2015): 1053–58.

Speck, Reinhard. "Cholera." In *Cambridge World History of Human Disease*, edited by Kenneth F. Kiple, 642–49. Cambridge etc.: Cambridge University Press, 1993.

Spierenburg, Pieter. *A History of Murder.* Cambridge: Polity Press, 2008.

Stallones, Reuel A. "The Rise and Fall of Ischemic Heart Disease." *Scientific American* 243, no. 5 (1980): 53–59.

Stapleton, Darwin H. "Lessons of History?" *Public Health Reports* 119, no. 2 (2004): 206–15.

Stearns, Stephen C., ed. *Evolution in Health and Disease*. Oxford etc.: Oxford University Press, 1999.

Steinberg, Benjamin A., *et al.* "Nine-Year Trends in Achievement of Risk Factor Goals in the US and European Outpatients with Cardiovascular Disease." *American Heart Journal* 156, no. 4 (2008): 719–27.

Steinbock, R. Ted. "Rickets and Osteomalacia." In *Cambridge World History of Human Disease*, edited by Kenneth F. Kiple, 978–80. Cambridge etc.: Cambridge University Press, 1993.

Stephenson, Patricia, *et al.* "Commentary: The Public Health Consequences of Restricted Induced Abortion - Lessons from Romania." *American Journal of Public Health* 82, no. 10 (1992): 1328–31.

Stevens, Emily E., Thelma E. Patrick, and Rita Pickler. "A History of Infant Feeding." *Journal of Perinatal Education* 18, no. 2 (2009): 32–39.

Stickley, Andrew, Yury Razvodovsky, and Michael McKee. "Alcohol Mortality in Russia: A Historical Perspective." *Public Health* 123, no. 1 (2009): 20–26.

Stiglitz, Joseph E. *The Price of Inequality*. New York etc.: W.W. Norton & Co., 2012.

Stokvis, Pieter R.D. *De Wording van Modern Den Haag*. Zwolle: Waanders, 1987.

Stolz, Yvonne, Joerg Baten, and Jaime Reis. "Portuguese Living Standards, 1720–1980, in European Comparison." *Economic History Review* 66, no. 2 (2013): 545–78.

Stroke Unit Trialists' Collaboration. "Organised Inpatient (Stroke Unit) Care for Stroke." *Cochrane Database Systematic Reviews*, no. 9 (2013): CD000197.

Stuckler, David, Lawrence King, and Martin McKee. "Mass Privatisation and the Post-Communist Mortality Crisis." *Lancet* 373, no. 9661 (2009): 399–407.

Sundin, Jan, and Sam Willner. *Social Change and Health in Sweden: 250 Years of Politics and Practice.* Stockholm: Swedish National Institute of Public Health, 2007.

Susser, Mervyn, and Zena Stein. "Civilisation and Peptic Ulcer." *Lancet* 279, no. 7221 (1962): 116–19.

Susser, Mervyn, and Ezra Susser. "Choosing a Future for Epidemiology: II. From Black Box to Chinese Boxes and Eco-Epidemiology." *American Journal of Public Health* 86, no. 5 (1996): 674–77.

Swaan, Abram de. *In Care of the State.* New York etc. : Oxford University Press, 1988.

Swaroop, S., and R. Pollitzer. "Cholera Studies: 2. World Incidence." *Bulletin of the World Health Organization* 12, no. 3 (1955): 311–58.

Szreter, Simon. "The Importance of Social Intervention in Britains Mortality Decline C. 1850–1914." *Social History of Medicine* 1, no. 1 (1988): 1–37.

Szreter, Simon. "The Idea of Demographic Transition and the Study of Fertility Change." *Population and Development Review* 19, no. 4 (1993): 659–701.

Szreter, Simon. "Economic Growth, Disruption, Deprivation, Disease, and Death." *Population and Development Review* 23, no. 4 (1997): 693–728.

Szreter, Simon. "The Prevalence of Syphilis in England and Wales on the Eve of the Great War." *Social History of Medicine* 27, no. 3 (2014): 508–29.

Szreter, Simon. "Treatment Rates for the Pox in Early Modern England." *Continuity and Change* 32, no. 2 (2017): 183–223.

Szreter, Simon, and Graham Mooney. "Urbanization, Mortality, and the Standard of Living Debate." *Economic History Review* 51, no. 1 (1998): 84–112.

Tangen, Catherine M., Marian L. Neuhouser, and Janet L. Stanford. "Prostate Cancer." In *Cancer Epidemiology and Prevention (Fourth Edition)*, edited by Michael Thun, Martha S. Linet, James R. Cerhan, Christopher A. Haiman and David Schottenfeld, 1–70. Oxford etc.: Oxford University Press, 2017.

Tanzi, Vito, and Ludger Schuknecht. *Public Spending in the 20th Century.* Cambridge etc.: Cambridge University Press, 2000.

Tapia Granados, Jose A. "Politics and Health in Eight European Countries." *Social Science & Medicine* 71, no. 5 (2010): 841–50.

Teleky, Ludwig. *History of Factory and Mine Hygiene.* New York: Columbia University Press, 1948.

Temkin, Owsei. "Zur Geschichte von 'Moral und Syphilis'." *Archiv für Geschichte der Medizin* 19, no. 4 (1927): 331–48.

Thomas, Kyla, and David Gunnell. "Suicide in England and Wales 1861–2007: A Time-Trends Analysis." *International Journal of Epidemiology* 39, no. 6 (2010): 1464–75.

Thun, Michael J., *et al.* "50-Year Trends in Smoking-Related Mortality in the United States." *New England Journal of Medicine* 368, no. 4 (2013): 351–64.

Thun, Michael J., *et al.* "Stages of the Cigarette Epidemic on Entering Its Second Century." *Tobacco Control* 21, no. 2 (2012): 96–101.

Timmis, Adam, *et al.* "European Society of Cardiology: Cardiovascular Disease Statistics 2017." *European Heart Journal* 39, no. 7 (2017): 508–79.

Timonin, Sergey, *et al.* "Reducing Geographic Inequalities in Access Times for Acute Treatment of Myocardial Infarction." *International Journal of Epidemiology* 47, no. 5 (2018): 1594–602.

Tkatchenko-Schmidt, Elena, *et al.* "Why Do Health Systems Matter?" *Health Policy and Planning* 25, no. 4 (2010): 283–91.

Tognotti, Eugenia. "The Rise and Fall of Syphilis in Renaissance Europe." *Journal of Medical Humanities* 30, no. 2 (2009): 99–113.

Tomasetti, Cristian, Lu Li, and Bert Vogelstein. "Stem Cell Divisions, Somatic Mutations, Cancer Etiology, and Cancer Prevention." *Science* 355, no. 6331 (2017): 1330–34.

Tomasetti, Cristian, and Bert Vogelstein. "Variation in Cancer Risk among Tissues Can Be Explained by the Number of Stem Cell Divisions." *Science* 347, no. 6217 (2015): 78–81.

Tomkins, Sandra M. "The Failure of Expertise: Public Health Policy in Britain During the 1918–19 Influenza Epidemic." *Social History of Medicine* 5, no. 3 (1992): 435–54.

Torrens, Marta, *et al.* "Methadone Maintenance Treatment in Spain." *Bulletin of the World Health Organization* 91 (2013): 136–41.

Toungoussova, Olga S., Gunnar Bjune, and Dominique A. Caugant. "Epidemic of Tuberculosis in the Former Soviet Union." *Tuberculosis* 86, no. 1 (2006): 1–10.

Trefilova, O.A., and I.M. Sechenov. "Nikolai Semashko: Social Activist and Health Care Organizer." *History of Medicine* 1, no. 3 (2014): 65–72.

Trowell, Hubert C., and Denis P. Burkitt. *Western Diseases, Their Emergence and Prevention.* Cambridge (Mass): Harvard University Press, 1981.

Tunstall-Pedoe, Hugh, *et al.* "Contribution of Trends in Survival and Coronary Event Rates to Changes in Coronary Heart Disease Mortality." *Lancet* 353, no. 9164 (1999): 1547–57.

Tunstall-Pedoe, Hugh, *et al.* "Estimation of Contribution of Changes in Coronary Care to Improving Survival, Event Rates, and Coronary Heart Disease Mortality." *Lancet* 355, no. 9205 (2000): 688–700.

Tuomilehto, J., *et al.* "Record-High Incidence of Type I (Insulin-Dependent) Diabetes Mellitus in Finnish Children." *Diabetologia* 42, no. 6 (1999): 655–60.

Turpeinen, Oiva. "Les Causes des Fluctuations Annuelles du Taux de Mortalité Finlandais entre 1750 et 1806." *Annales de Démographie Historique* (1980): 287–96.

Unal, Belgin, Julia Alison Critchley, and Simon Capewell. "Explaining the Decline in Coronary Heart Disease Mortality in England and Wales between 1981 and 2000." *Circulation* 109, no. 9 (2004): 1101–07.

Underwood, E. Ashworth. "The History of Cholera in Great Britain." *Processings of the Royal Society of Medicine* 41 (1948): 165–63.

Vacher, Léon C. "Statistique du Choléra de 1865 à 1867 en Europe." *Journal de la Société de Statistique de Paris* 9 (1868): 165–76.

Vahlquist, Bo. "Studies on Diphtheria. 1. The Decrease of Natural Antitoxic Immunity against Diphtheria." *Acta Paediatrica* 35, no. 1–2 (1948): 117–29.

Vallgårda, Signild. "Trends in Perinatal Death Rates in Denmark and Sweden, 1915–1990." *Paediatric and Perinatal Epidemiology* 9, no. 2 (1995): 201–18.

Vallgårda, Signild. "Addressing Individual Behaviours and Living Conditions: Four Nordic Public Health Policies." *Scandinavian Journal of Public Health* 39, no. 6 (Suppl) (2011): 6–10.

Vallin, Jacques, Domantas Jasilionis, and France Meslé. "Does a Turbulent History Lead to Turbulent Life Expectancy Trends?." *Historical Methods* 50, no. 4 (2017): 191–209.

Vallin, Jacques, and France Meslé. "Convergences and Divergences in Mortality: A New Approach of Health Transition." *Demographic Research* 2 (2004): 11–44.

Vallin, Jacques, *et al.* "A New Estimate of Ukrainian Population Losses During the Crises of the 1930s and 1940s." *Population Studies* 56, no. 3 (2002): 249–64.

Vandenbroucke, Jan P., H.M. Eelkman Rooda, and Harm Beukers. "Who Made John Snow a Hero?." *American Journal of Epidemiology* 133, no. 10 (1991): 967–73.

Vartiainen, Erkki, *et al.* "Thirty-Five-Year Trends in Cardiovascular Risk Factors in Finland." *International Journal of Epidemiology* 39, no. 2 (2009): 504–18.

Verbrugge, Lois M. "Longer Life but Worsening Health?." *Milbank Memorial Fund Quarterly. Health and Society* 62, no. 3 (1984): 475–519.

Vestreng, Vigdis, *et al.* "Twenty-Five Years of Continuous Sulphur Dioxide Emission Reduction in Europe." *Atmospheric Chemistry and Physics* 7, no. 13 (2007): 3663–81.

Vestreng, Vigdis, *et al.* "Evolution of NOx Emissions in Europe with Focus on Road Transport Control Measures." *Atmospheric Chemistry and Physics* 9, no. 4 (2009): 1503–20.

Viboud, Cécile, and Justin Lessler. "The 1918 Influenza Pandemic: Looking Back, Looking Forward." *American Journal of Epidemiology* 187, no. 12 (2018): 2493–97.

Vigarello, G. *Histoire des Pratiques de Santé: Le Sain et le Malsain depuis le Moyen Âge.* Paris: Éd. du Seuil, 1999.

Vishnevsky, Anatoly. "Mortality in Russia: The Second Epidemiological Revolution That Never Was." *Demographic Review (English Selection)* 1 (2014): 5–40.

Vishnevsky, Anatoly. "Demographic Consequences of the Great Patriotic War." *Demographic Review (English Selection)* 3, no. 2 (2016): 6–42.

Vitek, Charles R., and Melinda Wharton. "Diphtheria in the Former Soviet Union: Reemergence of a Pandemic Disease." *Emerging Infectious Diseases* 4, no. 4 (1998): 539–50.

Vlassov, Vasiliy V. "Russian Medicine: Trying to Catch up on Scientific Evidence and Human Values." *Lancet* 390, no. 10102 (2017): 1619–20.

Vogele, Jorg. "Urbanization, Infant Mortality and Public Health in Imperial Germany." In *The Decline of Infant and Child Mortality*, edited by Carlo A. Corsini and Pier P. Viazzo, 109–28. Dordrecht: Martinus Nijhoff, 1997.

Vries, Jan de. "The Industrial Revolution and the Industrious Revolution." *Journal of Economic History* 54, no. 2 (1994): 249–70.

Vynnycky, E., and P.E. Fine. "Interpreting the Decline in Tuberculosis: The Role of Secular Trends in Effective Contact." *International Journal of Epidemiology* 28, no. 2 (1999): 327–34.

Ward, John W., and Christian Warren. *Silent Victories.* New York etc.: Oxford University Press, 2006.

Warner, Jessica, *et al.* "Can Legislation Prevent Debauchery? Mother Gin and Public Health in 18th-Century England." *American Journal of Public Health* 91, no. 3 (2001): 375–84.

Waters, Hugh R., *et al.* "Health Insurance Coverage in Central and Eastern Europe: Trends and Challenges." *Health Affairs* 27, no. 2 (2008): 478–86.

Weber, Christian, and Heidi Noels. "Atherosclerosis: Current Pathogenesis and Therapeutic Options." *Nature Medicine* 17, no. 11 (2011): 1410–22.

Weber, Max. *Die Protestantische Ethik und der Geist des Kapitalismus.* Bd. XX & XXI: Archiv fur Soxialwissenschaft und Sozialpolitik, 1904–05.

Weehuizen, Rifka Maria. "Mental Capital: The Economic Significance of Mental Health." PhD thesis, Maastricht University, 2008.

Weindling, Paul. *Health, Race and German Politics between National Unification and Nazism, 1870–1945.* Cambridge etc.: Cambridge University Press, 1993.

Weindling, Paul., ed. *International Health Organisations and Movements, 1918–1939.* Cambridge etc.: Cambridge University Press, 1995.

Weindling, Paul. *Epidemics and Genocide in Eastern Europe, 1890–1945.* Oxford etc.: Oxford University Press, 2000.

Weisz, George, and Jesse Olszynko-Gryn. "The Theory of Epidemiologic Transition: The Origins of a Citation Classic." *Journal of the History of Medicine and Allied Sciences* 65, no. 3 (2009): 287–326.

Welzel, Christian. *Freedom Rising.* Cambridge etc.: Cambridge University Press, 2013.

Westerling, Ragnar, *et al.* "The Timing of Introduction of Pharmaceutical Innovations in Seven E Uropean Countries." *Journal of Evaluation in Clinical Practice* 20, no. 4 (2014): 301–10.

Wetherall, Karen, Kathryn A. Robb, and Rory C. O'Connor. "Social Rank Theory of Depression." *Journal of Affective Disorders* 246 (2019): 300–19.

Wheatcroft, Stephen G. "The Great Leap Upwards: Anthropometric Data and Indicators of Crises and Secular Change in Soviet Welfare Levels, 1880–1960." *Slavic Review* 58, no. 1 (1999): 27–60.

Wheatcroft, Stephen G. "Eastern Europe (Russia and the USSR)." In *Famine in European History*, edited by Guido Alfani and Cormac Ó Gráda, 212–39. Cambridge etc.: Cambridge University Press, 2017.

White Franklin, A. "Rickets." In *The History and Conquest of Common Diseases*, edited by Walter R. Bett, 189–203. Norman: University of Oklahoma Press, 1954.

White, Matthew. *Atrocities. The 100 Deadliest Episodes in Human History.* New York: W.W. Norton & Co., 2012.

Whitmee, Sarah, *et al.* "Safeguarding Human Health in the Anthropocene Epoch." *Lancet* 386, no. 10007 (2015): 1973–2028.

Wickes, Ian G. "A History of Infant Feeding: Part Iii: Eighteenth and Nineteenth Century Writers." *Archives of Disease in Childhood* 28, no. 140 (1953): 332–40.

Wijhe, Maarten van, *et al.* "Quantifying the Impact of Mass Vaccination Programmes on Notified Cases in the Netherlands." *Epidemiology & Infection* 146, no. 6 (2018): 716–22.

Wildman, Katherine, and Marie-Helene Bouvier-Colle. “Maternal Mortality as an Indicator of Obstetric Care in Europe.” *British Journal of Obstetrics and Gynaecology* 111, no. 2 (2004): 164–9.

Willemsen, Marc C. *Tobacco Control Policy in the Netherlands.* Palgrave Studies in Public Health Policy Research. n.p.: Palgrave Macmillan, 2018.

Willett, Walter C., *et al.* “Food in the Anthropocene.” *Lancet* 393, no. 10170 (2019): 447–92.

Willett, Walter C., *et al.* “Mediterranean Diet Pyramid: A Cultural Model for Healthy Eating.” *American Journal of Clinical Nutrition* 61, no. 6 (1995): 1402S-06S.

Williams, George C. “Pleiotropy, Natural Selection, and the Evolution of Senescence.” *Evolution* 11 (1957): 398–411.

Wilmoth, John R., and Shiro Horiuchi. “Rectangularization Revisited: Variability of Age at Death within Human Populations.” *Demography* 36, no. 4 (1999): 475–95.

Wilson, Edward O. *Half-Earth: Our Planet's Fight for Life.* New York & London: W.W. Norton & Co., 2016.

Wilson, Leonard G. “The Historical Decline of Tuberculosis in Europe and America.” *Journal of the History of Medicine and Allied Sciences* 45, no. 3 (1990): 366–96.

Wilson, Peter W.F., *et al.* “Prediction of Coronary Heart Disease Using Risk Factor Categories.” *Circulation* 97, no. 18 (1998): 1837–47.

Winegarden, Calman R., and John E. Murray. “The Contributions of Early Health-Insurance Programs to Mortality Declines in Pre-World War I Europe.” *Explorations in Economic History* 35, no. 4 (1998): 431–46.

Withington, Phil. “Utopia, Health, and Happiness.” *Lancet* 387, no. 10033 (2016): 2084–85.

Wohl, Anthony S. *Endangered Lives.* London etc.: Dent and Sons, 1983.

Wolfe, Ingrid. “Child Health.” In *Successes and Failures of Health Policy in Europe*, edited by Johan P. Mackenbach and Martin McKee, 115–34. Maidenhead: Open University Press, 2013.

Wolleswinkel-van den Bosch, Judith H. “The Epidemiological Transition in the Netherlands.” Erasmus University, 1998.

Wolleswinkel-van den Bosch, Judith H., *et al.* “Cause-Specific Mortality Trends in the Netherlands, 1875–1992.” *International Journal of Epidemiology* 26, no. 4 (1997): 772–81.

Wolleswinkel-van den Bosch, Judith H., *et al.* “Determinants of Infant and Early Childhood Mortality Levels and Their Decline in the Netherlands.” *International Journal of Epidemiology* 29, no. 6 (2000): 1031–40.

Wolleswinkel-van den Bosch, Judith H., *et al.* “Substandard Factors in Perinatal Care in the Netherlands.” *Acta Obstetricia et Gynecologica Scandinavica* 81, no. 1 (2002): 17–24.

Woods, Robert. *The Demography of Victorian England and Wales.* Cambridge etc.: Cambridge University Press, 2000.

Woods, Robert. *Death before Birth.* Oxford etc.: Oxford University Press, 2009.

Woods, Robert, and Chris Galley. *Mrs Stone & Dr Smellie: Eighteenth-Century Midwives and Their Patients.* Liverpool: Liverpool University Press, 2014.

Woods, Robert, Patricia A. Watterson, and John H. Woodward. "The Causes of Rapid Infant Mortality Decline in England and Wales, 1861–1921. Part I." *Population Studies* 42, no. 3 (1988): 343–66.

Woods, Robert. "The Causes of Rapid Infant Mortality Decline in England and Wales, 1861–1921. Part II." *Population studies* 43, no. 1 (1989): 113–32.

Woodward, Alistair, *et al.* "Climate Change and Health: On the Latest IPCC Report." *Lancet* 383, no. 9924 (2014): 1185–89.

World Health Organization. *Atlas of Mortality in Europe. Subnational Patterns, 1980/1981 and 1990/1991.* WHO Regional Publications European Series. Vol. 75, Copenhagen: WHO European Centre for Environment and Health, 1997.

World Health Organization. *Health Aspects of Air Pollution.* WHO Regional Office for Europe (Copenhagen: 2004).

World Health Organization. *European Status Report on Road Safety.* Copenhagen: WHO Regional Office for Europe, 2009.

World Health Organization. *Review of Evidence on Health Aspects of Air Pollution.* Copenhagen: WHO Regional Office for Europe, 2013.

World Health Organization. *Global Status Report on Alcohol and Health 2018.* Geneva: WHO, 2018.

Worobey, Michael, *et al.* "1970s and 'Patient 0' HIV-1 Genomes Illuminate Early HIV/AIDS History in North America." *Nature* 539, no. 7627 (2016): 98–101.

Wouters, Cas. "Formalization and Informalization: Changing Tension Balances in Civilizing Processes." *Theory, Culture & Society* 3, no. 2 (1986): 1–18.

Wrigley, E. Anthony, *et al. English Population History from Family Reconstitution 1580–1837.* Cambridge etc.: Cambridge University Press, 1997.

Wu, Kana, *et al.* "Cancers of the Colon and Rectum." In *Cancer Epidemiology and Prevention (Fourth Edition)*, edited by Michael Thun, Martha S. Linet, James R. Cerhan, Christopher A. Haiman and David Schottenfeld, 1–97. Oxford etc.: Oxford University Press, 2017.

Wu, Song, *et al.* "Substantial Contribution of Extrinsic Risk Factors to Cancer Development." *Nature* 529, no. 7584 (2016): 43–47.

Zanden, Jan Luiten van. *The Economic History of the Netherlands 1914–1995.* London and New York: Routledge, 1998.

Zatoński, Witold A., *et al.* "Liver Cirrhosis Mortality in Europe, with Special Attention to Central and Eastern Europe." *European Addiction Research* 16, no. 4 (2010): 193–201.

Zatonski, Witold, *et al.* "Tobacco Smoking in Countries of the European Union." *Annals of Agricultural and Environmental Medicine* 19, no. 2 (2012): 181–92.

Zatravkin, S.N., *et al.* *Заболеваемость Инфекционными Болезнями В Ссср. Сообщение 1. 1919–1949 Годы* [*The Incidence of Infectious Diseases in the USSR: Myths and Reality. Report 1: 1919–1949*]. Moscow: Semashko National Research Institute of Public Health, n.d.

Zatravkin, S.N., *Заболеваемость Инфекционными Болезнями В Ссср: Мифы И Реальность. Сообщение 2. 1950–1990 Годы* [*The Incidence of Infectious Diseases in the USSR: Myths and Reality. Report 2: 1950–1999*]. Moscow: Semashko National Research Institute of Public Health, n.d.

Zeitlin, Jennifer, Beatrice Blondel, and Babak Khoshnood. "Fertility, Pregnancy and Childbirth." In *Successes and Failures of Health Policy in Europe*, edited by Johan P. Mackenbach and Martin McKee, 91–114. Maidenhead: Open University Press, 2013.

Zeitlin, Jennifer, *et al.* "Declines in Stillbirth and Neonatal Mortality Rates in Europe between 2004 and 2010." *Journal of Epidemiology and Community Health* 70, no. 6 (2016): 609–15.

Zeitlin, Jennifer, *et al.* "Preterm Birth Time Trends in Europe: A Study of 19 Countries." *BJOG: An International Journal of Obstetrics & Gynaecology* 120, no. 11 (2013): 1356–65.

Zimmermann, Michael B., and M. Andersson. "Prevalence of Iodine Deficiency in Europe in 2010." Paper presented at the Annales d'Endocrinologie, 2011.

Zinsser, Hans. *Rats, Lice and History.* London etc.: Routledge [re-edition by Penguin Books in 2000], 1935.

Zuckerman, Molly K., ed. *Modern Environments and Human Health.* Hoboken: John Wiley & Sons, 2014.

Zwarte, Ingrid de. *De Hongerwinter.* Amsterdam: Prometheus, 2019.

Zylberman, Patrick. "Mosquitoes and the Komitadjis." In *Facing Illness in Troubled Times*, edited by Iris Borowy and Wolf Gruner, 305–43. Frankfurt am Main: Peter Lang, 2005.

Zylberman, Patrick. "A Transatlantic Dispute." In *Shifting Boundaries of Public Health*, edited by Susan Gross Solomon, Lion Murard and Patrick Zylberman, 269–297. Rochester: University of Rochester Press, 2008.

Index

In **bold**: major treatment of topic, often over several pages
In *italics*: term only occurs in a note

www.ingramcontent.com/pod-product-compliance
Lightning Source LLC
Chambersburg PA
CBHW070249260926
51849CB00001BA/72
* 9 7 8 9 0 0 4 4 2 5 8 2 8 *